'*Essential Oils* thoroughly elucidates the diverse ra
inform contemporary aromatherapy. Expertly anal
clinical rationale, Jennifer Rhind applies an astut
study. An indispensable handbook for the practi
Essential Oils succeeds as both a comprehensive re:

— *Gabriel Mojay, FIFPA, MBAcC, CertEd*

'This book is a breath of fresh air in written form. Jennifer's non-judgmental approach gives her the vision to encompass a wonderfully broad perspective. From the recent history of aromatherapy's development, to the potential uses of absolutes, to scientific validation for essential oil properties that were previously only "assumed" or "suspected", Jennifer brings us up to date by connecting clinical practice with biology in new and fascinating ways.'

— *Robert Tisserand, aromatherapy author, educator and consultant*

'Finally we have the "missing-link" text to facilitate the journey into the world of aromatherapy practice! This excellent book is well researched, detailed, up to date, relevant and completely accessible to student and qualified aromatherapists alike. It is rare to find a text that successfully combines holistic principles with practitioner-focussed evidence-based research. *Essential Oils* accomplishes this beautifully and is an ideal course text for all aromatherapy colleges.'

— *Rhiannon Harris, Editor,* International Journal of Clinical Aromatherapy

Praise for the first edition:

'A relevant, topical and highly readable text with very interesting ideas for today's practitioner.'
— *David Pirie, BSc, PGDip Herbal Medicine, M. NIMH, Dip Aromatherapy, Lecturer in Herbal Medicine, Edinburgh Napier University, UK*

'The information regarding classification of essential oils and blending approaches is both informative and extensive, and the knowledge contained within this text makes it essential reading for students, practitioners and lecturers of aromatherapy and indeed other complementary therapies. Dr Jennifer Rhind was an inspiration to me and I know that my copy of her book will never be far from reach.'
— *Lesley Ann Potter, BSc Complementary Therapies (Aromatherapy), Lecturer in Complementary Therapies, Moray College, Scotland*

'As a student I found Dr Rhind's book easy to use with a wealth of information about a wide range of oils. The suggestions for therapeutic blending are invaluable. As a practising aromatherapist, *Essential Oils* is still my first point of reference.'
— *Cath Boyle, MA (Hons) Sociology, BSc Complementary Therapies (Aromatherapy), PGCE, MIFPA*

Essential Oils

by the same author

Fragrance and Wellbeing
An Exploration of Plant Aromatics and their Influences on the Psyche
Jennifer Peace Rhind
ISBN 978 1 84819 090 0
eISBN 978 0 85701 073 5

Essential Oils

A HANDBOOK FOR AROMATHERAPY PRACTICE

2ND EDITION

Jennifer Peace Rhind

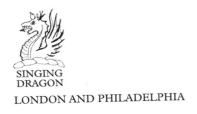

SINGING
DRAGON

LONDON AND PHILADELPHIA

First published in 2012
by Singing Dragon
an imprint of Jessica Kingsley Publishers
116 Pentonville Road
London N1 9JB, UK
and
400 Market Street, Suite 400
Philadelphia, PA 19106, USA

www.singingdragon.com

Library of Congress Cataloging in Publication Data
Rhind, Jennifer.
 Essential oils : a handbook for aromatherapy practice / Jennifer Peace Rhind with David Pirie. --
2nd ed.
    p. ; cm.
Includes bibliographical references and index.
ISBN 978-1-84819-089-4 (alk. paper)
I. Pirie, David. II. Title.
[DNLM: 1. Aromatherapy. 2. Oils, Volatile--therapeutic use. WB 925]
LC classification not assigned
615.3'219--dc23
                        2012000833

British Library Cataloguing in Publication Data
A CIP catalogue record for this book is available from the British Library

ISBN 978 1 848 19089 4
eISBN 978 0 85701 072 8

Printed and bound in Great Britain

For my husband, Derek, and Leeloo

Contents

Preface

Most of my earliest memories and significant memories have been linked in some way to scent. As a child, I was fortunate to have parents and grandparents who loved fragrant flowers, incense and perfumes, so from an early age using my sense of smell for pleasure became second nature. I recall joyful moments of being lifted by my grandfather to smell sweet pea blooms, and losing myself in the peppery scent and silky texture of peony blossoms. My father had a passion for roses, especially the old varieties and the sumptuous tea roses; my mother sought out lily of the valley every spring, not just for its delicate beauty, but for its fragrance. My personal favourite was the crushed leaves of artemisia, which I knew in those days as southernwood. Meanwhile, my grandmother had a taste for the exotic – she loved to burn incense, so the atmosphere in the home was often permeated by sandalwood, patchouli and the sweet, mysterious nag champa. So it is hardly surprising that, as an adolescent and young woman, I loved to explore the world of perfumery, developing what became a somewhat expensive habit.

I am sure that every one of us remembers their first exposure to the aroma of an essential oil. Mine happened in a shop in Byres Road in the West End of Glasgow, in the early 1970s. It was a place that sold incenses, oil-based perfumes, Indian carvings, silk scarves and embroidered clothing, herb teas and a few vegetarian and health foods. I opened a bottle that said 'Geranium essential oil' on the label, and held it to my nose. That was all it took. I had no idea where that moment would lead. At the time, I was a student studying microbiology, and aromatherapy was largely unknown outside France. However, during my later career in microbiology, quality assurance, food and flavours (sometimes involving the very peculiar smells of oriental fermented foods), my love of scents, flowers and plants and my longstanding interest in natural healing endured, and in some way sustained me, because I was not really fulfilled in my work. So it is not really surprising that I eventually became an aromatherapist and educator.

I wanted to tell this story because I hope to not only pass on information about essential oils and aromatherapy, but also to give a sense of the enormous pleasure and healing that can be brought about by these remarkable essences. You will get the most out of this book if you consciously engage with their odours, put aside preconceptions, and move on from the 'like or dislike' mindset. I often use meditations on essential oils with students, where we focus on the aroma alone to explore the odour profile and learn the vocabulary, perhaps linking this to the botanical origins or the chemical constituents. Then we allow ourselves to become immersed in the aroma, and see where it takes us. This allows deeper learning, and an immense respect for the sense of smell, not to mention experiencing the whole gamut of emotions!

In 2009 the first edition of this book was published – the result of a cross-faculty collaboration at Edinburgh Napier University, Scotland. In this revised and expanded second edition, you will find a greater selection of essential oils and absolutes, and more analysis of the theoretical and philosophical approaches to aromatherapy, with the evidence to support these.

As aromatherapy is such a multifaceted and multicultural subject – harnessing the senses of smell and touch, the traditional uses of plant aromatics and the biological actions of essential oils – it is easy to be travelling along one path and then find that you need to diverge and even change tracks several times to make sense of the whole. On this journey you will discover some good science, including animal studies (which make difficult reading for an animal lover who comes from a family of anti-vivisectionists), human studies and pharmacological studies, psychological and behavioural studies. However, in order to reach a fuller and more complete understanding of the contemporary practice of aromatherapy, Eastern philosophies of health and healing, such as the Chinese Five Elements and Ayurveda have been included. Although it may sometimes seem that there are irreconcilable differences between the Western 'scientific' and Eastern 'holistic' perspectives or indeed nineteenth-century 'vitalism', aromatherapy is one of the few contemporary healing modalities that can be practised within a holistic context, treating the person rather than the disease, whilst being supported by robust evidence derived from scientific research.

First, I would like to say thank you to all of the aromatherapy 'pioneers' who have captured my attention, made me think, and influenced my practice through their writings. I would also like to acknowledge and thank my many colleagues at Edinburgh Napier University who have supported and encouraged me, especially Dr Christine Donnelly, Dr Salma Siddique and Mairi Anderson. Special thanks to David Pirie for sharing his insights into Ayurveda. I am also indebted to our students, who always bring fresh perspectives and help me develop learning methods, and to our graduates, who will be the ones who help aromatherapy reach its full potential. Edinburgh Napier graduates have also helped with the literature search, especially Tamara Agnew, Audrey Quinn and Emma Allan – thank you for sharing the fruits of your labours.

The support at Jessica Kingsley Publishers has been excellent; for me, writing is always a pleasure, but Jessica Kingsley and her team – especially Emily McClave, Victoria Peters, Ruth Tewkesbury and Alex Fleming – have provided me with the best experience possible – thank you.

Finally, I extend my thanks to my husband Derek, who has always been there for me with love and understanding, not to mention his very practical as well as emotional support, as we have walked the 'road less travelled'.

PART I

Aromatherapy

Philosophical and
Theoretical Perspectives

CHAPTER I

From Historical Origins to the Present Day

The Philosophies of the Pioneers and Influential Thinkers

The exploitation of aromatic plants – from quintessence to essential oils

Aromatherapy could, very broadly, be described as the therapeutic use of the essential oils that are extracted from aromatic plants. Aromatic plant species have had an enormous impact on the life of the planet – from their ecological roles to their cultural uses, for healing and as medicines. These plants contain significant amounts of 'volatile oil' – which gives each of them their distinctive fragrances and tastes. Aromatic plants are found all over the temperate, subtropical and tropical regions of the Earth. However, only around 1 per cent of plant species on the planet are aromatic.

Early methods for extracting the fragrance included steeping plants in water, oils or fatty materials. Second- and third-century alchemists searched for ways in which to extract the fragrant *quintessence*, which they considered to be the 'soul' or 'spirit' of aromatic plants. In fact, the modern term 'essential oil' is derived from the word 'quintessence'. Later, in the sixteenth century, steam distilled essential oils became available in Europe, eventually becoming part of traditional medicine. Nowadays, essential oils can be extracted by both physical and chemical methods. These range from simple maceration to cold expression suited to citrus peel oils, and sophisticated steam distillation procedures and solvent extraction processes (Schnaubelt 1999). Most essential oils and aromatic extracts are destined for the flavour and fragrance industry. Aromatherapy is only a tiny part of the vast industry that has evolved around man's exploitation of the sense of smell.

Currently, around 80 per cent of essential oils are extracted by distillation (Williams 2000). Today the essential oil industry is huge, and a wide body of knowledge concerning the physical, chemical and biological nature of essential oils has been accumulated. However, modern uses of aromatic plants remain very similar to those of older cultures.

Throughout the history of mankind, and across all cultures, aromatic plants have been exploited – and they have played significant roles in many aspects of human life.

In ancient times, plant aromatics were used in ritual – as incenses, for purification, behaviour modification, and as meditation aids. They also had many varied culinary uses – herbs and spices were not only included for flavouring but also as preservatives. So as their use in food preparation developed, different cuisines became characterised and defined by their use of herbs and spices. Finally, aromatic plant extracts were widely used as perfumes, environmental fragrances, for personal care, grooming and well-being, and of course, as medicines (Classen, Howes and Synnott 1994). From this it is very apparent that, although technology has changed, and we can now extract, analyse and research essential oils in ways that older cultures could not even conceive of, we are still using plant aromatics in very similar ways. So although aromatherapy is a comparatively new discipline, it has ancient roots and an extensive, global tradition behind it. This must be acknowledged, and to put contemporary aromatherapy in its true context, its origins and recent evolution should be explored.

The cultural uses of plant aromatics in ancient and modern times

> Aromatherapy is shamanism for everyone. (Schnaubelt 1999, p. vii)

Aromatherapy means different things to different people. Popular conceptions vary, despite the best efforts of professional organisations to promote it as a therapeutic modality. Some associate it with an aromatic massage, while many in spas and the beauty industry consider it to be a relaxing or rejuvenating aesthetic treatment. Many understand that it involves the use of fragrant plant extracts – yet to some this simply means the use of naturally perfumed personal care products. Some aromatherapists will insist that aromatherapy is a therapeutic discipline based on the belief that odour affects the state of mind. Many aromatherapists who are attracted to a biomedical approach might view aromatherapy as a branch of herbal medicine, or as aromatic medicine in its own right. A growing number of therapists are exploring the energetic aspects of essential oils, and using ancient philosophical traditions to provide a new context for their practices.

A look at aromatherapy's historical roots and evolution will help to explain these anomalies. Aromatherapy's origins are inseparable from those of perfumery, as aromatic plants were used in both religious ceremonies and for personal use and adornment, long before recorded history. So this is a fitting place to start, before continuing to look at the development of modern aromatherapy from its inception in France in the 1930s.

The use of fragrance certainly dates from pre-Egyptian times, preceding 5000 BC. Since antiquity, scented flowers have been used for personal adornment. This long history of use is possibly grounded in the concept that the sense of smell is a form of communication in all species.

Other very early uses of plant aromatics were as incenses – sandalwood, cinnamon bark, calamus root, and resins such as myrrh, frankincense and benzoin were burned to release fragrant smoke and vapours. These aromatic incenses were used in religious ritual and ceremony. The root of the word 'perfume' is *per fumum*, the Latin expression meaning 'through smoke'; incense provided a link between the mundane and the divine. At an early stage it would have been recognised that different fragrances would elicit different effects on moods, feelings and states of mind during ritual practices. From this a tradition of using specific aromatics or combinations for specific purposes would have gradually developed.

In 1975 Paolo Rovesti (1902–1983), a chemist and pharmacist who became known as the 'father of phytocosmetics', discovered a terracotta distillation apparatus in the Indus valley, West Pakistan, which dates from around 3000 BC. Therefore we do know that the process of distillation was known as early as 3000 BC, and that the art and science of perfumery were well developed in ancient and Dynastic Egypt. A considerable array of aromatic products was available and was used for many purposes other than perfumery, including embalming the dead. It is acknowledged that not only the ancient Egyptians, but also the Assyrians, Babylonians, Chaldeans, Hebrews, Persians and Greeks used plant aromatics extensively as perfumes, incenses and medicines.

In the East, in China, perfumery and aromatic practices were evolving along similar lines. The Chinese also exploited animal-derived aromatics, including musk – a secretion of the small musk deer. They made extensive use of musk both as a medicine and as a perfume ingredient.

In India and Persia, the *attars* were, and are, the main forms of perfume for skin application. The term 'attar' has various meanings, including smoke, wind, odour and essence. Champaca flowers, jasmine and rose, and sandalwood, regarded as a holy fragrance, were common ingredients in attars. Vedic literature (c. 2000 BC) mentions hundreds of aromatics; the *Rig Veda* describes their uses in personal care and healing.

Around the same time, in Central America, the Incas, Aztecs and Maya also were using vast quantities of incense as religious offerings. The aromatics used in these cultures are perhaps less familiar to us, but reflected what was available in the environment, such as copal resin, copal wood and tobacco leaf. The remaining Maya in Guatemala continue to burn these incenses in support of prayers.

Perfumery in Japan developed with the practice of Buddhism. Incense was burned – in early days this was aloes wood, a rare and now costly aromatic. Later on, sandalwood, costus root, cinnamon bark, musk, ambergris, styrax and frankincense became part of the aromatic palette, and the personal use of fragrances in the form of powders, pastes and essences became popular.

The perfumers of Ancient Greece were highly skilled, learning from and basing their art on the work of Egyptian perfumers. Orris (iris root), rose, tuberose, violet, spices, herbs, woods and resins were extensively used in early Greek perfumes. Cosmetics were widely used by men and women too; a practice first popularised by the Egyptian Queen Nefertiti.

In Ancient Rome, perfumery was based on Greek practice, and further developed. Roman perfumers were afforded great respect, and even entire quarters of towns were populated by perfumery practices. By the time of Nero, aromatics were used extensively and extravagantly. Creativity, innovation and also an element of excess characterised Roman perfumery, and the strong links between scent and eroticism were also exploited. The Romans used many of the aromatic plants whose essential oils play an important role in current aromatherapy practice, including rosemary, sage, peppermint, aniseed, pepper and the more exotic floral oils of neroli, rose and jasmine. Herodotus was the first to write about the process of distilling turpentine from pine resin, and many other matters pertaining to the use of perfumes. After the fall of the Roman Empire the use of perfumes declined.

Islamic culture has a crucial role in the evolution of perfumery and aromatherapy. Circa 600 AD the Muslims were scholars and travellers, assimilating the knowledge of all the cultures they encountered. The eighth-century Persian pharmacist Jabir ibn Hayyan (the westernised name given was Geber) developed distillation processes for the production of aromatic waters, and by the thirteenth century these aromatic waters were widely used as medicines and perfumes. Ironically, the tiny droplets of an oily substance that floated on the surface of the distillation waters were regarded as impurities, and routinely discarded. This was, in fact, the essential oil. In the tenth century the Persian physician Ibn Cina (Avicenna) made wide use of distillation and indeed was initially credited as the first to do this. He certainly does appear to have invented steam distillation specifically for the preparation of rosewater and other scented floral waters.

Meanwhile, developments in Europe were taking place that also had an impact on the growth of the essential oil industry. Around 1150 AD the condenser was developed. As its name suggests, the purpose of the condenser was to condense the hot vapours of distillation, making the entire process more efficient, and the subsequent realisation of the nature and value of essential oils was the consequence.

Italy was the first European country to make perfumes with these essential oils, closely followed by Spain and Portugal. The perfume industry grew as new aromatic materials were introduced from newly discovered America. France had a perfumery industry by the thirteenth century. The area in the south, around Grasse, became renowned for the cultivation and extraction of flowers such as rose, tuberose, jasmine, mimosa and jonquil. Other areas of cultivation of aromatic plants became well established, notably Sicily for its citrus oils, Calabria for bergamot and southern Spain for citrus crops and herbs such as sage, rosemary and thyme.

Perfumery arrived in the British Isles with the Romans. However, the practice was slow to develop, and did not become popular until the time of Queen Elizabeth I, when fragrance became available in the forms of pomanders and incense; rosewater, too, became more widely available. Pharmaceutical chemists in England then began to distil aromatic waters of lavender, elderflower and rosemary. However, perfumery in England was not really established until after the Restoration of the Monarchy in 1660. By 1750, peppermint was being produced commercially in Mitcham, Surrey.

These aromatic materials also had pharmaceutical uses. Animal-derived aromatics, such as moschus (musk), were used as antispasmodics, and ambergris (a secretion of the whale) was used as an antispasmodic for the bowel and bronchial tubes, and as a nervine, narcotic, hypnotic and aphrodisiac. The aromatic lavender plant yielded *oleum lavandulae*, which was used as a stimulant and nervine in conditions such as headache and hysteria. Other aromatic balsams were used for apoplexy. So it can be seen that, although essential oils were originally produced for perfumery, they also very quickly found their way into pharmaceutical industry.

Modern use of essential oils and aromatic plant extracts for therapeutic purposes is based on long and varied traditional practices. However, this falls short of explaining how the discipline of aromatherapy actually came into being.

The pioneers of aromatherapy

Robert Tisserand, who should certainly be considered a pioneer of modern aromatherapy, edited the first English translation of the work of Gattefossé (1993) where he credits him with the creativity to develop a new therapeutic discipline.

> Rene-Maurice Gattefossé was not the first to use essential oils therapeutically, or to write about such use, both events having taken place thousands of years ago. However, he had an unprecedented vision. Not one of his predecessors, during the thousand years since the invention of distillation, had seen that the therapeutic application of essential oils constituted a discipline in its own right. (Tisserand 1993, p. v)

The modern approach to using essential oils for therapeutic purposes was indeed instigated by the French chemist and perfumer, René-Maurice Gattefossé. The respected Gattefossé family perfumery business had resurrected and reorganised the ailing essential oil crop growing and essential oil production industry in the south of France (Gattefossé 1992). The family also established a successful distillation industry in North Africa. Gattefossé completed a systematic study of indigenous and exotic essential oils, and after the First World War he began to investigate the medicinal potential of essential oils in collaboration with the medical profession. By 1923 his preliminary work was published, and he continued to collaborate with the medical and veterinary professions, researching essential oil applications in several fields, notably dermatology. His last two works were first published in 1937. One of these is entitled *Aromathérapie: Les huiles essentielles, hormones vegétales* – this is the first use of the term 'aromathérapie'.

Gattefossé's aromatherapy was influenced by the conventional medical approach – a far cry from the holistic discipline practised in the UK today. However, he was responsible for the concepts of synergy, the psychotherapeutic benefits of fragrance and the percutaneous absorption of essential oils – the key concepts that underpin current aromatherapy practice (Tisserand 1993; Schnaubelt 1999). Therefore, Gattefossé created the concept of aromatherapy, and because he presented his work in a medical and scientific way, aromatherapy initially developed in the medical domain. His work focused on the pharmacological activity of essential oils, specifically their active components and functional groups. However, as he was also cognisant of the potential of essential oils to have effects on the mind and nervous system, his contribution to aromatherapy has also influenced the holistic approach to practice.

In 1964 the French medical doctor Jean Valnet published *The Practice of Aromatherapy* (see Valnet 1982). This book is generally acknowledged to have been the main influence on the growing popularity of aromatherapy beyond France. Valnet founded the Association of Study and Research in Aromatherapy and Phytotherapy at a time when antibiotic use was rapidly increasing. His approach was similar to Gattefossé's, in that he selected essential oils on the basis of their active constituents, and he fostered the concept of relating the functional groups found in essential oil constituents with their potential therapeutic properties. He also created a system for essential oil prescription that still influences blending in modern holistic aromatherapy.

In France in the 1940s Marguerite Maury, a nurse and surgical assistant, became interested in the medical, cosmetic and holistic applications of essential oils. Unlike her predecessors, she was not scientifically or medically qualified, so she focused on the external applications of essential oils, as the internal prescription and medical use of essential oils was, and is, legally restricted or prohibited in most Western countries (Schnaubelt 1999; Bensouilah 2005). It was Maury who was largely responsible for reviving the practice of massage with aromatic plant oils, which was first advocated by Hippocrates, and for studying the effects of massage with essential oils (Tisserand 1977). She lectured throughout Europe on the subject, opened aromatherapy clinics and ran courses. Maury published *Le Capital Jeunesse* in 1961; the English version, *The Secret of Life and Youth*, was published in 1964. Two of her students, Micheline Arcier and Danièle Ryman, brought her holistic perspective on the subject to the UK in the 1960s. Nowadays, many UK aromatherapists use the philosophy and techniques derived from those developed by Maury (Ryman 1989).

As aromatherapy continued to develop in the clinical domain in France, Maurice Girault developed the 'aromatogram' in 1969, based on Schroeder and Messing's research (Girault 1979) work in 1949–1950. This is a laboratory technique that can elucidate the antimicrobial activities of specific essential oils in relation to specific microbial pathogens. The aromatogram does, because of the watery nature of agar, the matrix of the growth medium, favour the more water-soluble essential oil constituents, and can be seen as biased against the more fat-soluble ones. However, this paved the way for further investigation into the antimicrobial potential of essential oils and their application in the clinical arena.

Dr Paul Belaiche is seen as an instrumental figure in the development of clinical aromatherapy, specifically in the treatment of infection. In 1972, in conjunction with medical doctors Audhoui, Bourgeon, P. and C. Duraffourd, Girault and Lapraz, he used the aromatogram to study and develop treatments for a range of infectious diseases. Several of his colleagues in this study became well known in the field of aromatic medicine in France. In 1979 Belaiche published his best known and influential work, *Traité de Phytothérapie et d'Aromathérapie*. He also suggested that essential oils could be classified according their dominant functional groups. Earlier, the fragrance researchers Charabot and Dupont hypothesised that there was a link between these functional groups and odour, and Belaiche developed this suggestion for clinical application.

In the meantime, Daniel Pénoël, who had studied both medicine and naturopathy, was attracted to Valnet's work with essential oils. In collaboration with the chemist Pierre Franchomme (see below) he developed what they termed 'scientific aromatherapy', continuing the focus on treating infections with essential oils. Later on, in 1990, after several years of developing essential oil applications in a more holistic, but still clinical way, Franchomme and Pénoël published *L'Aromatherapie exactement*. This text eventually became the seminal work on medical aromatherapy. (It is worth noting that Pénoël reinforced the importance of the 'terrain' in clinical practice. Claude Bernard (1813–1878) was a physiologist who suggested that it was the condition of the body and its internal environment that determined the individual's healing capacity. For example, an infection could only develop if the conditions are favourable. Pénoël called this the 'terrain', and would treat the terrain in his aromatic interventions – hence developing a more holistic approach to aromatherapy practice in France, but keeping the biomedical model as the underpinning rationale.)

Pénoël became an educator too, influencing many English-speaking aromatherapy practitioners, writers and educators, such as Kurt Schnaubelt of the Pacific Institute of Aromatherapy, and Shirley and Len Price in the UK. He further developed Franchomme's 'functional group hypothesis' (see below) into what he called the 'molecular approach', and identified three ways of constructing synergistic blends of essential oils that have now found their way into holistic aromatherapy practice.

Pierre Franchomme is perhaps best known for his work with Pénoël; however, it was he who was largely responsible for the functional group hypothesis, which attempted to explain and predict the physiological and biological activities of essential oils. The hypothesis was based on an electrochemical experiment, where chemical constituents of essential oils were sprayed between electromagnetic plates. The results of this particular experiment (which is now generally regarded as 'bad science') led Franchomme and Pénoël to develop their molecular approach to selecting essential oils. Franchomme is also a proponent of using 'chemotypes', essential oils from plants bred or selected for their ability to produce significant amounts of key active constituents. Like Pénoël, he also became an aromatherapy educator, and founded the Institut des Sciences Phytomédicales in France.

At this point, it is worth mentioning Henri Viaud, who was a well-known distiller of essential oils in Provence. The main market for essential oils was the fragrance industry, but as clinicians in France began to use essential oils in the medical domain, Viaud developed guidelines for the production and quality of essential oils destined for therapeutic purposes. He advocated that such oils should be distilled from specified botanical species and chemotypes, and that the distillation should be slow, using low pressure (Lavabre 1990). He published these guidelines in 1983. At the time of writing, there are many essential oil quality standards and grades; however, there is no such thing as a therapeutic grade.

The 1980s and 1990s were the decades of real growth for aromatherapy in France. Philippe Mailhebiau published *La Nouvelle aromathérapie* in 1994, where he emphasised the importance of the terrain in aromatherapy practice. His concept of the terrain was quite wide, embracing genetic, physical, physiological and psychological aspects of the individual, maintaining that if the terrain was not balanced, pathologies could develop. He published *Portraits in Oils* in English in 1995. Mailhebiau also ventured into the education sector, and was the editor of the short-lived journal *Les Cahiers d'aromathérapie*.

Christian Duraffourd and Jean Claude Lapraz are medical doctors who originally specialised as oncobiologists in Paris. They founded the French Society for Phytotherapy and Aromatherapy in 1980. They are the directors of The Phyto-Aromatherapy Institute, and they further refined the concept of the terrain and its importance. Duraffourd and Lapraz published a paper in the *British Journal of Phytotherapy* in 1995, where they postulated that the terrain is governed by the endocrine system. This would appear to have been quite influential in the development of aromatic medicine, both within France and in other countries. Lapraz disputed the value of chemotypes, proposing the 'law of all or nothing', where the entire essential oil is of importance, not individual constituents. Duraffourd and Lapraz, who originally worked on the aromatogram too, developed the 'endobiogenic concept', which addresses the root causes of pathology and the terrain of the patient to establish the optimum phytotherapeutic treatment. Duraffourd and Lapraz currently organise post-graduate education for clinicians and pharmacists around the world, although not in the UK.

Robert Tisserand published *The Art of Aromatherapy* in 1977 – the first book written in English on the subject. It joined Valnet and Maury, and other writers such as Lavabre, on the bookshelves of the curious public and aromatherapists. This marked the beginning of widespread interest in the subject in the UK, initially within the beauty industry, and shortly followed by aromatherapy schools and professional associations for the non-medical practice of aromatherapy – often termed holistic aromatherapy or clinical aromatherapy, to distinguish it from aesthetic aromatherapy.

Tisserand also founded and edited the long-running and influential *International Journal of Aromatherapy*, which had contributions from most of the leading proponents and writers at the time. This journal was also the vehicle for research in other related disciplines, such as the psychology of fragrance, to reach the aromatherapy audience. Since the 1970s there has been considerable research into the psychology of perfumery, and the social and behavioural effects of odour, but odour was a somewhat neglected aspect of aromatherapy at that time, as the focus tended to be on the clinical applications of essential oils. So the work of perfumers Paul and Stephan Jellinek, fragrance researchers Alan Hirsch, Susan Knasko, Craig Warren and many others, got exposure in the aromatherapy world. The journal opened up the road for practitioners to write about alternative approaches to aromatherapy too, including Peter Holmes and Gabriel Mojay, who were bringing the perspectives of Eastern medicine to aromatherapy practice. The effect of the journal was to widen the philosophical basis of aromatherapy and challenge and open up new avenues for practice, as well as to provide some evidence for aromatherapy. The result was an increased 'respectability' for the profession.

Bob Harris and Rhiannon Harris (now Lewis) were the founders of Essential Oil Resource Consultants and editors of the *International Journal of Essential Oil Therapeutics* and the *International Journal of Clinical Aromatherapy*, respectively. The Harrises have studied the French approach to aromatherapy practice, bringing this to the English-speaking world, and they are well-respected educators. Although there was an attempt in the 1980s to bring aromatic medicine education to the UK, via Daniel Pénoël, this was largely unsuccessful, and fraught with insurance issues. However, the Harrises have adopted the principles – such as the concept of the terrain, the biological and physiological activities of the essential oils – and some of the practices, such as delivery by pessaries, suppositories and oral delivery, and adapted these for incorporation into holistic practice. At the time of writing, although holistic aromatherapists can use relatively high concentrations of essential oils on the skin (if their education has addressed this type of use), they cannot be insured for delivery by pessaries, suppositories or by the oral route.

From this short history, it can be seen why perceptions of aromatherapy, and indeed its contemporary practices, are so varied. It is also clear that at the very heart of aromatherapy is the sense of smell and the fragrance of plant aromatics, and this is why it has remained an integral part of our lives and healing practices – be they clinical or otherwise.

Contemporary aromatherapy – scope of practice

In the UK and the English-speaking world, aromatherapy practice ranges from the purely aesthetic to holistic, clinical and olfactory domains.

In the UK aromatherapy was initially embraced within the beauty profession. Marguerite Maury's adherents and educators, such as Danièle Ryman and Micheline Arcier, found that, in the UK, aestheticians were in a good position to deliver aromatherapy treatments. They already used plant-based products, scent and massage in their practice, and aromatherapy was seen as a welcome extension of what could be offered. Consequently, beauty-training establishments, such as Eve Taylor's Institute of Clinical Aromatherapy began to develop the modality, embracing the clinical element. Within a few years, as the numbers of aromatherapy practitioners grew, some aromatherapists began to view the 'beauty' aspect as disadvantageous and diminishing the clinical credentials of the therapy (Bensouilah 2005).

Despite this division, aromatherapy has flourished within the beauty profession, and is practised across the UK in salons and spas. The emphasis in aesthetic aromatherapy is on well-being, relaxation and skin care. It generally commands quite a high price and is perceived by many as a luxury, not an alternative medicine. Full body aromatherapy massage, often using pre-blended essential oils, is commonplace. Clients will usually be offered a choice of blends – some will be asked to self-select according to how they would like to feel, or the therapist will make a selection following a consultation and assessment. Many phytocosmeceutical companies will offer a sophisticated range of aromatherapy massage products, but the choice is often (disappointingly) between 'relaxing', 'stimulating' or 'reviving' or 'energising' and 'detoxifying' variants. If the product is of good quality and appealing to the client, and the massage is well executed by a dextrous and empathetic therapist, the therapeutic result can be excellent – even producing an 'altered state of consciousness'. In these circumstances, and as a short-term, de-stressing intervention, the description of the treatment as aromatherapy is perfectly appropriate. However, research conducted by the sociologist Livingstone (2010), who has extensive experience in the field of beauty therapy and spas, revealed that in many Scottish spa hotels (excluding 'destination' spas), this was not the case. Often, the therapists had very poor product knowledge and limited psychomotor skills, resulting in a disappointing experience.

Many skin care manufacturers incorporate essential oils in their face and body care ranges. Often these are used in salons and spas as part of aesthetic aromatherapy. The essential oils in their formulae are often credited with properties that are beneficial to the skin and general well-being, and very often this is underpinned with research. For example, soothing formulae often contain essential oils of lavender, rose or Roman chamomile, which are noted for their anti-inflammatory properties; and formulae for blemishes and excess sebum may include geranium, bergamot and ylang ylang or tea tree, which are antibacterial, cicatrising and astringent. So it could be argued that this is aromatherapy too – in the hands of a skilled therapist using skin care products that are supported by in-house research. Is it aromatherapy when the client purchases these phytocosmeceuticals to use at home?

The division between 'aesthetic aromatherapy' and 'clinical aromatherapy' has become more significant over the years. This is apparent in education, practice and regulation. It is not the intention to explore education and regulation here, but the reader should be aware that these distinctions do exist in the UK today (Jenkins 2006).

'Clinical aromatherapy' was the original designation used to distinguish between practitioners of aesthetic aromatherapy and those practising aromatherapy outside the beauty profession, where the emphasis was on tailoring the treatment to address physical, physiological and emotional concerns. A detailed consultation that addresses well-being, medical and social concerns, the selection and blending of essential oils to meet the needs of the individual, the application of appropriate massage techniques and the preparation of products for home use, are central to clinical aromatherapy practice. Clinical aromatherapy practitioners do not usually make claims to treat disorders, as this is against their code of conduct. However, they will often offer therapeutic interventions to ill and compromised client groups, in conjunction with medical support and/or consent.

Many clinical aromatherapy practitioners are self-employed, and practise either from their own premises or from multi-disciplinary clinics. Often they will undertake additional education, and specialise in, for example, aromadermatology (Bensouilah and Buck 2006), cancer care, care of the elderly, and dementia, palliative, mental health, fertility, pregnancy and maternity care (Price and Price 2007), sports therapy and sports injuries (Harris 2009; Quéry 2009), musculoskeletal and nervous system disorders.

with the main focus being the promotion of physical and emotional well-being rather than the treatment of disease. Here, aromatherapy is practised (mainly) by non-medical therapists, and is regarded as complementary to orthodox health care. Aromatherapy is generally recognised as being of considerable value in the prevention and alleviation of stress, and the numerous adverse effects of stress on well-being. Its full potential has yet to be achieved or recognised.

In the English-speaking countries, essential oils are administered dermally and by inhalation. This style of aromatherapy was called 'Anglo-Saxon' aromatherapy (Harris 2003), to distinguish it from the practice of aromatic medicine. In this book we will refer to this type of practice simply as 'aromatherapy'. It is because the essential oils are introduced to the body via these routes that massage therapy is often included in the therapeutic intervention. In fact, in the UK and other English-speaking countries, the principal style of aromatherapy practice has become inextricably linked with massage. Again, this is largely a consequence of Maury's promotion of aromatherapy as an external therapy in the 1960s (Harris 2003).

A holistic approach that integrates the use of essential oils with massage, the beneficial effects of odour on both physical and emotional well-being, and the great potential of essential oils as healing agents come together to make aromatherapy a unique but inherently complex therapy. Therefore, since the 1960s, aromatherapy writers and practitioners, life and social scientists have proposed theories that might explain how aromatherapy exerts its effects.

The theoretical basis of aromatherapy

> Aromatherapy is a shadowy world of romantic illusion, its magic easily dispelled by the harsh light of science. (King 1994, p. 413)

> Aromatherapy needs to develop a theory to explain and predict its effects. (Schnaubelt 2003, pp. 8–10)

The above statements were made some time ago, in response to the general image of aromatherapy as portrayed in the prevailing popular literature at that time, and criticism from scientific quarters. Aromatherapy was not seen as having a strong evidence base, and it was certainly not viewed as being scientific, so it was, and still is, the subject of some criticism by the scientific community. Also, because of the level of education of many practitioners, unfortunately many were, and still are, not able to defend their practices. At the same time, in 2003, this led Bob Harris to comment in an editorial that:

> It is no longer valid to state that aromatherapy just 'works' or that it is the intrinsic energy of the oils that exerts an effect. There is the possibility that

you will not be taken seriously. It would be a pity if aromatherapy were to be dismissed out of hand simply because representatives of the therapy are unable to present it in a conventionally acceptable and understandable manner. (Harris 2003, p. 57)

In order to explain how aromatherapy might work, from a Western, scientific perspective, various mechanisms could be considered. These include the physical and physiological effects of essential oils via transdermal absorption, inhalation and olfaction, the effects of essential oils via the limbic system, and the physical, physiological and psychological effects of massage.

Authors such as Holmes (1997, 1998, 2001) and Mojay (1996, 1998, 1999) have applied traditional Eastern concepts to aromatherapy practice, suggesting that the beneficial effects of aromatherapy on health and well-being could also be explained in terms of correspondences with traditional Chinese medicine. This philosophy gives aromatherapy an energetic dimension, and underpins the holistic nature of the therapy. Practitioners and writers such as Davis (1991), who developed 'subtle aromatherapy' and explored the use of essential oils for spiritual well-being, incorporating vibrational healing, crystals and chakra energy, and Holmes (1997), who developed 'fragrance energetics', have essential oil energetics as their core philosophy. This is more difficult to explain in Harris's (2003) 'conventionally acceptable and understandable manner'; but despite this, many practitioners have adopted this way of practising aromatherapy. The majority of writers who embrace the energetic models also state that it is very important for aromatherapists to understand the chemistry and pharmacokinetics of essential oils – perhaps in order to maintain respectability in our culture where science is highly respected. These energetic philosophies, however, have also led to criticism about aromatherapy from scientific circles, and can be found in blogs such as that of Professor David Colquhoun FRS (www.dcscience.net 2011).

With cognisance of the controversial backdrop, an exploration of aromatherapy philosophy and hypothesis/theory follows. We will explore the energetic philosophy, but first we will look at the more conventional science-based hypotheses, and the body of research and evidence around these. For information about the chemical constituents mentioned, please refer to Appendix A.

The pharmacological hypotheses

By this, we mean the hypotheses that consider the biological actions of essential oils. These include some of the central hypotheses of aromatherapy, such as the transdermal absorption of essential oils, absorption via inhalation, pharmacokinetics and pharmacodynamics.

Absorption through the skin

One of the central beliefs in aromatherapy is that the skin is an important route for the application of essential oils (often with massage), as essential oils applied to the skin are absorbed and enter the body fluids.

From the aromatherapy perspective, it is generally accepted that essential oil molecules diffuse through the skin. Essential oils can also gain access via hair follicles, sweat ducts and sebaceous glands. It is likely that, and it is believed that, larger molecules pass through more slowly than smaller ones. Substances with a molecular weight greater than 500 have great difficulty passing through the skin; however, all essential oil constituents have molecular weights well below this. Most terpenoids have a molecular weight of around 150 and sesquiterpenoids around 225.

Fat-soluble (lipophilic) compounds are able to cross the skin better than water-soluble (hydrophilic) ones. However, the outer layer of the skin, the stratum corneum, is partly hydrophilic and partly lipophilic. A highly fat-soluble substance will have trouble getting through the hydrophilic components of the stratum corneum, whereas a molecule that has high solubility in water will be unable to pass through the lipid-rich regions. Essential oils are composed largely of fat-soluble molecules, but there are also essential oil molecules that are hydrophilic, so essential oils certainly possess the characteristics of substances that can pass easily through the skin. Metabolism can commence in the skin due to the presence of metabolic enzymes in skin cells – including those known as P450s.

Essential oils have diverse characteristics – some contain high proportions of volatile molecules ('top notes') whilst others are more viscous, composed of larger molecules (often 'base notes'). The different chemical components will have varying abilities to cross the skin – so rates of transdermal absorption will vary, depending on the chemical composition of an essential oil.

The upper layer of skin cells could act as a 'reservoir', holding the molecules for unknown periods of time. Meanwhile, the more volatile molecules can evaporate and be lost into the air. The effects of viscosity on essential oil absorption are likely to be complex, because for a slightly viscous oil, such as sandalwood, absorption is likely to be slower than for a highly mobile liquid oil, such as sweet orange, and evaporation and loss of molecules to the atmosphere is likely to be slower as well.

To optimise absorption of the essential oils through the skin, the massage blend of essential oils in fixed vegetable 'carrier' oils is applied to as large an area of skin as possible at the very start of the treatment, and then the body should be fully draped. Throughout the ensuing massage, only the area being treated should be exposed. Other factors affecting absorption are warmth, massage, occlusion and hydration of the skin (Tisserand and Balacs 1995).

The possible 'reservoir' property of the top layers of the stratum corneum could be significant in some topical essential oil treatments. For example, a topical antifungal application of essential oils such as tea tree may benefit from the addition of oils such as sandalwood or vetivert, which may act like the 'fixatives' in perfumery, and allow the active principles to remain in contact with the skin cells for longer periods.

Tisserand and Balacs (1995) certainly hold the view that the skin is an efficient way of introducing essential oils into the body, because essential oils components are largely lipophilic (they will dissolve in fatty substances), and of small molecular weight, and so they can pass through the skin and enter the body. They cite a personal communication (from Hotchkiss, a toxicologist at St Mary's Hospital, London) and two published studies (Bronaugh et al. 1990; Jäger et al. 1992) which led to this conclusion, and they state 'we know that, after application to uncovered skin, between 4 per cent and 25 per cent of the essential oil is absorbed' (Tisserand and Balacs 1995, p. 24).

Price and Price (2007) and Bowles (2003) also cite Jäger et al. (1992) and some studies that explore the ability of some essential oil components, such as nerolidol and some terpenes, to increase skin permeability by acting on the lipid bilayer (Cornwall and Barry 1994; Takayama and Nagai 1994).

Buck's 2004 paper on the barrier function of the skin cites Jäger et al. (1992), Cornwall and Barry (1994) and Fuchs et al. (1997) to support the principle; however, Buck does acknowledge that there is some dispute regarding the pharmacological significance of the small amounts absorbed.

Bensouilah and Buck (2006) write about transdermal permeation of essential oils and identify that the stratum corneum is the rate-limiting barrier to skin penetration, and that there are three ways in which molecules can cross this barrier. These are the intercellular, intracellular and shunt routes (via hair follicles and sweat glands, although other exocrine glands could be included here). Like the other writers mentioned, they cite the older papers by Jäger et al. (1992) and Fuchs et al. (1997) as evidence of skin permeability to essential oils.

The objective of a more recent study conducted by Fewell et al. (2007) was to establish if d-limonene could be detected in the blood after an aromatherapy massage with sweet orange oil (d-limonene is a major component of this oil). Their study led to the conclusion that although d-limonene was absorbed and detected in the blood, less than 10 per cent of the d-limonene applied was taken up by the skin, and that the levels were too low (less than 0.008 µg/ml) to exert any pharmacological (in this case sedative) effects. Chen, Chan and Budd (1998) estimated that 0.28 µg/ml d-limonene is the level required to initiate sedation in mice – this is 30 times higher than the levels detected in the Fewell et al. (2007) study.

More recent studies have investigated the potential of essential oils to decrease skin barrier resistance and enhance the skin penetration of topical drugs. In a review by Adorjan and Buchbauer (2010), six animal studies are cited, all carried out since 2007. All of the studies demonstrated that the essential oils under investigation, many of which are part of the Chinese materia medica but unfamiliar in Western aromatherapy (with the exception of basil oil, which is used in aromatherapy), had penetration enhancing effects. Earlier, Williams and Barry (2004) had suggested that essential oils could interact with the liquid crystals of skin lipids, so this is a possible explanation of how this may happen.

So although this aromatherapy principle is perfectly reasonable and logical, the body of 'hard' scientific evidence is not extensive. We now need to consider another route of absorption – inhalation.

Inhalation

Essential oils are volatile, so their molecules can enter the body via inhalation and they can have direct effects on tissues via the respiratory tract. Essential oil vapours are carried with the inspired air via the nose to the respiratory tract. The molecules may be absorbed throughout the respiratory tract, ending at the alveoli, where they are easily transported into the bloodstream. Absorption via the nasal epithelium could also be considerable – it is very thin and has an extensive capillary supply allowing rapid access to the circulation. As the nasal epithelium is located close to the brain, the essential oil molecules have the potential to access the central nervous system and arterial circulation.

Therefore, the importance of absorption via inhalation in aromatherapy should not be underestimated. The client will be the recipient of the beneficial effects of the essential oils on mood via the limbic system and central nervous system, and also of any effects on the respiratory tract. However, it is not only the client who will be affected – there is the potential for therapists to experience psychotropic effects (mood changes), stimulating and sedative effects and respiratory changes during and after treating clients. There is anecdotal evidence for this phenomenon.

Most scientific studies are concerned with the uptake via inhalation of essential oil constituents, including the commonly occurring monoterpenes such as α-pinene and d-limonene, and the oxide 1,8-cineole that is found in many eucalyptus oils. Falk-Filipsson et al. (1993) demonstrated that in human volunteers, the relative pulmonary uptake of d-limonene was in the region of 70 per cent, with 1 per cent of this being eliminated unchanged in exhaled air. Jäger et al. (1996) investigated blood concentrations of 1,8-cineole during prolonged inhalation, finding that approximately 750 ng/ml plasma was the peak concentration after 18 minutes.

It has indeed been demonstrated that some essential oil components have physiological effects upon inhalation. For example, inhalation of 1,8-cineole, the major constituent of many eucalyptus oils, increases cerebral blood flow (Buchbauer 1996).

Some essential oils have direct effects on the tissues of the respiratory tract, notably those containing ketones, such as menthone and carvone, and the oxide 1,8-cineole. Mucolytic and expectorant effects – where the secretions become thinner as the activity of the cilia and goblet cells is increased – have been investigated in the past. *Eucalyptus globulus*, fennel, pine and thyme oils are all noted for this action (Price and Price 2007).

Since it is a reasonable assumption that essential oil constituents can gain entry via the skin and the respiratory system, we then need to consider what happens to them once they are in the body. This takes us to the subject of *pharmacokinetics* (how the body deals with *xenobiotics*, or foreign substances) and *pharmacodynamics* (what xenobiotics do to the body). Both Tisserand and Balacs (1995) and Bowles (2003) give comprehensive accounts of these processes in relation to aromatherapy. A summary based on these sources is presented below.

Distribution – an overview of current hypotheses

Research into the distribution of essential oil components after absorption is limited; however, it is generally acknowledged that they are distributed in a similar way to fat-soluble drugs. Distribution, like absorption, depends on the characteristics of the molecules, the most important being their solubility in fats and water.

It could be expected that the more highly lipophilic essential oil molecules will tend to be taken up by fatty tissues, such as the brain (some lipophilic molecules found in essential oils can pass though the protective 'blood–brain barrier') and nervous tissue and the liver; they move more slowly to adipose tissue, as it has a poor blood supply. However, the adipose tissue, with its low metabolic rate, could act as a reservoir – attracting, accumulating and storing the lipophilic molecules.

The more hydrophilic components will tend to be found in the blood and some organs that receive a high blood flow – including the adrenal glands, kidneys and muscles. As the majority of essential oil molecules are lipophilic, however, they will tend to leave the blood for the muscle and adipose tissue fairly quickly.

Blood contains a soluble protein called 'plasma albumin'. Many electrically charged substances are able to bind to the plasma albumin; this is a reversible process. If a substance binds to the albumin, it is not available to other tissues via the circulation. Some essential oil components – ketones, esters, aldehydes and carboxylic acids – are electrically charged in the internal body environment and are thought to bind to the plasma albumin. Plasma albumin levels can be low in patients with kidney or liver disease – hence the need to reduce the amount of essential oils administered in aromatherapy treatment in order to avoid higher blood concentration levels of essential oil components. Binding to plasma proteins could go some way to explaining potential interactions between essential oil components and some drugs.

Metabolism – a summary of key events

All substances that enter the body – xenobiotics – are metabolised. The liver is the most important organ in the process, but the skin, nervous tissues, kidneys, lungs, intestinal mucosa and blood plasma all have metabolic activity. The most important concept of metabolism in relation to essential oils is that the molecules undergo *biotransformation* to make them less fat-soluble and more water-soluble, in order that they can be excreted via the kidneys in urine.

In simple terms, this process occurs in two distinct biochemical processes, known as Phase I and Phase II reactions.

1. *Phase I reactions* – these biochemical reactions (oxidation, reduction and hydrolysis, depending on the chemical being metabolised) are often referred to as the 'prelude' to making the molecules more water-soluble. They are also often described as 'detoxification' reactions, rendering toxic molecules less so. However, a few molecules, including the relatively non-toxic estragole found in basil essential oil, are initially metabolised into toxic metabolites – the carcinogenic 1'-hydroxyestragole in this example.

2. *Phase II reactions* – these are conjugation reactions where the metabolites from Phase I are joined to specific atomic groups in preparation for excretion. These molecules are called conjugates. There are three types of conjugation reactions – glucuronide conjugations, oxidations and glutathione conjugations. Alcohols and phenols will probably be excreted as glucuronides. The cytochrome P450 enzymes catalyse these reactions. It is thought that some of the aldehydes, such as citral and citronellal, are oxidised and converted to carboxylic acids. The terpenes are oxidised to alcohols, then carboxylic acids, prior to excretion. Glutathione is a chemical in the liver that conjugates with reactive, toxic molecules, rendering them safe. If glutathione levels are low, these reactive metabolites can cause serious liver damage. A few essential oil components could cause glutathione depletion; however, the amounts used in aromatherapy are not likely to pose any risk.

Excretion of essential oils and their metabolites

If essential oils have entered the bloodstream, they will be metabolised and excreted by the kidneys. Most of the terpenes will be oxidised to alcohols, then carboxylic acids, and water-soluble conjugates – all excreted in the urine. Some alcohols, such as geraniol, are converted into carboxylic acids and excreted in the urine, while others, for example linalool, are excreted as glucuronides. Aldehydes such as citral and citronellal are converted to carboxylic acids before excretion; cinnamaldehyde is converted to cinnamic acid, which is then conjugated and excreted as a glucuronide. Esters are easily hydrolysed, and are excreted as water-soluble glucuronides and acids.

As essential oil molecules are volatile, small amounts will also be lost through exhalation and sweat. For example, the oxide 1,8-cineole can be eliminated, unchanged, via the breath. If the essential oils have been ingested, they will also be eliminated in the faeces.

Pharmacodynamics – the biological effects of essential oils

For some years there has been anecdotal information concerning the potential therapeutic actions of essential oils, such as their anti-inflammatory, sedative and analgesic effects, and there is also some scientific evidence (Bowles 2003). Price and Price (2007) describe an extensive range of properties, some of which are backed up by research. For a summary, please see Table 2.1.

Table 2.1 Therapeutic effects of essential oils (adapted from Price and Price 2007)

Therapeutic property	Comments	Aromatherapy application
Antibacterial	Research to support this Aromatograms	Synergistic blends may minimise resistance, air disinfection, skin and respiratory tract infections, MRSA
Analgesic	Traditional medicine, e.g. clove oil for dental pain, peppermint for headaches Anecdotal evidence Specific research lacking Complex mechanisms, psychological aspects	Chronic pain Headaches Joint and muscle pain
Antifungal	Research to support this	Fungal infections and yeast infections

Anti-inflammatory	Abundant anecdotal evidence. Some research on specific components, e.g. α-bisabolol and chamazulene	In synergistic blends for clients where appropriate, e.g. pain, infection, irritation, etc.
Antipruritic	Abundant anecdotal evidence. One clinical study has confirmed that a blend of lavender and tea tree in jojoba and sweet almond oil has antipruritic effects	Skin irritation and itching
Antitoxic	Limited studies have suggested that oils such as chamomile can inactivate bacterial toxins	Incorporation of chamomile in blends where infection by *Staphylococcus* spp. and *Streptococcus* spp. could cause pain and irritation
Antiviral	Anecdotal evidence and limited scientific evidence Possibly due to lipid solubility	Support for clients with viral infections, *Herpes simplex*
Deodorant	Anecdotal evidence and limited scientific evidence	Disease processes that generate unpleasant smells, e.g. burns, wounds Personal care products for underarms and feet
Digestive	Traditional uses of aromatics – spices, citrus and oils from the Apiaceae – to increase gastric secretions, stimulate secretions from the gallbladder, stimulate peristalsis, improve liver function Research to support this property, but not specifically in the context of holistic aromatherapy	Appetite stimulation, support for digestive process, constipation
Diuretic	Some writers attribute this property to essential oils especially juniperberry (specifically terpinen-4-ol) but others disagree	Fluid retention Encourage excretion process

cont.

Table 2.1 Therapeutic effects of essential oils (adapted from Price and Price 2007) *cont.*

Therapeutic property	Comments	Aromatherapy application
Energising	Essential oils can correct deficits or blockages in energy Difficult to back up with scientific research, but nevertheless an important property in aromatherapy	Synergistic blending using the energetic approaches
Granulation promoting or cicatrisant	Anecdotal evidence (beginning with Gattefossé) Studies support this property for some oils (hypericum, chamomile)	Healing the tissues, e.g. lavender for minor burns Price and Price (2007) recommend geranium
Hormone-like activity	Claim that some oils can normalise endocrine secretions via hypophysis, but no research to support this Anecdotal evidence and folk medicine Sclareol, viridiflorol and *trans*-anethole – oestrogen analogues? *Pinus sylvestris* – cortisone analogues? Stimulants of suprarenal glands, modulants of adrenal cortex, thyroid stimulation and regulation Franchomme and Pénoël support hypothesis; limited research	Dysmenorrhoea and amenorrhoea Pain relief Stress Allergic reactions Thyroid
Hyperaemic	Primary irritation of skin results in release of mediators, e.g. bradykinin which causes vasodilation; humoral reactions result in an anti-inflammatory effect	Poor circulation, warmth, comfort, pain relief
Immuno-stimulant	Niaouli may have an immunostimulant effect by increasing level of immunoglobulins – Pénoël, not 'proven' Probably conferred by a range of physical and psychological effects	Debility Convalescence Stress
Mucolytic expectorant	Supported by studies	Improve function of lungs, bronchodilation, bronchitis, congestion, chest infections

Sedative	Anecdotal and scientific evidence supports this property	Calming, stress, anxiety, insomnia
Spasmolytic	Research supports the antispasmodic activity of some oils in smooth muscle Anecdotal evidence supports spasmolytic activity in skeletal muscle	Digestive or skeletal muscle spasm Cramp Muscular tension

Some research is beginning to elucidate the mechanisms behind these therapeutic actions. For example, one of the most significant therapeutic effects attributed to some essential oils is the anti-inflammatory effect. Pro-inflammatory leukotrienes are derived from the metabolism of arachidonic acid; the enzyme 5-lipoxygenase (5-LOX) is the first enzyme involved in its oxidation. Some essential oils are thought to inhibit this enzyme, and this could go some way towards explaining how they have anti-inflammatory action.

Baylac and Racine (2003) conducted an *in vitro* assessment of a wide range of essential oils, absolutes and nature identical fragrances to establish their ability to inhibit 5-LOX, and thus potential anti-inflammatory activities. In some cases, such as that of myrrh and sandalwood, it is clear that their ability to inhibit 5-LOX is related to their reported anti-inflammatory properties. However, other oils such as Himalayan cedar and the citrus oils (lemon, sweet orange and mandarin) have similar ability to inhibit 5-LOX, yet these are not commonly described as possessing anti-inflammatory actions. Their main component, *d*-limonene, also showed good inhibitory activity. The sesquiterpenes β-caryophyllene and α-bisabolol showed strong inhibitory potential, and it was suggested that oils rich in *trans*-nerolidol and *trans-trans*-farnesol will also show the ability to inhibit 5-LOX. Conversely, anti-inflammatory actions are usually attributed to Roman chamomile, yet it is a weak inhibitor. Therefore, this oil must have another mode of action. Some absolutes and resinoids also showed inhibitory activities – notably ambrette seed (*Hibiscus abelmoschus*), myrrh resinoid and *Immortelle stoechas*. Jasmine, one of the more widely used absolutes in aromatherapy, only showed weak inhibitory activity.

However, since 2007 a considerable amount of scientific research concerning essential oils has been published. Adorjan and Buchbauer's 2010 updated review on the biological properties of essential oils, and Dobetsberger and Buchbauer's 2011 updated review of the actions of essential oils on the central nervous system present some high quality research. These reviews bring together the very best of the studies, leaving no doubts as to the therapeutic actions of some essential oils and their constituents. For a summary, please refer to Tables 2.2 and 2.3.

Table 2.2 Biological properties of essential oils (adapted from Adorjan and Buchbauer 2010)

Action	Comments	Therapeutic potential
Anti-nociceptive effect (the peripheral nervous system)	This is a reduction in pain sensitivity made within neurones when a substance, e.g. an opiate or endorphin, combines with a receptor Several studies indicated that essential oils and their constituents have anti-nociceptive effects, and a few of these studies explored the molecular mechanisms for this activity. This effect is often found in combination with analgesic and anti-inflammatory activity Many of the studies concerned essential oils that are not familiar to aromatherapy, but are obtained from aromatic plants used in folk medicine, including *Eugenia uniflora* (the Brazilian cherry tree) and *E. pitangueira*, *Zingiber zerumbet*	Constituents with anti-nociceptive potential include β-pinene, β-caryophyllene, β-myrcene, sesquiterpenes including α-humulene, 1,8-cineole with β-pinene, synergistic potential with 1,8-cineole and morphine, linalool, linalyl acetate, furano-sesquiterpenes in *Eugenia uniflora* Essential oils with anti-nociceptive potential include *Eucalyptus camadulensis* (1,8-cineole and β-pinene) some *Salvia* spp., including *S. officinalis*, *Rosmarinus officinalis*, *Citrus bergamia*, *S. sclarea*, *Thymus vulgaris* CT linalool, *Mentha villosa* (piperitone oxide), *Phlomis* spp.
Anti-cancer activity	*In vitro* studies using human tumour cell lines indicated that some essential oil constituents potentiate the effects of anti-cancer drugs by stimulating accumulation and crossing the cell membrane. One study indicated that *Tanacetum gracile* (alpine aromatic herb) essential oil could induce apoptosis via the mitochondrial pathway The ethnobotanical use of *Anemopsis californica* root to treat uterine cancer led to a study of its essential oil with lung, breast, prostate and colon cancer lines – demonstrating its ability to inhibit the proliferation of these cell lines *In vivo* animal studies have indicated that the toxic effects of some anti-cancer drugs on the male reproductive system are in part due to the formation of free radicals, and that the antioxidant potential of essential oils such as *Satureja khuzestanica* could offer protection	Most studies highlighted the anti-cancer activities of monoterpene alcohols or sesquiterpene hydrocarbons Constituents include β-caryophyllene, which potentiates anti-cancer effects of α-humulene, *iso*-caryophyllene, and paclitaxel; linalool improved the activity of anthracyclines against breast cancer cells There may be a synergistic relationship between thymol, piperitone and methyleugenol in *A. californica* essential oil *Eucalyptus sideroxylon* and *E. torquata* essential oils were active against a breast cancer cell line but not a hepatocellular carcinoma line *Cymbopogon flexuosus* showed anticancer activity by activating apoptosis and reducing tumour cell viability (*in vitro* and *in vivo*, via injection)

Anti-phlogistic activity	There were many *in vivo* and some *in vitro* studies exploring the anti-inflammatory potential of essential oils and their constituents, and both acute and chronic inflammations were addressed	Thymoquinone from *Nigella sativa* supressed induced rheumatoid arthritis in rats
	Several of the studies cited concern the essential oils and their components of aromatic plants used in folk medicine, and unfamiliar to aromatherapy, e.g. the fruits of *Heracleum persicum* are used as a painkiller in traditional Iranian medicine, and the essential oil was shown to have significant anti-inflammatory and analgesic effects	*Thymus vulgaris* and *Origanum vulgare* in combination can reduce the production of pro-inflammatory cytokines
		A combination of α-humulene and *l-trans*-caryophyllene (isolated from *Cordia verbenacea*), given in an oral dose or via injection, might be useful in the management of inflammatory diseases
	The anti-inflammatory activity of essential oils and their constituents has more or less been ascertained, in that they act upon inflammation mediators as well as enzymes such as kinases	*Rosmarinus officinalis* essential oil has anti-inflammatory and anti-nociceptive potential (*in vivo* study)
		Ocotea quixos (*trans*-cinnamaldehyde and methyl cinnamate) has striking anti-inflammatory action, and does not damage gastric mucosa, shown *in vitro* and *in vivo*
		Cymbopogon citrates may inhibit cytokine production *in vitro*, thus the oil may have anti-inflammatory activity
		In vivo studies showed that α-bisabolol has a gastro-protective effect, and that an alcohol extract of *Origanum majorana* has potential for healing and protecting against the formation of gastric ulcers
		Citrus aurantium essential oil and the main component limonene also have protective effects on gastric mucosa; possibly due to stimulating an increase in mucous production

cont.

Table 2.2 Biological properties of essential oils (adapted from Adorjan and Buchbauer 2010) *cont.*

Action	Comments	Therapeutic potential
Penetration enhancement	Several studies have explored the potential for essential oils to improve transdermal drug delivery (known as penetration enhancers, sorption promoters or accelerants). Several of the oils investigated were from plants significant in the Chinese materia medica	Potential to improve drug delivery; could lead to the administration of lower doses with perhaps fewer side effects, e.g. in cancer treatments. Essential oils include *Camellia oleifera* – NSAIDs (Nonsteroidal Anti-inflammatory Drugs); *Fructus evodia* and *Radix saposhnikoviae* – ibuprofen; *Ocimum basilicum* – labetalol hydrochloride (an alpha and beta blocker used to treat hypertension)
Insect repellent activity	This research revolves around the prevention of pathogenic reactions after insect bites. Some essential oils had repellent activity, but usually these were less effective than DEET (N, N-diethyl-meta-toluamide)	Geraniol appears to be the most promising constituent in this area, especially in combination with DEET Essential oils are too volatile to have a lasting effect
Antiviral activity	Several studies have looked at the antiviral potential of essential oils against *Herpes simplex* virus (HSV) 1 and 2 The *in vitro* activity of several Lebanese oils against SARS (Severe Acute Respiratory Syndrome)-CoV and HSV 1 was explored *Eucalyptus globulus* was investigated with regard to its activity against strains of respiratory bacteria and viruses, including flu viruses, and the mumps virus. Results were varied, and only mild activity against mumps was observed	*Artemisia arborescens* showed activity against HSV1 and 2, it inactivated the virus and inhibited cell-to-cell virus diffusion *Eugenia caryophyllata* and *Cedrus libani* showed varying degrees of activity against strains of HSV 1 and 2 *Laurus nobilis* showed promising activity against SARS *Juniperus oxycedrus* was effective against HSV 1 *Matricaria recutita* was effective against HSV 2 *Pimpinella anisum*, *Pinus pumila* and *Matricaria recutita* affect

| Actions on relaxation, sedation and sleep | Relaxation is defined here as the absence of arousal caused by rage, anxiety or worry; a condition of low tension. Sedation is a medical procedure to calm down the functions of the CNS with the aid of sedative drugs. There is overlap in the terms 'sedative' and 'hypnotic'. Benzodiazepines are often used as sedatives and hypnotics. Nearly all of the studies cited demonstrated the beneficial effects of essential oils and their constituents in relation to relaxation and the treatment of insomnia | Dermal application of rose oil, whilst preventing olfactory stimulation, can cause a significant decrease in breathing rate, blood oxygen saturation and blood pressure, compared with the placebo; emotional responses include feeling more relaxed and calm, but less vigilant. This study supports the use of rose oil in the treatment of depression or stress

Japanese incense ingredients (agarwood oil and spikenard oil) were investigated in regard to their sedative actions if inhaled. The oils were effective; however, the main constituents were isolated, and these too had sedative effects – in lower concentrations than found in the oils

The rhizome oil of *Kaempferia galangal* was shown to have strong sedative and relaxant properties, as did its main constituents ethyl *trans-p*-methoxycinnamate and ethyl cinnamate, supporting the use of the rhizome in folk medicine to treat stress, anxiety and improve sleep

Rosewood essential oil, with its high linalool content, is used in Brazilian folk medicine as a sedative. A study demonstrated that the oil has sedative actions and can reduce neuronal excitability

A study focusing on the use of sweet orange oil in aromatherapy massage found that the dermal uptake of *d*-limonene was higher if higher concentrations (4%) had been administered, but even then, the blood concentration was low, as it had possibly been metabolised to perillic alcohol and its derivatives. It was concluded that any sedative effects were due to olfactory/cognitive influences rather than direct systemic action

Several essential oils (cinnamon, coriander and clove) could, if co-administered, increase the sleeping times induced by phenobarbital, possibly by binding to gamma aminobutyric acid (GABA) receptors). A later study included single isolated fragrance constituents (terpinen-4-ol, 1-octen-3-ol) which also produced anti-stress effects

Inhalation of spikenard essential oil was shown to have strong sedative activity, as was its volatile component valerena-4,7(11)-diene. It was suggested that this is a non-harmful method for the treatment of insomnia and attention deficit hyperactivity disorder (ADHD) in children

The effects of a range of odorants (lavender, vanillin, vetivert and the unpleasant ammonium sulphide) on sleep did not enhance arousal or wake-up, but did transiently reduce inhalation and enhanced exhalation for up to six breaths |

cont.

Table 2.3 Essential oils and the central nervous system (adapted from Dobetsberger and Buchbauer 2011) *cont.*

Biological action	Comments	Therapeutic potential
Anticonvulsive action	Epilepsy might be caused by excessive neuronal activity and a reduction in the seizure threshold in the CNS. Perhaps neurones are able to release the neurotransmitter glutamate in large amounts and thus cause excessive release of calcium by post-synaptic cells. Or, mutations may lead to ineffective GABA (a neurotransmitter inhibitor) action. Epilepsy can be controlled but not healed by conventional medicine. All of the studies were animal studies with mice, snails and pigeons	All of the oils and their constituents investigated showed potential as an alternative therapy. These included safranal (from *Crocus sativus*), terpinen-4-ol, nutmeg, anise (*Pimpinella anisum*), sweet basil (which had a depressant influence on the CNS and anticonvulsant properties due to interactions with GABA receptors), halfabar (*Cymbopogon proximus*, with major constituent piperitone, was a cardiovascular depressant, and an antiemetic as well as an anticonvulsant) and bergamot However, it was emphasised that nutmeg oil should be avoided in those with myoclonic and absence seizures, and that anise oil should be used with caution as it caused neuronal hyper-excitability in snails
Actions on dementia and Alzheimer's disease	Alzheimer's disease is a common form of neurodegenerative disease which is characterised by a deficit in cholinergic mediated neurotransmission in the synaptic cleft. This impairs cognitive functions and causes progressive loss of memory Drug therapies often have side effects	Narcissus absolute was investigated as a potential cholinesterase inhibitor; inhibition was observed at 0.1 mg/ml (*in vitro*). It is not certain that narcissus absolute has a therapeutic application; however, it did have behavioural effects and therefore could have a place in the cognitive domain Lavender and melissa essential oils were shown to reduce agitation So far, essential oils and their constituents have only shown symptomatic alleviation in Alzheimer's disease

Despite some of the potential uses of essential oils identified in these papers, it is not usually the role of the aromatherapist to treat specific conditions, such as infections. However, a therapist can include appropriate oils in a holistic context, and can offer aromatherapy preparations for home use.

It is a reasonable belief that essential oils possess a fairly wide spectrum of therapeutic effects, many of which have now been investigated. Despite the wealth of anecdotal evidence regarding the therapeutic efficacy of essential oils, the scientific studies and a reasonable working hypothesis regarding the actions and modes of action of essential oil components, there is still uncertainty over a few aspects – notably the amounts of essential oils reaching the cells, tissues and organs when applied via massage, and indeed, whether this is sufficient to exert significant, systemic pharmacological effects.

It is also possible that very small 'doses', in some cases, are as effective as larger doses. For example, an early study conducted by Boyd and Pearson (1946), which investigated the expectorant action of lemon oil, established that the optimum dose was 50 mg/kg, but that even 0.01 mg/kg was effective. Doses within that range were less effective. More recently, Balacs (1995) made a comparison of blood plasma concentrations of lavender essential oil constituents with the effective levels for a range of psychoactive drugs (see Table 2.4). He commented 'the oft-quoted opinion that during treatment, essential oils reach the blood in amounts too small to have pharmacological effects, is not supported by the evidence.'

However, there is another important element in aromatherapy to explore – the use of the sense of smell to enhance or modify the emotions, and in turn positively affect behaviour. Balacs (1995) suggested that although essential oil molecules may interact with receptors for neurotransmission and with enzymes in the central and peripheral nervous systems, their psychoactive effects would be modified by olfaction.

Table 2.4 Blood plasma concentrations of essential oil constituents following massage and effective levels of some psychoactive drugs (adapted from Balacs 1995)

Essential oil constituents	Blood plasma concentration
Linalool and linalyl acetate (in lavender oil)	100 ng/ml (Jäger *et al.* 1992)
Psychoactive drug	**Effective level in blood plasma**
Amitriptyline (antidepressant)	200 ng/ml
Chlorpromazine (major tranquilliser)	100 ng/ml
Clonazepam (minor tranquilliser)	25 ng/ml
Morphine (narcotic analgesic)	65 ng/ml

Around the same time, Kirk-Smith (1995) suggested that pharmacological mechanisms may play an important part in some essential oil actions such as sedation, and that even ambient odours could have effects along the lines of intranasal drug treatments. For example, inhalation of lavender oil can lead to a light sedative or anaesthetic effect (Buchbauer et al. 1991, 1993). The main chemical components of lavender oil (linalool and linalyl acetate) can interact with cell membranes, damping cell electrical activity by closing ion channels. The inhalation of lavender oil can lead to effects similar to intravenous injection, due to rapid absorption by both nasal and lung mucosa (Buchbauer et al. 1991). These studies also revealed that some essential oil components may have the potential to interfere with drugs; for example, the compound iso-eugenol found in clove essential oil could interact with caffeine.

In 2007 Hongratanaworakit and Buchbauer suggested that both pharmacological and psychological effects could be active simultaneously. In their investigation into the effects of transdermal absorption of sweet orange oil, in which they prevented the human subjects from actually smelling the oil, they found that autonomic arousal was decreased, but the subjects actually felt more cheerful and vigorous at the same time. They concluded that their research was evidence to support the use of sweet orange oil for the relief of depression and stress.

Hongratanaworakit (2009) also investigated the effects of the transdermal absorption of rose, while avoiding olfactory stimulation. He measured the human subjects' blood pressure, rate of respiration, blood oxygen, pulse and skin temperature, and used rating scales to measure emotional responses. Rose oil produced a significant decrease in breathing rate, blood pressure and blood oxygen saturation, compared with the placebo group. The rose group reported that they felt more relaxed, although less vigilant, than the responses recorded by the placebo group. Again, his findings support the aromatherapeutic use of rose oil for relaxation and stress reduction.

It would seem that aromatherapy is at a stage where some of the pharmacological hypotheses and therapeutic claims are underpinned by evidence, yet the discipline is still struggling to gain credibility. This is perhaps because much of the research remains relatively inaccessible to practising aromatherapists.

Olfaction and aromatherapy

Having considered the hypotheses and evidence for the entry of essential oils into the body via transdermal absorption and inhalation, and their biological effects and therapeutic potential, we will now consider the effects of the fragrance of plant aromatics on the mind, emotions and behaviour.

found for several organic molecules, such as anisole, camphor and benzaldehyde. It is possible that OBPs bind to the odorants in the mucus at the olfactory epithelium, increasing their concentration and facilitating transport across the olfactory membrane. They may also have a protective function, preventing excessive amounts of an odorant reaching the receptors (Jacob 1999a).

There are families of odour receptors, which are encoded by possibly as many as 1000 genes. The odour receptors are known as '"7-pass" transmembrane proteins'. This name has been given because each protein contains seven regions of hydrophobic alpha helix, which allows a molecule to pass back and forth through the plasma membrane seven times. Also, many of the hydrophobic, lipophilic odorant molecules can easily enter the lipid bilayer of the plasma membranes of the cilia, without the aid of the transmembrane proteins. When an odorant molecule binds to the receptors on the cilia, this initiates a cascade of events that result in the generation of an olfactory signal, which is conducted along the olfactory nerve to the brain (Leffingwell 1999).

In 1999 Buck and Malnic of Harvard Medical School, with Hirono and Sato of the Life Electronics Centre, Amagasaki, Japan, demonstrated that single receptors can recognise multiple odorants, that a single odorant is typically recognised by multiple receptors, and that different odorants are recognised by different combinations of receptors (Malnic et al. 1999). They proposed that the olfactory system used a combinatorial coding scheme to encode the identities of odours. This explains why 1000 receptors can describe many thousands of odours (Leffingwell 1999).

So instead of the traditional steoric theory that one type of odour receptor is dedicated to a specific odour, the combinatorial diversity theory proposes that the olfactory system uses *combinations* of receptors, analogous to musical chords, or computer processing, to greatly reduce the number of actual receptor types that are required to detect a vast number of odorants.

> Each receptor is used over and over again to define an odour, just like letters are used over and over again to define different words. (Buck, cited in Howard Hughes Medical Institute 2004)

Malnic et al. (1999) demonstrated that even slight changes in chemical structure activate different combinations of receptors, and that a large concentration of an odorant binds to a wider variety of receptors than smaller amounts of the same odorant. This would explain why substances with traces of some chemicals such as indole, found in tiny amounts in some floral oils and absolutes, have a pleasant floral odour, yet large amounts are said to smell faecal (Leffingwell 1999). In 2004 Axel and Buck were awarded the Nobel Prize in Physiology and Medicine for their discovery of 'odorant receptors and the organisation of the olfactory system' (Miller 2004).

Earlier, Dyson (1938) had suggested that infrared resonance (IR) could be associated with odour, as IR could measure a molecule's vibrational frequency. As the frequency of many odours was in the IR range, their resonance could be associated with their smell. In the 1950s Wright was able to make such correlations, and commenced the classification of odorants on this basis. However, there were problems inherent in this theory, such as the fact that optical isomers have identical IR spectra, yet can smell different. Eventually, this theory was rejected (Leffingwell 1999).

However, in 1996 Luca Turin, a biophysicist at University College, London, proposed his 'vibrational induced electron tunnelling spectroscope theory'. Turin claimed that central to the process of olfaction was the frequency at which the bonds of an odorant molecule vibrate. He proposed that olfactory receptors are tuned to the vibrational frequency of odorants. When an odorant binds to the receptor protein, electron 'tunnelling' occurs across the binding site if the vibrational mode is equal to the energy gap between filled and empty electron tunnels (Turin 1996). The detail of this rather complex concept is worthy of exploration, especially the involvement of zinc in electron transfer aspects – as the olfactory sense diminishes drastically in cases of zinc deficiency.

However, no theory as yet has provided all of the answers, and the vibrational theory should not be discounted. The answers probably have an element of all of the above.

Personal differences

There are varying degrees of sensitivity to odours between individuals. This is probably genetic, as variations in ability to perceive odours have also been found between peoples of different ethnic origins. 'Hyposmia' is a reduced olfactory capability, while 'hyperosmia' is enhanced olfactory capability. An extreme example of this is related in Oliver Sacks' (1985) *The Man who Mistook his Wife for a Hat*. The case concerns a medical student who took a cocktail of recreational and hallucinogenic drugs, and had a vivid dream that he was a dog. On waking, he had a profound experience of hyperosmia that lasted for three weeks. His sense of smell was so heightened that he experienced his environment and relationships in a way that he likened to the way a dog might – '...*and now I awoke to an infinitely redolent world – a world in which all other sensations, enhanced as they were, paled before smell*' (p. 149). When he returned to his previous level of olfactory sensitivity, he reported feeling a sense of loss.

'Anosmia' is the loss of the sense of smell. This can be temporary – for example, caused by an upper respiratory tract infection – or permanent, caused by, for example, damage to the olfactory organ as a result of a head injury. Again,

Sacks (1986) describes the distress of a man whose olfactory tract was damaged because of a head injury.

> 'Sense of smell?' he says, 'I never gave it a thought. You don't normally give it a thought. But when I lost it – it was like being struck blind. Life lost a good deal of its savour – one doesn't realise how much 'savour' is smell. You smell people, you smell books, you smell the city, you smell the spring – maybe not consciously, but as a rich unconscious background to everything else. My whole world was suddenly radically poorer...' (Sacks 1986, p. 152)

Congenital anosmia is not common; however, if the sense has been missing since birth, it is less likely to cause stress and depression than anosmia resulting from injury. 'Hyposmia', the partial loss of the sense, can sometimes be treated if the underlying cause is mucous or swelling. 'Parosmia' is more common, and often occurs in anosmics. This term relates to the illusion or hallucination of a smell – usually a bad odour such as drains or faeces (Douek 1988). Specific anosmia is the inability to perceive a particular odour. This condition is most often associated with the synthetic musks in perfumery, and sandalwood constituents; also with some perfumery materials such as ambergris and methyl ionone. Olfactory fatigue occurs if an individual is exposed to a particular odour for a period of time, and the ability to perceive that particular odour is temporarily lost. Some perfumery materials cause this phenomenon very rapidly, such as violets, ionones and irone, and synthetic musks (Perfumery Education Centre 1995).

Our perception of, and reaction to, odours is affected by 'hedonics' – we respond in a way that is influenced by our personal and cultural experiences (Engen 1988; Jellinek 1994, 1997). Babies do not discriminate between pleasant and unpleasant odours; hedonic discrimination is learned behaviour. Classical conditioning – also known as Pavlovian conditioning – relates to the linking of a neutral object with an emotional and/or physiological reaction. King (1983) demonstrated that odour could be linked with a positive emotional state, using unconscious conditioning, and that future exposure to the odour could produce the same emotion. Around the same time a group of researchers at Warwick University published their research, which indicated that it was possible to link an odour with a negative emotional state (in this case a stress response), and that the emotion could be evoked at a later stage in response to the odour (Kirk-Smith, Van Toller and Dodd 1983). Another example of this phenomenon is discussed by Kirk-Smith (1995), citing the work of Shiffman and Siebert (1991), which demonstrated that a pleasant, 'neutral' apricot fragrance, paired with a relaxed state, could trigger a state of relaxation at a later time. More recently, Chu (2008) conducted a study on underachieving schoolchildren, which showed that olfactory conditioning could not only positively influence behaviour, but also enhance performance. It was concluded that, in broad terms, if ambient odours become associated with significant emotions, they can influence conscious behaviour.

Several further studies have shown that classical conditioning techniques, using odour, could be used to increase the immune response. Kirk-Smith (1995) suggested that this may reflect a link between the olfactory and immune systems, and the importance of this for species survival. In 2001 Milinski and Wedekind explored the link between perfume preferences and the major histocompatibility complex (MHC), which is a set of genes that is important in immune function. It had already been demonstrated that mice and humans prefer the body odour of partners who have a dissimilar MHC genotype; this could potentially produce heterozygous offspring and contribute to genetic diversity. Their study supported the hypothesis that perfumes that are self-selected for personal use in some way amplify body odours that resonate with the individual's immunogenetics.

The actual mechanisms of odour memory are not understood, yet odours leave a very powerful and indelible imprint on our psyche. Odours quickly become linked with emotional meanings, which can be personal and unique to the individual (King 1988). Therefore, using odour as an evocative agent has potential clinical applications. For example, could children with learning difficulties (Sanderson, Harrison and Price 1991), and the elderly and individuals who experience difficulties with sensory, motor and cognitive tasks, benefit from the therapeutic use of odours?

Odour and psychological effects

Jellinek (1997) proposed four mechanisms that could explain how odours have their psychological effects, summarised below:

- The *quasi-pharmacological* mechanism – this is the mechanism by which essential oils enter the body via the nose, and enter the blood stream via the nasal or lung mucosa, and thereby exert effects on nervous tissue. The quasi-pharmacological mechanism would imply that specific odours would elicit the same responses in everyone (apart from individual idiosyncrasies).

- The *semantic* mechanism – odours are experienced in the context of life situations; so each odour will carry an emotional memory, the impact of which will lead to physiological changes such as an increase in blood adrenalin. Unlike the quasi-pharmacological mechanism, this is a very personal mechanism, but it is environment dependent.

- The *hedonic valence* mechanism – where the effects depend on the subject's state of pleasure or displeasure; in other words, if an individual finds an odour pleasing, the perceived effect on the psyche will be positive and vice versa. This is also a personal mechanism; however, there can be an element

assigned to three groups and asked to undertake a word memory test, without the presence of any odour. The first group (negative expectancy) was then told that Spanish sage would impair their memory, the second group (positive expectancy) was informed that Spanish sage would positively influence their memory and the third group (control) was not given any information about Spanish sage. The subjects then undertook a second word test similar to the first. The negative expectancy group scored lower than in their first test and the positive expectancy group performed better – as expected. The control group performed as in the first test. This demonstrates that the manipulation of expectations will have a very strong influence, and that great care should be taken to avoid this in research with human subjects. Expectation undoubtedly will play a part in aromatherapeutic interventions.

However, if the factor of expectation is eliminated, changes in cognition can still be observed. For example, exposure to a novel smell has been shown to reduce decision-making capacity. Overman *et al.* (2011) explored the effect on the cognitive abilities of males undertaking a gambling task that involved decision making, concluding that the poor performance when exposed to the odour was possibly due to the stimulation of the emotional areas of the brain, reducing rational capacity.

Social and psychological perspectives

The effects of odour on self-perception and the perception of others has been explored and speculated upon. A therapeutic implication is the use of odour to improve self-esteem and self-confidence. It is difficult, however, to make generalisations about the social effects of fragrance, as so many factors will influence responses (Kirk-Smith 1995).

In 1997 Knasko reviewed studies concerning the effects of ambient odour on task and approach behaviours, particularly in the context of the controversial practice of scenting ambient air to elicit responses in a variety of settings, such as hotels, offices and shops. At that time, there had only been a limited number of studies on task performance, with mixed results, possibly because the many variables had not been addressed in the methodologies. However, studies concerning approach and avoidance behaviours had indicated that odour congruency and odour hedonics were important factors in some situations and not in others.

More recently Hirsch *et al.* (2007a) conducted research into the effects of odour on men's perception of women's weight. This is an extremely complex area; however, it was found that if a women was wearing a floral-spice odour, the perceived weight could be reduced by as much as 7 per cent. They concluded that the use of a hedonically positive scent could increase self-esteem and, on a behavioural level, encourage socialisation.

However, subtle aromas in the environment can also influence behaviour. This can be seen in many areas of daily and social activities. For example, Schifferstein, Talke and Oudshoorn (2011) investigated the influence of ambient odours of activating aromas such as peppermint, orange and 'seawater' on behaviour in a nightclub – and observed that the attendees danced and partied for longer, and rated the music as better than did those in the control experiment. Another study by Holland, Hendriks and Aarts (2005) revealed that the aroma of a citrus-scented household-cleaning agent increased the cleaning activities of students, although the majority reported that they had been unaware of a smell.

Aroma-chology

The science of aroma-chology is relatively new. In 1982 Annette Green of the Fragrance Foundation coined the term, which is also a 'service mark', to denote the science that is:

> ...dedicated to the study of the interrelationship between psychology and fragrance technology to elicit a variety of specific feelings and emotions – relaxation, exhilaration, sensuality, happiness and well-being – through odours via stimulation of olfactory pathways in the brain, especially the limbic system. (Fragrance Research Fund 1992, cited in Jellinek 1994, p. 25)

However, despite the obvious similarities, there are distinctions between aromatherapy and aroma-chology. The main point is that aroma-chology is concerned with the temporary effects of natural and synthetic fragrances (not just essential oils), but not their therapeutic potential. A variety of methods have been used in aroma-chology studies (Jellinek 1994), including the following:

- measurement of electrical brain activity, e.g. evoked potentials, contingent negative variation (CNV), brainwaves

- physiological measurements, e.g. systolic blood pressure, micro vibration, peripheral vasoconstriction, heart rate, electro-dermal activity (EDA), skin potential level, pupil dilation/constriction and the startle probe reflex

- examining behaviour modification, in controlled environments – for example, performance in sustained tasks, reaction times, sleep latency, learning and recall, memory retrieval, creative task solving, evaluation of ambiguous stimuli, miscellaneous cognitive tasks

- examination of odours and sleep, in laboratory/controlled environments

- examination of behaviour modification, for example shopping, gambling

- measurement of mood and emotion changes, such as reduction of stress and anxiety, effects on perceived health, conditioned mood changes.

As a consequence of aroma-chology and the associated research, our understanding of this aspect of aromatherapy has deepened, and the potential of the therapeutic effects elicited by the aroma of essential oils has widened. Perfumery itself has influenced our understanding of the specific psychotherapeutic effects of different odour types and characteristics.

Psychotherapeutic effects of odour types and characteristics

Paul Jellinek, in *The Practice of Modern Perfumery* (1959), first proposed that there were eight mood effects, which were linked to odour types and characteristics (see also Williams 1996). Robert Tisserand (1988) later devised a scheme which classified essential oil aromas in relation to correspondences with mood states and the Greek Four Elements/Humours. Tisserand refers to his scheme as a 'mood cycle', identifying eight positive moods, and opposing negative moods that we can all experience at different times. For example, the positive mood of clarity (associated with the transition from winter to spring, and the elements of Water and Air) is paired with the fresh scent of peppermint, so using the mood cycle, the fresh fragrance type of peppermint, exemplifying clarity, could be used to counteract the opposing mood of confusion (associated with the transition from summer to autumn, and the elements of Fire and Earth).

As we will discuss later in this chapter, following these ideas of Jellinek and Tisserand, several models have been proposed linking odour types to specific responses. These models are usually associated with semantic, hedonic valence and placebo mechanisms of action. However, an animal study conducted by Akutsu *et al.* (2002) highlighted the stress-reducing effects of inhaling a 'green odour' (in this context, the scent of deciduous trees, such as oak leaves) on rats with stress-induced hyperthermia. They concluded that the volatile plant constituents were having direct pharmacological effects on the rats' behaviour and physiology. We could, therefore, hypothesise that distinct odour types could elicit specific responses in humans.

Craig Warren, at International Flavours and Fragrances (New Jersey), has studied the effects of fragrance on mood for many years, using both psychological and physiological methods. In 1993 Warren and Warrenburg made some significant observations:

- Fragrance-evoked mood changes are small, but beneficial to our well-being.

- Fragrance can be used to reduce the stress response in human beings, but its physiological effects on a non-stressed subject are minimal and difficult to measure.

- Measurement of fragrance-evoked mood change by psychological methods is feasible and yields intriguing results.

Warren and Warrenburg (1993) developed the Mood Profiling Concept (MPC), which is of particular interest to aromatherapists. The MPC uses psychological self-reporting to measure subjective mood changes evoked by fragrance. The odours used were all 'pleasant', and synthetic in origin ('living flower' reproduction fragrances).

In the MPC, eight mood categories were identified; four were classed as positive and four as negative. The words used to describe the positive moods states were 'stimulation', 'sensuality', 'happiness' and 'relaxation'; the negative moods were 'stress', 'irritation', 'depression' and 'apathy'. In Warren and Warrenburg's study, exposure to different fragrances either intensified or reduced these mood states, and profiles of the effects of specific fragrances were constructed, and presented in graphical format.

It was found that the floral muguet (lily of the valley) fragrance increased both stimulation and relaxation, and lowered depression, apathy and irritation. The effect was reported as producing a heightened sense of calm, with an increase in awareness and energy.

The fresh, coniferous/pineapple-like/lemony Douglas fir fragrance decreased all of the negative mood categories. It was reported as being distinctly relaxing, the effects being similar to those of meditation.

The fruity, raisin-like osmanthus fragrance increased stimulation and happiness, and prominently reduced apathy and depression.

Finally, the cool, floral-green hyacinth fragrance increased all of the positive mood categories and decreased all of the negative categories.

However, it is difficult to align specific essential oils precisely with specific psychotherapeutic effects, partly because of the lack of data on the subject (and the influences described earlier, such as hedonics and expectations). At the 'scientific' end of the scale, there are lists of stimulants and sedatives, activators and deactivators (Tisserand 1988); also studies of more specific circumstances (Lawless 1994). However, in reality, it can be difficult to relate this information to the practice of holistic aromatherapy. Martin (1996), in a paper on 'olfactory remediation', is highly critical of aromatherapy, mainly because of the poor quality of research carried out by its practitioners. He suggests that:

> ...future studies examine closely their methodology: they need to accrue an adequate subject sample, to measure objectively the subject's state of mind (if the study is claiming to look for olfactory effects on anxiety, for

stress reduction have focused on the essential oils with a reputation for these actions, such as lavender, neroli, rose and citrus peel oils like bergamot, sweet orange and lime. Researchers look to oils that are often described as stimulating and activating for studies exploring cognitive functions, vigour and alertness – especially rosemary, peppermint, eucalyptus and jasmine. Again, the studies cited support the established aromatherapeutic uses of these oils in conjunction with transdermal absorption and massage.

A pharmaco-physio-psychological mode of action

In this chapter the theories and hypotheses that underpin aromatherapy have been explored, including:

- the pharmacological hypothesis:
  - transdermal absorption
  - inhalation
  - pharmacokinetics and pharmacodynamics
- olfactory hypotheses:
  - the brain and the limbic system
  - the quasi-pharmacological mode of action
  - the semantic mode of action
  - the hedonic valence mode of action
  - the placebo mode of action
- the physiological responses to massage:
  - direct mechanical effects on the soft tissues
  - indirect reflexive effects via the nervous system
  - psychological effects.

There is one study in particular that illustrates all of the above. Dobetsberger and Buchbauer (2011) cite research conducted by Xu *et al.* (2008) comparing the effects of *Shirodhara* with and without essential oil of lavender. *Shirodhara* is an Ayurvedic treatment where herb-infused sesame oil is dripped onto the forehead over the region related to the 'third eye' or *ajna chakra*. This is reputed to produce profound relaxation, or even an altered state of consciousness. The study demonstrated that Shirodhara with plain sesame oil has an anxiolytic effect (concurring with other studies), but that Shirodhara with lavender and sesame oil has a greater effect. They concluded that the psycho-physiological effects were due to three mechanisms working in parallel: the relaxing effect of lavender via olfaction, the pharmacological action of the substances absorbed through the skin and the physiological effects elicited by the dripping action on the thermosensors and pressure sensors via the trigeminal nerve (a somato-autonomic reflex). Xu *et al.* call this a 'complicated pharmaco-physio-psychological action' (p. 956) and they suggest that it could be a useful model for future therapies. Indeed, this single study provides some evidence for the aromatherapy theories explored in this chapter, and supports the hypothetical modes of action that underpin aromatherapy.

PART II

Approaches to Creating Essential Oil Synergy

CHAPTER 3

Synergy and Antagonism

Blending essential oils to create a synergy, an individual aromatic prescription, is at the very core of contemporary aromatherapy practice. However, apart from one paper published by Harris in 2002, there has been little written specifically about this topic. Discussions with teachers of aromatherapy in further education in Scotland, and personal experience as a tutor in higher education, have led me to the conclusion that, although students of aromatherapy appear to understand the basis of the practice of blending, few are able to explain synergy in this context.

The holistic approach to aromatherapy treatment entails the synthesis of a synergistic prescription of essential oils for an individual, not simply for a collection of symptoms. As aromatherapy practice has developed, several distinct approaches to selecting and blending essential oils have emerged. The original, holistic approach advocated by Maury (the 'individual prescription' or IP) includes the core elements that are considered important by many contemporary aromatherapists. However, a more clinical approach, used by practitioners of aromatic medicine such as Franchomme and Pénoël, is based on the molecular structure and functions of essential oil constituents. This offers a more 'scientific' way of thinking that is increasingly being adapted for use by aromatherapists. Psycho-olfactory approaches appeal to therapists who adhere to the philosophy that it is the aroma of the essential oils that contributes most significantly to the therapeutic outcomes, while other therapists and writers, such as Mojay and Holmes, advocate an energetic approach, based on Chinese medicine principles.

Synergy and antagonism

Harris (2002) gives a very succinct explanation of essential oil synergism, which can form the basis of further exploration:

> The synergistic rationale for using combination products looks to producing a dynamic product that has multiple modes of action, respecting the principle that the action of the combined product is greater than the sum total of known and unknown chemical components. (Harris 2002, p. 179)

Each essential oil has a range of therapeutic actions; therefore it may be indicated for use in many circumstances. However, a particular essential oil can possess a whole array of therapeutic actions that make it particularly useful in very specific instances. All essential oils may have actions on the physical, physiological and psychological levels – but it seems likely that some oils have more pronounced, or evidence-based, actions in just one or two of these realms.

An essential oil is composed of many chemical constituents, each contributing to a greater or lesser extent to the effects of the essential oil. Some constituents enhance each other's effects; therefore the effect of the whole essential oil is greater than that of its individual chemical components. This is called synergy. For example, two of the main constituents of true lavender oil, linalyl acetate and linalool, are credited with sedative action, and these components work together to give true lavender oil its sedative properties. Adorjan and Buchbauer (2010) comment that some studies have demonstrated that essential oils sometimes have more pronounced actions than their main constituents have singly.

Sometimes, constituents in an essential oil may in fact have opposing actions, and the overall effect of the oil will depend on the relative proportions of antagonistic components. For example, rosemary essential oil contains 1,8-cineole and α-pinene. 1,8-cineole has been shown to have spasmolytic effects on tissues, while α-pinene has distinct spasmogenic effects (Buchbauer 1993). Therefore varying extents of spasmolysis can be observed, depending on the 1,8-cineole content of rosemary oil. This in turn depends on the plant variety, origin and time of harvest.

There is some evidence to support the concept of synergy and antagonism in essential oil combinations (Harris 2002). One of the few studies to explore the aromatherapeutic potential of synergistic blending is by Hongratanaworakit (2011). It was hypothesised that a synergistic blend of essential oils could be used to treat depression or anxiety. A combination of lavender and bergamot was used in abdominal massage, and a range of autonomic parameters and emotional responses were analysed. Compared with the placebo group, the lavender and bergamot blend caused significant decreases of pulse rate and systolic and diastolic blood pressure, indicating a decrease in autonomic arousal. This treatment group also reported that they felt 'more calm' and 'more relaxed' than the control, suggesting a decrease in subjective behavioural arousal.

In holistic aromatherapy practice, where endless possibilities for essential oil combinations exist, largely unsupported by any hard evidence, synergy and antagonism within blends are virtually impossible to assess. However, based on current knowledge, Harris has drawn some pertinent conclusions, and produced some sound guidelines for formulating potentially synergistic blends of essential oils for aromatherapy practice. These are summarised below.

- The therapeutic purpose of the blend should be the focus – and one formula should not encompass too many goals.

- The selected essential oils should be complementary to one another in terms of activity, direction and chemistry.

- The number of essential oils in the blend should be restricted to between three and seven, to ensure that the final blend remains high in active components.

- The base (carriers) should be chosen with care, as this is also part of the synergy/antagonism issue (see Appendix D).

- The dose should be appropriate for the application.

- There should be an awareness of the potential synergistic/antagonistic therapist/client relationship.

- The psychological effect of the odour of the selected essential oils will either contribute to or detract from the synergistic potential of the prescription.

- If massage is used as part of the intervention, the psychological and physiological effects of the massage routine will also impact on the treatment outcome; this should also inform the choice of essential oils and the treatment plan.

Regardless of the approach selected, the above guidelines will apply. Part II of this book will explore and give examples of how to apply a diverse range of approaches to blending essential oils, from intuitive blending to functional group theory, from East to West, from the energetic domain to the physical domain, from the mind–body–spirit perspective to aromatic medicine. First, we will look at what is meant by holism in the context of aromatherapy, and then we will examine synergistic blend construction, prior to exploring the original approach to blending essential oils for aromatherapy – Maury's 'individual prescription'.

CHAPTER 4

Maury's Individual Prescription and its Derivatives

Holistic intent

When a client presents for aromatherapy treatment, much may be learned during the consultation and assessment stage by close observation and careful listening. Approaches to client assessment vary. Some therapists will use a *biomedical* approach, which has a focus on dysfunction and disease, and the identification and characterisation of presenting symptoms. Others may incorporate a humanistic element, and concentrate on human needs such as those identified by Maslow. Maslow produced a model to assist understanding of human behaviour. Using the visual analogy of a pyramid, he suggested that the most basic human needs of water, food and shelter were found at the base of the pyramid. The next level up was safety and freedom from stress, then social needs such as friendship and love. The higher levels were self-esteem and confidence, and at the top was self-actualisation, or reaching full potential. Each level needs to be achieved, or the higher levels cannot be reached. The *humanistic* approach will focus on the client's lived experiences, and will be geared to helping the client reach their full potential. A few will focus on an *energetic* approach. This builds on the humanistic approach, but embraces the concept of spirituality and interconnectedness and the principles of uncertainty, non-locality and non-objectivity. Those who choose to take this approach will have an insight into their own level of awareness, and will aim to help their client in the search for meaning and purpose in life.

When asked to describe holistic intent, the majority of therapists will mention 'mind, body and spirit'. The three broad approaches outlined above could meet this description. The objective biomedical approach equates to the 'body' or the physical and material world. The more subjective humanistic approach equates to the 'mind' and the cognitive and social domains. Finally, the energetic approach equates to the 'spirit' and the non-material realm. So if the therapist is to prepare a holistic essential oil prescription, the assessment should really incorporate all three realms – albeit the emphasis may be on one or two, depending on the therapist and the client.

Blend construction

Often, student aromatherapists have difficulty in sifting out their clients' priorities, given the amount of information divulged and any tensions or coherences with their own observations and impressions. It can often be a case of 'not seeing the wood for the trees'. In this event, a therapist should not try to come up with one prescription that will achieve everything. It is preferable to agree the short- and medium-term aims of the treatment, focus on one or two issues at any one time, and, if possible, try to find the root of any problems and address these rather than the symptoms.

In addition to clarifying the aim(s) of the prescription, the overall 'direction' should be clear. For example, this may mean that the prescription is directed to a body system by including essential oils (or constituents) that are known to have effects on a specific system, or directed towards overall stimulation or sedation, activation or deactivation, or psychoactivation, producing an enhanced mood or an altered state of consciousness, for example. Looking at the essential oils in terms of their chemical constituents or their expected therapeutic actions or energetic activity can reveal the synergistic/antagonistic potential of a prescription.

Emotional responses to fragrance

The overall fragrance of the prescription is also important – a client should react positively to this, unless of course it is a purely clinical prescription. For this reason, odour preferences and dislikes should be addressed during the consultation. This is another area where student aromatherapists often encounter difficulties. These can easily, although not quickly, be overcome by becoming familiar with the odours of essential oils and recognising odour types and characteristics, so that communications about aromas with clients are conducted from a sound knowledge and understanding, but above all from experience. Turin and Sanchez are absolutely right when they comment that 'direct experience is the only experience. You can't reproduce smells in books or digitise them' (Turin and Sanchez 2009, p. 4). This is true for those who want to learn about perfume, and it is equally valid for those studying essential oils. The scents of different constituents within oils can also be recognised, and these can also be related to potential therapeutic actions. See Appendix B for more information.

Despite the many studies that have asked subjects to report their emotional reactions to odours using tools such as the established and reliable Geneva Emotion and Odour Scale (Chrea et al. 2009), the verbal measurement of odour-evoked feelings had not, until recently, been developed for consumer preferences for fragranced products. Porcherot et al. (2010) used the following words in their revised, quick and efficient questionnaire summarised here:

- pleasant feeling – happiness, well-being, pleasantly surprised

- sensuality – romantic, desire, in love

- unpleasant feeling – disgusted, irritated, unpleasantly surprised

- relaxation – relaxed, serene, reassured

- sensory pleasure – nostalgic, amusement, mouth-watering

- refreshment – energetic, invigorated, clean.

It is reasonable to suggest that this vocabulary could be utilised within the client–aromatherapist relationship when exploring essential oil aroma preferences.

Perfume construction principles and applications in aesthetic blending

The principles of perfume construction can also shed some light on the aesthetic aspects of blending. Perfumes contain top, middle and base notes. Perfumes also will contain fixatives, or fragrance retarders, which are slow to evaporate and can hold the other components together, so that the top notes will contain some of the body notes and the base contains some of the middle notes. A fragrance should not 'break up' or 'fall apart' and the changes over time should be imperceptible (Müller 1992). Lavabre (1990) also uses the note concept, in conjunction with his own concept of blend modifiers, enhancers and equalisers.

Modifiers or *personifiers* are intense fragrances that have a major impact on the fragrance of the blend – even in tiny amounts – and can be found in top, middle and base categories. They give a blend real personality and can be used to improve 'flat' blends. Generally they should be used sparingly to avoid totally dominating a blend. Examples are clove, cinnamon, peppermint, thyme, German and Roman chamomiles and patchouli.

Enhancers also have strong presence, but they are not as overpowering as the modifiers. Consequently, they can be used in greater proportions within a blend than the modifiers. Examples are bergamot, cedarwood, geranium, clary sage, lavender, lemon, lime, may chang, palmarosa, sandalwood, ylang ylang, jasmine, rose, neroli and myrrh.

Finally, *equalisers* are the essential oils that help improve harsh blends, dampen down unwanted intensity of over-dominant notes, fill 'gaps' and help the blend flow. They should not have an effect on the overall personality. Equalisers are context dependent. Lavabre maintains that rosewood and wild Spanish marjoram are universal equalisers. Orange and tangerine can be used with neroli, petitgrain and bergamot, and citrus oils act as equalisers with spice oils such as clove, cinnamon and nutmeg, and also with florals such as ylang ylang, rose, jasmine and geranium. He also comments that fir and pine can improve blends containing oils of the *Myrtaceae* and the order *Coniferae*.

Therapeutic positions

Mojay (1996) identified three levels of blending, namely aesthetic, clinical and psychological/spiritual. He created a clear and imaginative method of constructing a synergistic, clinical prescription, using the idea of essential oils occupying 'therapeutic positions' in a blend. Using terminology borrowed from Chinese medicine (the 'Officials'), he suggested that each prescription should contain an Emperor, a Minister, Assistant(s) and a Messenger, where:

- The Emperor brings all-round benefits to the condition.

- The Minister reinforces one or more properties of the Emperor.

- The Assistant enhances one or more benefits of the Emperor–Minister combination.

- The Messenger directs the blend.

So having established what is meant by holistic intent, and by blend construction, an exploration of Maury's writings and some of her prescriptions will help illustrate further the principles of holistic blending.

Maury's Individual Prescription

Marguerite Maury developed the concept of preparing a mixture of aromatic essences based on what she termed 'the physiological and psychic identity of the individual'. Here, the word 'psychic' refers to the psyche, an overarching term for the cognitive, emotional and non-physical domain. She called this mixture of aromatics the 'individual prescription' or IP (Maury 1989 [1961]). Maury's philosophies were influenced by her studies of Tibetan medicine, which contains elements of both Chinese and Ayurvedic medicine. She claimed that:

> The individual mixture is designed to reflect the weaknesses and violence of an individual; it has to compensate for the deficiencies and reduce the excesses. It serves above all to normalise the rhythm of the functions. The latter risk, either by inveigling the body into excessive expenditure of energy or by an over-accentuated slowing down, preventing it from satisfying the demands made on it. For these reasons the individual mixture may be compared to the negative of a film with its reversed shadows and light. (Maury 1989 [1961], p. 95)

The intent of the IP should always be to restore balance. When Maury's examples of IPs are examined, it becomes apparent that, in broad terms, essential oils classed as base notes impact on the physical and cellular level, middle notes affect function and rhythm, and top notes impact on the limbic system. She was adamant that the balance of essences in the mixture was a very important factor. During a course of aromatherapy treatments, Maury would modify the mixture when appropriate, saying that:

> We should like to point out that an I.P. is only correct and effective when it has become a combination and has not merely remained a simple mixture. (Maury 1989 [1961], p. 100)

Maury's holistic approach can be seen in the case of a male client who was suffering from mental strain and insomnia. She noted great anxiety, exhaustion and melancholy. He also had an irregular heartbeat, his blood circulation was susceptible to 'blockage', his kidney function was poor and his heart was not compensating. Maury believed that melancholy has 'a murderous effect on cellular life' and that in keeping with Chinese doctrine 'sorrow attacks the kidneys' and 'lack of love hardens the heart'. Maury's IP for this client contained rose, sandalwood, lavender, geranium and 'benzoic' (benzoin). She reasoned that these essences would compensate for his deficiencies and 'hardening' and would help with his rehabilitation and restore balance. Benzoic would help dispel his anxiety and promote euphoria, creating a safe 'padded zone' to encourage healing. Rose and sandalwood could compensate for his cardiac and renal difficulties, while lavender normalised the kidney function and geranium normalised the psyche.

It could be argued that although the language may be a little outdated, and perhaps some of the nuances have been lost in translation, this IP is also appropriate when examined from a contemporary aromatherapy perspective. Rose and geranium are often used to combat anxiety and lift the mood, while sandalwood and lavender are calming and indicated for insomnia. The scent of benzoin is still regarded as having a comforting effect. Sandalwood is often regarded as a tonic for the urinary system, and rose for the heart. We can also examine the synergistic potential by considering the therapeutic positions of the component oils. Rose may well be the Emperor, as it is, above all, a relaxing oil with euphoric qualities, and has a reputation as a cardiotonic. Geranium, the Minister oil, supports rose, as it is also uplifting and notably anxiolytic. The Assistants to this combination are sandalwood and lavender, with their affinity for the urinary system and relaxing properties. The Messenger is benzoin – it reinforces the relaxing and uplifting oils and creates a 'padded zone', directing the blend so that the overall effect is one of warmth, safety and comfort. Maury did insist that this IP was 'powerless to cure pathological lesions', so the prescription is not clinical in focus. A contemporary aromatherapist would have the same aim, as aromatherapy is not claimed to be curative. Not all aromatherapists are conversant with Chinese or Tibetan medicine; however, this holistic ethos can easily be incorporated into Western practice. The following present-day example can illustrate how this might be achieved.

A female client presented as a well-groomed, intelligent, professional individual who was apparently plagued by anxiety and low self-esteem. This was verbalised but also apparent in her general demeanour, body language and especially her tone of voice and speech patterns. The anxiety was causing disturbed sleeping patterns and consequent feelings of tiredness and 'low energy levels'. Her digestive system was affected too, as she admitted to comfort eating and frequent bouts of indigestion as a consequence. She also complained of fluid retention, which had been a source of aesthetic concern for many years, and there were no clinical reasons underlying this complaint. Above all, this client needed to relax and rediscover a feeling of well-being. The IP that was devised aimed to restore balance to the psyche while supporting the physical aspects that were also under stress, and contained essential oils of sandalwood, jasmine, black pepper, coriander seed, grapefruit and bitter orange. Here we can see that these essential oils have multiple overlapping therapeutic qualities. Jasmine and the citrus oils were included to counteract her low mood and poor self-image, and to encourage relaxation while improving focus and outlook. Grapefruit and bitter orange can support digestion while promoting a feeling of well-being. Meanwhile, the spice oils, black pepper and coriander seed also support digestion, while counteracting fatigue. Sandalwood with black pepper is a relaxing and 'grounding' combination, which can help individuals who perhaps feel out of control of their feelings. Finally, sandalwood, coriander seed and grapefruit are all indicated for fluid accumulation and lymphatic system support. Most important, as with Maury's IPs, there were no claims that this would have specific curative effects.

The majority of aromatherapists will adopt this type of approach to synergistic blending – finding one or two essential oils that address most of the therapeutic aims, and then building a prescription on these foundation oils. Maury's influence has indeed been far reaching, and it was only in the early 1990s that an alternative, more scientific way of thinking was embraced by aromatherapists, especially those who felt that this would give more credibility to their practice. This was what has become known as the 'molecular approach'.

CHAPTER 5

Functional Group Influence and the Molecular Approach

Functional group hypothesis

'Functional groups' are small groups of atoms on a molecule that are important in determining how that molecule will behave and react. Charabot and Dupont were fragrance researchers who, in the course of their investigations, suggested that many of the properties of essential oils, including their odours, could be explained in terms of their chemical composition and especially by the presence of functional groups on molecules (Schnaubelt 2000). This is an example of the 'structure determines function' phenomenon witnessed in many fields. We know that Gattefossé and Valnet considered the influence of functional groups on the therapeutic potential of essential oil molecules; however, it was the proponents of French medical aromatherapy, Franchomme and Pénoël, who applied the concept to help explain the therapeutic properties of essential oils and developed this in the context of aromatic medicine. Please see Table 4.1 for an overview of the common functional groups found in essential oil molecules and their potential actions.

It is very reasonable to believe that there is a relationship between the chemical structure of odour molecules and their physiological and pharmacological properties. The influence of functional groups has been linked with rather specific properties and actions. However, there has been a tendency to overgeneralise this concept, and consequently many erroneous assumptions have been made with regard to both toxicity and therapeutic properties. For example, some ketones, such as thujone found in sage essential oil, can be toxic, especially with regards to the nervous system, but not all ketones are neurotoxic – especially at the low levels found in most essential oils. Another example is in relation to therapeutic actions, where the monoterpene alcohol found in lavender, *l*-linalool, is sedative, but not all monoterpene alcohols have been shown to be sedative – even its isomer *d*-linalool found in coriander seed oil may not have this particular action. These isomers have the same molecular formula, but the orientation of the atoms within the molecule is subtly different. This is called 'chirality'.

Table 5.1 Molecular approach – the influence of functional groups (summarised from Bowles 2003)

Chemical group	Effects – general and specific	Examples – specific
Monoterpenes	General tonic and stimulant. Decongestant – mucous (exocrine glands)	α- and β-pinenes
	Cancer prevention and treatment Hormone-like properties – action on the pituitary/adrenal system – adrenalin production	Limonene
	Analgesic	Myrcene, *para*-cymene
Sesquiterpenes	Anti-inflammatory – counter-histamic reactions	Chamazulene, β-caryophyllene
	Hormonal effects	Farnesene
Monoterpene alcohols	Antibacterial Vasoconstrictive Local anaesthesia	
	Tonifying and stimulant	Menthol
	Sedative	Terpinen-4-ol
	Spasmolytic	*l*-linalool
		l-linalool
Sesquiterpene alcohols	General tonic (<monoterpene alcohols) Phlebotonic	
	Cardiotonic	Viridiflorol, cedrol
	Neurotonic	Santalol
	Oestrogenic	α- and β-eudesmol
	Anti-inflammatory	Viridiflorol
	Anti-cancer effects	α-bisabolol
		Farnesol, nerolidol, α-bisabolol
	Antiviral	Santalols
	Antimalarial	Nerolidol
Phenols	Tonics and general stimulants Antimicrobial	Thymol and carvacrol
	Analgesic	Eugenol
Aldehydes	Calming to CNS Anti-inflammatory Antimicrobial	Citral Cinnamaldehyde (aromatic)
	Antifungal	Citral, cinnamaldehyde

Ketones	Mucolytic Wound healing Antihaematomal Antiviral (papilloma, herpes)	Methone Italidiones
Esters	Antispasmodic Sedative	Linalyl acetate Esters in Roman chamomile, linalyl acetate
Oxides	Expectorant Antispasmodic	1,8-cineole, linalool oxide
Ethers	Antispasmodic Analgesic Euphoric	*Trans*-anethole Methyl chavicol Phenyl ethanol (alcohol)
Lactones	Mucolytic Expectorant Analgesic	Alantolactone, *iso*-alantolactone Nepetalactone

A good case for the structure/function relationship can be seen in the study conducted by Kuroda *et al.* (2005), examining the effects of *d*- and *l*-linalool in the scents of jasmine tea and lavender essential oil. The odours of the isomers are different; the *d*-isomer has a sweet floral note, while the *l*-form is woody and reminiscent of lavender. In the experiment the linalool odours were undetectable, although the jasmine tea and lavender odour was noticeable. It was found that *l*-linalool decreased heart rate and improved mood, and *d*-linalool increased heart rate and did not improve mood.

An earlier study conducted by Heuberger *et al.* (2001) investigated the effects of the inhalation of *d*- and *l*-limonene, and *d*- and *l*-carvone on autonomic nervous system (ANS) parameters and mood. The study revealed that both *d*- and *l*-limonene increased systolic blood pressure, but only the *d*-form caused subjective alertness and restlessness; the *l*-form had no effects on psychological parameters. It was also found that *l*-carvone increased pulse and diastolic blood pressure and evoked restlessness, while *d*-carvone increased both systolic and diastolic blood pressure. Correlational analysis of the results showed that changes in ANS and self-evaluation were related to subjective evaluation of the odours, and that both pharmacological and psychological mechanisms contribute to the effects. They concluded that chirality of odour molecules is an important factor in determining biological activity.

Therefore, it could be argued that the functional group hypothesis does provide a useful starting point for synergistic blending, but only if it is remembered that ultimately each molecule must be considered as a whole, not just as a functional group; that each essential oil contains many different types of molecules; and that the whole oil must be considered. Schnaubelt (1999) noted the synergies that exist within essential oils, in terms of their functional groups, thus restoring a more naturalistic and holistic view of the functional group hypothesis. He called this the 'kaleidoscope principle'. An example is the monoterpene/terpene alcohol/ cineole synergy that can be witnessed in essential oils such as ravintsara, niaouli and *Eucalyptus radiata*. This is described as the 'cold and 'flu' synergy, where the components act together to impart a characteristic 'medicinal' aroma associated with their antiseptic and expectorant properties. However, these components can be found in other combinations in other oils, and different 'internal' synergies will result.

Medical aromatherapy and the molecular approach

Pénoël (1998/1999) identified that medical aromatherapy, using what he termed the 'molecular approach', may have curative purpose, preventative action, or even be applied for an evolution search. By this he means 'I feel well, but I want to feel even better and improve my potential in general and/or specific areas.' He also considers that 'aromatic care' can be emergency, intensive or regular, for chronic states.

The molecular approach to creating a synergistic prescription relies on knowledge of the likely properties of functional groups, and combining essential oils with this in mind. The molecular approach can be applied in aromatherapy for constructing potentially synergistic blends. Essential oil blends can be created for either 'horizontal' or 'vertical' synergistic actions (Pénoël 1998/1999).

Horizontal synergy

'Horizontal synergy' may be found in a blend of several essential oils containing similar functional groups, for a single specific purpose. For example, an antimicrobial blend of several monoterpene alcohol-rich essential oils such as palmarosa (geraniol), tea tree (terpinen-4-ol), common thyme CT (thujanol) and Moroccan thyme (borneol) would demonstrate horizontal synergy, where these molecules enhance each other's antimicrobial actions. Horizontal synergy would be considered if treating a client with a specific aim in mind – for example, to treat an infection. However, aromatherapists cannot claim or offer to do this. So although the intent of this blend could be to combat infection, the combination could benefit a client in other ways, as each essential oil possesses a spectrum of activity.

Vertical synergy

'Vertical synergy' may be found in a blend of essential oils containing different functional groups, intended for more than one purpose. For example, an antimicrobial monoterpene alcohol combined with a mucolytic monoterpene ketone and an antispasmodic ester would demonstrate vertical synergy. In this case, the essential oils could be palmarosa (geraniol) with peppermint (menthone) and lavender (linalyl acetate). Vertical synergy is usually more appropriate in holistic aromatherapy practice, where usually clients present with more than one need. Even a single disease normally entails several different pathophysiological processes, such as inflammation and pain. As each essential oil in the blend will contain more than one type of functional group, there is scope for further overlap of properties.

The molecular approach debate

Since the early 1990s there has been an ongoing debate about the validity of the molecular approach, especially when the concepts are applied to aromatherapy practice. Schnaubelt (2000) comments on the Franchomme and Pénoël hypothesis that the properties of an essential oil are determined by the functional groups of its constituent molecules, especially in relation to the over-generalisation of this hypothesis:

> If functional group therapy is seen as a rigid dogma (e.g. all aldehydes are sedative), it is self-contradictory. I might venture to say that this certainly was not the intent of those who originally put forward this concept. However if functional group therapy is understood as an attempt to understand the physiological effects of essential oils, it certainly contributes to the therapeutic utilisation of essential oils. (Schnaubelt 2000, p. 62)

He also argues that:

> One dimensional pharmacology can only do so much to explain its [aromatherapy's] benefits. Do we even need this type of research at all if its main purpose is to simply legitimise aromatherapy as a healing modality to mainstream scientific experts? I cannot suppress the notion that the more aromatherapy strives to be accepted by the medical profession, the more it is likely to copy its mistakes and failures. (Schnaubelt 2000, p. 63)

The molecular approach, when applied to aromatherapy, has indeed a few drawbacks. First, evidence for the some of the pharmacological actions attributed to essential oil functional groups/molecules (originally in Franchomme and Pénoël's *L'Aromatherapie exactement*) remains empirical, because independent researchers have not yet investigated them. Second, the physiological effects attributed to many essential oil molecules or whole oils are often based on oral/rectal administration, not transdermal absorption at the low levels used in aromatherapy. Therefore it may not be correct to assume that an approach used in aromatic medicine is equally valid for aromatherapy. Finally, the essential oils are considered largely in terms of their possible pharmacological actions – giving little or no consideration to the psycho-olfactory influence that is so important in aromatherapy. For some examples of this approach to essential oil prescribing, please see Appendix C.

Around the same time that the molecular approach began to influence essential oil prescribing in the aromatherapy domain, there was a growing interest in what might be considered the antithesis of the molecular approach. This is the psycho-sensory approach, which encompasses different philosophical frameworks, but at its heart is the emotional response to the fragrance of essential oils.

CHAPTER 6

Psychosensory Approaches

Aromatic typology

Philippe Mailhebiau developed the concept of the '*characterologie*' of essential oils, linking the olfactory characteristics and 'personalities' of essential oils with the olfactory affinities and temperament of the individual. He uses this concept to refine and personalise his aromatherapy treatments so that they not only address symptoms or complaints, but also aim to restore balance and equilibrium. In his book *La Nouvelle Aromathérapie: caractérologie des essences et tempéraments humaines* (published in the UK in 1995 as the abbreviated form *Portraits in Oils*), he explores the idea of aromatic typology and the psychosensory impact of essential oils. His approach was intuitive in origin, and as such has been compared to the work of Hahnemann, the founder of homeopathy (Clerc 1995).

Mailhebiau maintains that aromatherapy is a specialised medical field. His work is firmly grounded in aromatic medicine; however, there is much in his writing that could influence psycho-olfactory prescribing in aromatherapy. He claims that

> From a therapeutic point of view, this approach opens the door to personalised treatments which go beyond the scope of symptomatic aromatherapy by combining efficient physiochemical action with a decisive psycho-sensory effect. (Mailhebiau 1995, p. xi)

He explored the interactive bond between feelings and odours, olfactory affinities and organoleptic actions of plant essences. This culminated in his '*characterology of essences*', which presented the archetype (a symbolic character) of each essence. These archetypes relate to contemporary personalities as well as mythological characters from the East and West.

Clerc (1995) translated Mailhebiau's example of the aromatherapeutic treatment of insomnia, by considering the characterologies of *Lavandula vera* (true lavender), *Ocimum basilicum* (basil) and *Citrus aurantium* leaf oil (petitgrain).

- *Lavandula vera* is characteristic of 'the disturbed sleep of a child upset by his mother's physical or emotional absence; it corresponds to a nervous and emotional sleeplessness; to the fear of the dark.'

- *Ocimum basilicum* would be suited to treat 'the sleeplessness of people "digesting" their concerns during the night, i.e. a sleeplessness resulting from stress or overeating.'

- *Citrus aurantium* corresponds with 'the sleeplessness of a mature person suffering from emotional turmoil, upset by a separation, and who cannot sleep alone at night.'

Mailhebiau states, however, that 'nuances are imperative in assigning a patient a specific characterology' and that the characterology model is not a 'simplistic classification directory'. Most aromatherapists do not consciously use characterology. However, the concept does emphasise the importance of what could be considered an 'inside knowledge' or even an intuitive understanding of the nature of essential oil aromas – and the ability to produce personalised aromatic prescriptions based on a genuinely holistic client assessment.

The sensory impact of botanical aromas

Michel Lavabre has also suggested that the psychosensory philosophy should be central to aromatherapy practice. His *Aromatherapy Workbook* (1990) contains some interesting ideas, not least the concept of Sheldrake's 'morphogenetic fields', Lovelock's Gaia hypothesis, and his own *'evolution–involution'* concept for essential oil biogenesis (see p. 64). Mojay (1996) holds the view that it is the fragrance of essential oils that has the 'most immediate and generalised effect on the body and mind'.

So to use the psychosensory approach (or indeed any other approach) in aromatherapy, it is vital to engage directly with the essential oils in terms of their scents, experiencing the diverse fragrances of essential oils from roots, stems and leaves, grasses, woods, resins, flowers, fruits and seeds. This requires the active use of the sense of smell, and allows the individual to gain tangible insights into the oils' interactions with us.

However, Lavabre suggests that we should develop an appreciation of the aromatic plants – their morphology, physiology and growth habits – as these also give insight into their nature and fragrances. For some suggestions of the botanical sources and the feelings their aromas can engender, please see Table 6.1. These suggested effects are subjective but commonly reported reactions to the aromas of these essential oils.

Table 6.1 Essential oil sources, scents and reported responses

Botanical and anatomical source	Essential oil	Reported responses to scent
Zingiber officinalis, rhizome of erect leafy perennial	Ginger	Grounded, fortified, energised, warmth and clarity, strength
Nardostachys jatamansi, rhizome and rootlets of aromatic herb	Spikenard	Emotional and spiritual release, at ease with transition, freedom from grief and emotional pain, calmness
Vetiveria zizanoides, rootlets of grass	Vetivert	Feeling grounded, at peace, at ease, safe and secure
Ocimum basilicum, leaves of herb	Basil	Restores the mind, clarity, strength, calm
Eucalyptus globulus, leaves of blue gum tree	Eucalyptus	Mental clarity and focus, room to breathe, vitality
Origanum majorana, aerial parts of herb	Marjoram, sweet	Mental clarity, emotionally calm, able to give and receive, able to feel loss then move on
Melissa officinalis, aerial parts of herb	Melissa	Serenity, uplifting, cheering, restores the spirits
Mentha × piperita, aerial parts of herb	Peppermint	Alertness, sharpens the senses, clarity, vision
Thymus vulgaris, aerial parts of herb	Thyme	Revived and restored, warmth, stimulated, energised, strength
Cymbopogon citratus, leaves of grass	Lemongrass	Relaxed, sustained, focused and positive
Cymbopogon martinii v. *martinii*, leaves of grass	Palmarosa	Emotional security and adaptability, gentleness, ability to go with the flow, compassion
Cedrus atlantica, wood of conifer	Cedar, Atlas	Capacity for risk assessment, good judgement, self-possessed, self-reliant, self-confidence, steady drive
Cupressus sempervirens, leaves (needles) of conifer	Cypress	Ability to manage transition, inner strength, release of fear

cont.

Table 6.1 Essential oil sources, scents and reported responses *cont.*

Botanical and anatomical source	Essential oil	Reported responses to scent
Pinus sylvestris, leaves (needles) of conifer	Pine, Scots	Vitality, exhilaration, open mind, strong identity
Aniba rosaeodora, wood of tree (*Lauraceae*)	Rosewood	Calm, uplifted, refreshed and relaxed
Santalum album,* wood of tree	Sandalwood	Tranquil, still, peace, centred
Styrax benzoin, resin from shrubby tree	Benzoin	Feeling supported, nourished, centred, stable, sense of belonging, assimilation, letting go
Boswellia carterii, oleoresin from small shrubby tree	Frankincense	Feeling calm and peaceful, promotes insight, self-understanding and acceptance
Ferula galbaniflua, oleogum secretion of perennial herb	Galbanum	Refreshed, centred, in touch with the senses
Commiphora myrrha, oleoresin from small shrubby tree	Myrrh	Feeling grounded and uplifted, free of negativity, soothed, tranquil and at peace
Anthemis nobilis, flowers of creeping perennial daisy	Chamomile, Roman	Soothed, balanced, calm and in control, patient
Jasminum officinale, flowers of evergreen climber	Jasmine	Joy, exhilaration, creativity, warmth, in touch with the senses, liberation, confidence
Citrus aurantium v. *amara*, flowers of bitter orange tree	Neroli	Calm, cheerful, harmony, clear consciousness and self-identity, creative spark
Rosa centifolia, *R. damascena*, flowers of shrub	Rose	Uplifted, comforted, soothed, emotionally healed
Cananga odorata v. *genuina*, flowers of tropical tree	Ylang ylang extra	Relaxed, uplifted, emotional flow, in touch with the senses

Elettaria cardamomum, fruits/seeds of rhizomatous perennial herb	Cardamom	Feeling alert, animated, balanced, co-ordinated, clear sensations, inspired, high self-esteem, feeling complete
Citrus genus	Bitter orange Lemon Lime Grapefruit Mandarin Sweet orange	A sense and vision of your path in life, patience, understanding that everything unfolds at the right pace, easy-going, ability to think ahead and plan, but also be flexible, general contentment with the status quo, expansive, innovative energy
Coriandrum sativum, seeds of tall annual herb	Coriander seed	Happy, creative, revitalised
Foeniculum vulgare v. dulce, seeds of large biennial herb	Fennel, sweet	Putting ideas into action, self-resolve, courage, self-expression, purity and clarity
Juniperus communis, small fruits of coniferous shrub	Juniperberry	Purified, let go of negativity, move forward with confidence
Piper nigrum, small fruits of perennial vine	Pepper, black	Stimulated, fortified, strength, stamina, warmth

*At the time of writing *Santalum album* is scarce or unavailable, and is often substituted with *S. spicatum* or *S. austrocaledonicum.*

Essential oils from roots

Roots anchor the plant to the ground, and water and nutrients enter the plant via its root system. In some plants the roots also act as an organ of food storage. Ginger, spikenard and vetivert are examples of essential oils obtained from roots. Typically, and as might be expected, essential oils from roots have grounding, nurturing and warming qualities. There are times in our lives when we may feel uneasy, insecure, scared or out of touch. These oils can help us get in touch with our 'roots' and feel anchored or grounded.

Essential oils from stems and leaves

The stems and leaves are the aerial parts of the plant – the very obvious dynamic, living part of the plant. Not only do they form the main structure, they are also where photosynthesis and gas exchange occur. Plants use carbon dioxide as a carbon source and give off oxygen into the atmosphere. Many essential oils are obtained from leaves and stems – in some cases the entire aerial parts of a plant, sometimes the leaves and twigs, and sometimes just the flowering tops of herbaceous plants. Essential oils obtained from leaves often have an affinity with the respiratory system. Such oils can be helpful not only with physical problems in this system, for example infections, but also on an emotional level, when we find it difficult to breath effectively due to stress and anxiety. Leaf oils can also be useful when we find it difficult to 'let go' or release feelings that are affecting our well-being, or when our minds are cluttered and we need mental clarity.

Essential oils from grasses

The types of plants known as grasses belong to a large botanical family called the *Poaceae*. This is a diverse family, whose members are widespread over the Earth. They have extensive fibrous root systems (vetivert is a member of this family), and the aerial parts are characterised by long, narrow, linear leaves. Grasses are economically an important family, containing the cereals – man's staple diet. However, they are also grown as pasture and animal fodder. A few grasses have aromatic leaves and are sources of essential oils like lemongrass and palmarosa. Their essential oils are useful antimicrobials that are supportive of the immune system. However, they are derived from a family that is, in essence, about nurturing. They can also strengthen our physiological balance and immune systems by imparting emotional support, as their aromas comfort and relieve anxiety. Oils from the grasses are very useful for debility, lethargy or fatigue – both mental and physical.

Essential oils from woods

Some plants, such as trees and shrubs, have woody stems. Woody tissues are often aromatic and yield a wide range of essential oils. Woody essential oils can be found in a range of botanical families. The conifers, which are found in colder and temperate climates, yield oils that are typically warming and restorative, perhaps reflecting the characteristics they need to survive. Others, such as those from the *Lauraceae* and *Santalaceae* families, grow in tropical and subtropical climates. Therefore it is not easy to generalise about woody oils. However, like the leaves and stems, woody essential oils often have affinities with the respiratory system. Woody essential oils tend to help the individual find balance and equilibrium – they are good aids to meditation. So if the aim is to feel centred, and to open the consciousness, they are a good choice.

Essential oils from resins

Some woody plants produce aromatic resins and gums, which have been used in incenses, in perfumery and as astringents (to control secretions from exocrine glands) and healing agents for thousands of years. Some of their oils are used in aromatherapy. Like the woody oils, they are very well suited for times when there is a need to find your core and seek inner peace, perhaps along with meditation or contemplative practice.

Essential oils from flowers

Flowers are the reproductive parts of the plant. Not all flowers contain enough volatile oil to make extraction a viable process, and even when the oil can be extracted, the yield of essential oils from flowers is usually very low. Often solvent extraction is the most efficient method – producing an 'absolute'. Echoing the biological role of their source, the flower oils usually have intense, sometimes sensual aromas, associated with all aspects of creativity. At times of emotional shock the flower oils can bring comfort and they can help allay anxieties – especially those related to the social domain, such as poor self-image, shyness and lack of confidence. They are useful when there is lack of imagination, creative drive or even the urge to have fun, or play, as some have quite pronounced euphoric effects.

Essential oils from fruits and seeds

Fruits are the structures that develop to protect the seeds that form from the fertilised ovules in flowers. Essential oils can be extracted from different types of fruit, from the small fruits used as spices, to the large citrus fruits whose peel contains fairly large amounts of volatile oils. In some cases it is the seeds contained within the fruit that are the source of the oil. Fruit and seed oils have an affinity with the digestive system – not just on a physical level but also on a mental level. All of the citrus oils have refreshing odours that will usually impart happy feelings, while the spicy oils derived from either the seeds or the entire fruits tend to confer the energy contained within their source and have stimulating, revitalising and strengthening effects. As their effects on the digestive system are via reflex action, they can be very useful at times of low mood or loss of appetite (for food, or even for life itself). The citrus oils are also described as useful 'detoxifiers', especially grapefruit and lemon, and can be useful if there is a desire to clear out and make a fresh start.

Fragrance energetics

Peter Holmes (1997) developed the concept of 'Fragrance Energetics' – a system linking the scent of essential oils to their impact on the psyche. Essentially, this is a psychosensory approach; however, he suggests that it is the energetic dimension of a fragrance that elicits responses within an individual, that manifest on cognitive, emotional and spiritual levels. Holmes suggests that if the root of a disease is in the psyche, the fragrance of essential oils will work via the psychoneuroendocrine pathway, thus healing the physical dimension, and vice versa.

In fragrance energetics there are three fragrance parameters – *tone* (the quality of an odour), *intensity* and *note* (the evaporation rate), with tone being the most significant. There are also six fragrance categories, aligned loosely with perfumery but adapted to include the most common odour types and characteristics found in essential oils. These are *spicy, sweet, lemony, green, woody* and *rooty*. Holmes proposes that these fragrance characteristics can bring about specific psychotherapeutic effects.

For example, 'high/top tone' oils such as those from the citrus group, the *Myrtaceae* family typified by eucalyptus, ravintsara, niaouli, the floral ylang ylang extra, and the soft, floral, woody lavender, and mimosa absolute will have a stimulating, uplifting effect. Conversely, 'low/base tone' oils, including vetivert, patchouli, sandalwood and also the floral/caramel tuberose, the cut grass odour of hay and woody oakmoss absolute, most pine oils, and the spicy cinnamon bark, will have a depressing, sedating effect. Holmes suggested that:

- *Spicy* oils are stimulating, invigorating, intensifying, awakening, opening and dispersing.

- *Sweet* oils are relaxing, calming, harmonising, regulating, moistening, dissolving, nourishing and regenerating.

- *Lemony* oils are clearing, clarifying, sensitising, focusing, energising and invigorating.

- *Green* oils are balancing and regulating, cooling, relaxing, clearing and clarifying.

- *Woody* oils are centring, contracting, grounding and strengthening.

- *Rooty* oils are stabilising, grounding, solidifying, tonifying, desensitising and calming.

Each of these energetic odour effects can then be selected to counteract negative mood states. For example, 'woody' essential oils such as sandalwood, which has centring and contracting properties, can be used to help with feelings of insecurity and loss of boundaries.

Holmes, in his work *Clinical Aromatherapy* (2001), explored the application of essential oils using Chinese medicine philosophy, giving correspondences in terms of their warm/cool qualities and their meridian tropisms, as well as their relationships with the Chinese Five Elements and the *Zang Fu* (Chinese organ) models. He also extends this to acupoint applications, where the essential oils are applied with a Q-tip directly onto the point before the needle is inserted.

Chinese Five Element theory and prescribing essential oils

Mojay, in his introduction to *Aromatherapy for Healing the Spirit* (1996), explains that this approach encompasses the botanical, traditional and energetic aspects of essential oils and Oriental medicine to define their unique healing potential. At the outset he defines *qi* as the energy that manifests in our vital substances (such as blood and body fluids), but extends this to essential oils, which can also be viewed as vital substances produced in aromatic plants.

> All essential oils have the power to affect us both emotionally and spiritually. Only those that are right for the individual – at that moment in their life – will possess the subtle potential to transform. (Mojay 1996, p. 132)

Mojay's words not only convey the impact of essential oils on the psyche, but also the importance of the individuality of an essential oil prescription. He uses the framework of the Chinese Five Elements to explore the fragrance energies of essential oils, proposing that Five Element theory allows the therapist to align the actions of essential oils with holistic therapeutic intentions that encompass the body, emotions and spirit.

The theory of the Five Elements is central to Chinese medicine. The Five Elements are symbolic of phases or movements of *yin* and *yang* energy, and can be observed in myriad manifestations in the natural world, including the seasons, the climate and human emotions. The Five Elements are named Earth, Metal, Water, Wood and Fire; they are interrelated, and these relationships are described symbolically by the *sheng* cycle and the *ke* cycle. The *sheng* cycle is a cycle of generation where Wood creates Fire by burning, Fire creates Earth from ashes, Earth creates Metal (ore) by hardening, Metal creates Water by containment or condensation and Water creates Wood by nourishment. The *ke* cycle is one of protective control, or restraint, where Fire controls Metal by melting, Metal controls Wood by cutting, Wood controls Earth by covering, Earth controls Water by damming and Water controls Fire by extinguishing.

Within an individual, if any one of the Five Elements becomes out of balance, this will have an effect on all of the Elements, and will be observed in the emotions, facial colour, tone of voice and even personal odour (Hicks, Hicks and Mole

2011). It is invariably a complex scenario, and it is important to be able to find the root of the disharmony and focus the prescription on that aspect.

Another aspect of Five Element theory that permeates Mojay's work is that of the *shen*, or the spirit. The word 'spirit' has many connotations, often religious or mystical in nature. The *shen* equates to the psyche – the emotional, mental and spiritual aspects of a human being. The spirit is expressed in many emotions, such as love and compassion, joy when witnessing beautiful natural phenomena, or being moved by music. If the health of the spirit is adversely affected by stress, there is a knock-on effect that can result in mental and physical illness. So the health of the spirit is of vital importance (Mojay 1996; Hicks, Hicks and Mole 2011).

Just as there are five elements, there are five aspects of the *shen*, and these are also associated with the *yin* organs of the body. The five *shen* are:

- *hun* (the ethereal soul and the Liver, and Wood)
- *po* (the corporeal soul and the Lungs, and Metal)
- *shen* (the mind/spirit and the Heart, and Fire)
- *zhi* (the will, drive, the Kidneys, and Water)
- *yi* (the intellect, thought and intention, the Spleen, and Earth).

Each element and *shen* also have an associated root emotion.

- Earth (*yi*) is associated with over-thinking, worry, pensiveness and need for sympathy.
- Metal (*po*) is associated with grief, difficulty in letting go, feeling a void within.
- Water (*zhi*) is associated with fear.
- Wood (*hun*) is associated with anger.
- Fire (*shen*) is associated with overexuberance.

So for example, the *yi* allows us to manifest our ideas, so that our projects are successful. If the individual is consistently unable to do this, the *yi* is weak, and this would point to an imbalance in the Earth element. Or, if a person has experienced intense grief and loss, the *po* and the Metal element will be affected, and this should perhaps be the focus of treatment to restore balance.

By aligning fragrance energies with the Five Elements, Mojay has devised a system for essential oil prescribing, relevant mainly to the treatment of psychological conditions. He gave an outline of taste energies in Oriental medicine, before putting fragrance energies in this context (Mojay 1998).

- *Sweet* taste reinforces nourishes the Spleen-Pancreas and supports Earth.

- *Pungent-spicy* taste stimulates the Lungs and revitalises Metal.

- *Salty* taste nourishes the Kidneys and reinforces Water.

- *Sour* taste benefits the Liver and regulates Wood.

- *Bitter* taste benefits the Heart and supports Fire.

Chinese Five Element theory also aligns specific personal odour characteristics with the elements (Hicks, Hicks and Mole 2011):

- Earth has a cloying, sickly, *sweet* odour that permeates a space.

- Metal has a *rotten* odour, perhaps like rotten meat or decomposing garbage, that irritates the inside of the nose.

- Water has a *putrid* odour, like stagnant water or stale urine – male cat's urine – a sharp, aggressive smell like ammonia.

- Wood has a *rancid* odour, like rancid butter or decomposing grass cuttings.

- Fire has a *scorched* odour, like burning toast or the smell of a hot iron on clothing.

Considering the odour types and energetic qualities of the essential oils of aromatherapy, Mojay made the following correspondences:

- *Sweet-resinous* oils settle, and *lemony-citrus* oils clarify, Earth.

- *Camphoraceous* and *coniferous* oils revitalise Metal.

- *Woody* and *rooty* oils strengthen and anchor Water.

- *Sweet-herbaceous* and *fruity-citrus* oils smooth and regulate Wood.

- *Spicy* oils invigorate, and *floral* oils harmonise, Fire.

Therefore, if the practitioner can make an assessment in terms of the Five Elements, essential oils may be prescribed that can support or balance the affected elements. When blending oils to restore emotional and mental balance, it is suggested that no more than three oils constitute the blend, because the 'unique and subtle influence of each oil will only emerge if the blend is kept relatively simple' (Mojay 1996, p. 133). Mojay gives numerous examples of this process, lists of essential oils and their Five Element correspondences, and some eloquent essential oil profiles. However, it must be emphasised that Chinese Five Element assessment is based on detailed observations and an understanding of the underlying theory, and it is only with this perspective that a practitioner could construct a philosophically sound individual prescription.

The Greek Four Element framework has not been exploited to the same extent in contemporary aromatherapy. However, the Four Humours or Temperaments are derived from this model, and these are central to some healing traditions. Here, we will consider the Four Elements as a potential model for a psycho-sensory approach to essential oil prescribing.

The Four Elements as a model for prescribing essential oils

Empedocles was a Greek philosopher who, in his Doctrine of the Four Elements (*Tetrasomia*, c. 5 BC) proposed that all matter was composed of the elements of Fire, Air, Earth and Water, and that they had both physical and spiritual manifestations. His influences included the Pythagoreans (a brotherhood which followed the teachings of Pythagoras), and ancient Greek mystery traditions such as the cults of Hades and Dionysus. However, it is the dynamic of 'Love' and 'Strife' that is at the heart of Empedocles' treatise on the Four Elements – an ongoing cycle of joining and dissolution known as the 'Vortex' – that can be witnessed in all aspects of existence. He suggested that in the beginning all was Love, and that the Elements were distinct and equal, but held as one in a Sphere, divided in quarters. In time, Strife dissolved the Sphere and then became the dominant force. However, in turn, Love became stronger and the elements would gather again under its influence, eventually forming the Sphere again – and the cycle is repeated (O'Brien 1969).

Hippocrates and Aristotle also developed their own interpretations of the concept of the Four Elements. Aristotle proposed a fifth element, *Aether*, a divine substance that gives form to the stars and planets. He also added the dimensions of hot, cold, dry and moist to the Four Elements. He maintained that moistness was fluid and flexible, and thus able to adapt, and in contrast dryness was rigid and less flexible, more structured and defined. Aristotle suggested that Air was hot and moist, Fire was hot and dry, Earth was cold and dry, and Water was cold and moist.

Hippocrates viewed the elements as 'humors', or bodily fluids, with associated temperaments, as follows:

- Air was associated with yellow bile, and an irritable personality – the *choleric* type.

- Fire was associated with blood, and an enthusiastic personality – the *sanguine* type.

- Earth was associated with phlegm, and an apathetic personality – the *phlegmatic* type.

- Water was associated with black bile, and a pensive personality – the *melancholic* type.

These concepts devised and developed by the Greeks in an attempt to explain the nature of the universe, our planet and ourselves influenced thinking over the centuries in many areas, eventually being rejected by science but embraced in alchemy, astrology and many spiritual traditions. Over time, the Four Elements became imbued with myriad qualities – natural manifestations (air, sun, land and sea), subtle anatomy (the mental, astral, etheric and physical bodies) and aspects of the psyche, personal growth and transformation.

The psychologist Carl Jung used the symbolism of the Four Elements in his work and writings. Jung (1875–1961) was one of the creators of modern depth psychology or analytical psychology. Central to his work were the concepts of the personal unconscious and the collective unconscious, symbolism and the concepts of the archetype, persona, shadow, anima and animus, and also personality typology.

Jung used the symbolism of the Four Elements in his classification of eight personality types. He paired the polarities of introversion and extroversion with his concepts of the four personality types – thinking (Air), intuiting (Fire), sensing (Earth) and feeling (Water). Today some well-known personality assessments such as the Meyers-Briggs test are based on this. Jung's writing on the symbolism of the Four Elements has also influenced modern psychological astrology, as the Four Elements are the cornerstones of Western astrology.

Stephen Arroyo, a well-respected astrologer/psychologist, gives a contemporary perspective on the symbolism in his work *Astrology, Psychology and the Four Elements* (1975), suggesting that 'the Four Elements represent specific areas of consciousness and perception, and the ability to relate to different realms of life experience and vitalising forces.' In addition to this, he gives his view that 'The Four Elements could also be described as energetic atunements. Each individual's relationship with each dimension can be in harmony or discord, but we all have the choice of making creative use or misuse of our energetic atunements.'

Using this as a basis, we can start to apply Four Element philosophy to essential oil prescribing. Just as the Five Elements of Chinese medicine have interrelationships and correspondences, so do the Four Elements. The interrelationships between them are best described by analogies with the natural world. Air is confined by Earth, saturated by Water and stimulated by Fire. Fire is smothered by Earth, extinguished by Water and fanned by Air. Earth is parched by Fire, disturbed by Air and refreshed by Water. Water is all-conquering because it is yielding. Water is heated by Fire but escapes by turning to steam, then condensing back to Water; it is stirred up and channelled by Air but saturates and dampens Air and then returns to a calm state; and Water is given form by Earth but can wash away Earth or flow around it.

The qualities ascribed to the Four Elements begin to reveal resonances with essential oil fragrance qualities:

- *Air* is associated with the spring, the mental realm and Jung's personality type 'thinking'.

- *Fire* is associated with summer, the realm of the spirit and Jung's 'intuiting' personality type.

- *Earth* is associated with autumn, the material/physical realm and Jung's 'sensing' personality type.

- *Water* is associated with winter, the realm of the emotions and Jung's 'feeling' personality type.

Accordingly, *Air* would resonate with cephalic oils, oils that support breathing, decongestant oils, uplifting and stimulating oils, and oils that stimulate creativity and mental faculties. The fragrance types and characteristics that elicit these effects tend to be green, herbal, minty, coniferous, anise, cineolic, camphoraceous, pine-like, sharp/citrus, fresh, penetrating and diffusive.

Fire is like Air, in that it shares the same quality of 'levity'. However, Fire is more aligned to action. So essential oils that are associated with Fire are stimulating, invigorating and uplifting oils that may also support the nervous system (action) and the digestion (often associated with 'fire'). The fragrance types and characteristics of essential oils that resonate with Fire are spicy, caryophyllaceous (clove-like), floral/fruity, peppery, pungent, rich and warm.

Earth, as would be expected, is associated with 'gravity' rather than levity. Therefore calming, comforting, grounding, sensual and nurturing oils and those that support the musculoskeletal system are associated with the qualities of Earth. Balsamic, caramel, earthy, rooty, sweet/citrus, soft, heavy, musty, rich, smooth, sweet and warm, sensual essential oil fragrances could be expected to impart these types of responses.

Finally, *Water* shares the association with gravity, but with the quality of movement and permeability. Calming, anchoring oils that promote a sense of ease and adaptability, anxiolytic oils, oils that balance and oils that support the lymphatic and urinary systems and metabolism are associated with the qualities of water. The fragrances of the essential oils that are associated with these qualities are citrus/sweet, rosy, floral/sweet, floral/green, fruity/green, agrestic/hay/grass, woody/fresh and woody/soft. As might be expected, with its permeable nature, Water scents combine characteristics found in the other three elements' scents, but with subtle variations.

The Four Elements do not form a cycle in the same way as the Chinese Five Elements – and they are usually depicted within a quadrant structure. If an element were under-emphasised in an individual, we would look to remedies that resonate with, or support that element. However, when an element is overemphasised in the individual, balance can be restored by looking to the opposite element, using the idea attributed to Hippocrates – the 'remedial power of opposites', which is also found in homoeopathic theory.

For example, if there is an overemphasis on Air, we would observe someone with an overactive mind, who is living 'in the head', whose mind 'runs away', or whose 'head is in the clouds'. This individual may not like to get involved with the world of emotions; he or she may dabble in ideas but does not develop anything, because the will is paralysed – although this would depend on the status of Fire too. In extreme cases, there may be no sense of reality, they will be out of touch with their body and their physical and emotional needs, they may be showing signs of nervous exhaustion, or even eccentricity, with a strong dislike of, or dismissive attitude to practical limitations. Applying the remedial power of opposites, we would look to essential oils that resonate with Earth, which is the opposite of Air, and depending on the individual's other characteristics, we might also include Water oils.

Staying with the Air element as an example, we may also observe an underemphasis on Air qualities. In this case, we might find someone who is too involved in action (Fire), feelings (Water) or material (Earth) concerns. There may be a lack of perception, an inability to reflect or analyse self, and a mistrust of those who place importance on thinking and ideas. This person may also be overly subjective, and psychosocial problems might be an issue. We would consider using Air oils to help redress the balance, while also considering any overemphasis on the other elements.

As is the case with all approaches that are essentially symbolic in nature, it is vital to have a good understanding of the underpinning philosophy in order to make best use of the system. In the case of the Four Elements, this will certainly involve an exploration of Jungian psychology.

We will now explore an ancient healing system that includes aromatic oils: Ayurveda – and how this too can relate to contemporary aromatherapy. We have already seen how essential oils can successfully be incorporated in some Ayurvedic practices such as *Shirodhara* (see p. 71). Some aromatherapists study Ayurveda in order to incorporate their aromatherapy practice within this system of healing; others will use some of the philosophical principles to gain an understanding of their clients and inform essential oil prescription. In the latter case, it is usually the concepts of the *doshas* and the *chakras* that can be related to the psychosensory approach to essential prescribing, and it is these that we will focus on in the following section.

Ayurveda and aromatic oils

Ayurvedic medicine of the Indian subcontinent originates from the ancient Sanskrit sacred texts, known as the *Vedas* (Caldecott 2006). The four books that comprise the *Vedas* date from around 3000 BCE and give detailed instructions on how a human being should live a spiritual life – a path with heart, which will ultimately lead to enlightenment. Ayurveda, meaning 'the knowledge of life', forms one strand of the intricate brocade of the *Vedas*, and details how humans can live healthily in body, spirit and mind through an understanding of their own nature and their interactions with the world. This is a system of medicine that is completely individualised; and although it gives great therapeutic detail on the treatment of illness through herbs, oils, massage, diet, etc., it is more about prevention of disease through correct living. There is a rich history of the use of aromatic oils in the prevention and treatment of disease in Ayurveda.

The Vedic theory of the origins of the universe talks of inertia coming from the void – this is the will of 'pure consciousness' desiring to become matter. The vibrations of this desire gave rise to Ether, which through movement became Air. The Air, as it circulated and moved with restless energy, created friction that inevitably produced heat, or Fire. The great burst of heat expanded out in all directions, consuming, driving forward. As it spread, the energy of Fire started to cool and condense into fluids, and Water was formed. Water further cooled and condensed into matter, or Earth, which makes up all the physical things in the universe. The Earth then gave birth to all living things (Pole 2006). This account demonstrates how the Vedic theory of the origins of the universe give rise to the Five Elements (*mahabuttas*) of Ayurveda – Ether, Air, Fire, Water and Earth. These Five Elements represent processes, not absolutes, and all things in the universe are composed of a combination of all Five Elements. As we humans are part of nature, we must too be made of the Five Elements.

In the Ayurvedic texts, these Five Elements are combined into pairs, creating three *doshas* – *Vata* (Ether and Air), *Pitta* (Fire and Water) and *Kapha* (Water and Earth) (Frawley and Lad 1986). Each and every human being, as part of nature, has their own particular mix of the three *doshas*, which gives rise to that individual's unique constitution, or *pakriti* (Svoboda 1984). Our *pakriti* is set at the time of our conception, when our very first cells came into being, and is dependent on our spiritual past lives and the health and well-being of our parents and all our ancestors. In the philosophical treatise of the *Vedas*, humans are beings of spirit manifest as matter. The spirit or soul is on a journey of enlightenment to reunite with pure consciousness. In that journey, the human spirit manifests as matter on the planet, to learn the great spiritual lessons that it has forgotten – love, compassion, etc., in order to bring about the uniting or yoking (*yoga*) with the unknown (Svoboda 1984). This may take many, many lifetimes and explains why life can be so hard for us, or, if we decide to follow the 'true' path, why life can become so simple and easy – for all is provided. So the soul on its journey chooses how it manifests in this world in order to learn those lessons. In other words, we, as individual spiritual beings, choose our parents, and our human form, and therefore our unique doshic balance.

We have our own unique combination of all three *doshas* – for we all need the principle of motion that is Air, the principle of illumination that is Fire and the principle of cohesion that is Water and Earth (Pole 2006). However, our constitution or *pakriti* will generally be dominant in either one or two of the doshas – rarely there is an individual with balance of all three *doshas* – a tridoshic individual. The *doshas* have behavioural, emotional, cognitive and physical/ physiological correspondences; a good practitioner of Ayurvedic medicine will recognise that each of the doshic predominances will generally display differing emotional responses.

Here we will focus on these aspects rather than the physical/physiological ones, so that we can apply a psychosensory approach when prescribing essential oils.

The doshas

- If *Vata* is dominant:

  o Characteristics will manifest as someone who is always 'on the move', full of creative energy and ideas, with a sharp intellect, usually full of enthusiasm.

  o Tastes and qualities suitable for a *Vata* type are sweet, salty and sour, and ones that aggravate are drying, bitter and pungent.

  o Oils suitable for a *Vata* constitution would be ones that are of the Earth: warming and grounding. As there is a tendency to cold and dry, the oils chosen should be warming and moistening.

  o Consider oils that would be beneficial to the nerves, lungs, colon, skin and the bones, particularly in old age.

  o The following therapeutic actions may prove useful – nervines of all classes, carminatives, expectorants, vulneraries, and tonics for the lungs, digestion and nerves.

  o Oils to be avoided are ones that are drying and pungent.

  o As all fixed oils nourish the nervous system, a wide range can be used internally and externally – flax, hemp, sesame, ghee, olive, sunflower, and evening primrose, borage, and fish oils.

  (adapted from Pole 2006)

- If *Pitta* is dominant:

  o This will manifest as someone with passion, direction, force and drive, who likes to be in control and who likes action, adventure, with a keen intellect and good memory. There will be a tendency to work and play hard.

- ○ Tastes and qualities suitable for the *Pitta* type are bitter and sweet, and ones that aggravate are pungent, salty and sour as they will heat.

- ○ Oils suitable for a *Pitta* constitution would be ones that are of the Water and Earth; sweet, cooling and moistening, because there is a tendency towards hot and moist.

- ○ Consider oils that would be beneficial to the cardiovascular system and digestive system, including the liver.

- ○ The following therapeutic actions may prove useful – cardiac tonics, vasodilators, nervines, anti-inflammatories, digestives, aperients, carminatives.

- ○ Oils to be avoided would be ones that are pungent.

- ○ Fixed oils suitable for *Pitta* include flax, hemp, ghee, olive, sunflower, and evening primrose, borage and coconut. Oils that should be avoided because they increase heat are sesame, almond and corn oil.

(adapted from Pole 2006)

- If *Kapha* is dominant:

  - ○ This will manifest as a nurturing, caring, home-loving, grounded yet versatile individual, who is cool in a crisis. There will also be a tendency to enjoy their creature comforts, and be somewhat lazy; the intellect may seem slower than that of the other *doshas*, but knowledge, once acquired, may be deep.

  - ○ Tastes and qualities that are suitable to counteract the heavy *Kapha* constitution, which is cold and moist, would be ones that are light and airy.

  - ○ As there tends to be fluid build-up and stagnation with *Kapha*, warming, stimulating, pungent and drying oils would be useful.

  - ○ You might also consider oils that would be beneficial to the lungs, and mucous membranes – especially tonics.

  - ○ The following therapeutic actions might be useful – astringent, circulatory stimulant, expectorant, immune stimulant, and in the case of infections, antibacterial.

  - ○ The *Kapha* constitution, however, is already well lubricated, and in general the use of oils internally and externally should be kept to a minimum.

  - ○ Oils that are suitable would be flax, corn and sunflower.

(adapted from Pole 2006)

Aromatics in Ayurveda

Herbs and spices used in Ayurveda are often the sources of essential oils that we use in aromatherapy. These include:

- Anise – pungent and bitter; controls *Vata* and *Kapha* and increases *Pitta*.

- Black pepper – pungent and hot; decreases *Kapha* and *Vata* and increases *Pitta* slightly. It is mixed with ginger and long pepper into *Trikatu* – the 'Three Pungents' – for increasing digestive fire, treating cold fevers and relieving respiratory congestion.

- Caraway – pungent and bitter; controls *Vata* and *Kapha*, and increases *Pitta*.

- Cardamom – sweet and pungent taste, and hot; however, it does not increase Pitta – it decreases all three *doshas*. It is added to coffee to relieve acidity.

- Cinnamon – it is the bark that is used; however, the leaf oil will share the pungent, sweet, bitter and hot qualities that control *Vata* and *Kapha*, without aggravating *Pitta*.

- Coriander – leaves and seeds are used; neither are pungent and both are very cooling, they can relieve *Vata* and *Kapha* and remove heat from the system.

- Cumin – pungent and slightly hot; controls *Vata* and *Kapha*, without aggravating *Pitta* unless used in excess. It is often used with coriander and fennel.

- Dill – the seeds are pungent and bitter, and hot; and they are used in poultices too.

- Fennel – the seeds are sweet, pungent and bitter, slightly cooling and used to decrease all the *doshas*; it is a decongestant.

- Ginger – is sometimes called the 'universal remedy'; pungent, sweet, hot and used to control the three *doshas*, although in excess it can increase *Pitta*. It is used to increase digestive fire, relieve bloating and digest toxins, and promote the circulation.

- Lime – sour, bitter, astringent and cooling; it does not aggravate normal *Pitta*, but might aggravate elevated *Pitta*. It is claimed that there is no disease that this fruit does not have the potential to treat.

- Nutmeg – pungent, bitter, astringent and hot; reduces *Vata* and *Kapha* and increases *Pitta*.

- Turmeric – bitter, astringent and pungent, hot; balances the *doshas*, but in excess can aggravate *Vata* and *Pitta*. It is used to purify and protect, and as an antiseptic.

Other aromatics used in Ayurvedic medicine, with which we are familiar in aromatherapy, include:

- *Centella asiatica* – we use this as a carrier oil; it is bitter and cool, and balances all three *doshas*.

- Camphor – is used to increase flow; it is excreted in the breath so is used for respiratory complaints.

- Inula – in Ayurveda, it is elecampane that is used; however, we might consider using sweet inula. It decreases *Kapha* and *Vata* and increases *Pitta*, targeting the chest and lungs.

- Myrrh – is considered to be drying; it balances all three *doshas*, but can aggravate *Pitta* in excess.

- Rose – bitter, pungent and astringent, sweet and cool; used to cool and soothe, balance all three *doshas* and eliminate *Pitta* from the mind and eyes. Rose attar (with sandalwood) is said to be cooling and tonic to the sex organs and the mind.

- Sandalwood – bitter, sweet, astringent, cool; controls the *doshas*, but has more physical effects on *Pitta*. It is used to lighten and concentrate the mind.

- Spikenard – balances all three *doshas*; promotes awareness and strengthens the mind.

- Tulsi (holy basil) – pungent and bitter, hot; controls *Vata* and *Kapha* but can increase *Pitta*. It has many uses, including purification and elimination of toxins, expulsion of mucus, and the reduction of spasm. Sweet basil is also used in this way.

- Vetivert – bitter, sweet and very cooling; strongly reduces *Pitta* and reduces *Kapha*. In the hot season, bundles of the roots are soaked in drinking water to stay cool and prevent Pitta 'flare up'. The incense and essential oil are used to cool the mind and improve concentration (Svoboda 2004).

The chakras

The *Vedas* describe humans as spiritual made physical. We are fields of energy manifest as matter (Bhagwan Dash 1989). This is congruent with many ancient belief systems – from the Taoists of ancient China, to shamans from as far apart as Siberia and North and South America, and ancient seers of Aboriginal Australia and Africa – peoples who lived very closely with nature.

Our energy bodies are described clearly in the Vedic texts. Energy circulates throughout the body keeping us healthy, and accumulates in a vortex at certain points known as *chakras* (the Sanskrit for 'wheel'). There are hundreds of tiny vortices in the human body found along certain paths or *marmas*. These points were utilised in a system of acupuncture not unlike that of ancient China, to open blockages and ease energy flow.

There are seven major *chakras* in the human being, found in the midline of the human body and extending about a foot outwards to the front and back (Angelo 1997). The seven major chakras largely correspond to the physical position and function of the glands of the endocrine system. Rising from the base, the seven chakras are Root, Sacral, Solar Plexus, Heart, Throat, Brow and Crown. Each of the seven chakras corresponds to certain emotions, and the path to enlightenment can only be achieved when all are open and free.

Essential oils and the chakras

- The Root *chakra* is our link with nature and the Earth, and deals with the physical and our instinct for survival; sex, food, aggression and self-defence. If out of balance we may become over-aggressive, over-materialistic; or in the opposite direction we may lose our sense of connectedness with the Earth and nature. Often those seeking a spiritual path can fall into the latter category.
  - Oils useful for the Root *chakra* are ginger, lotus and spikenard.

- The Sacral *chakra* is connected with issues of creativity and sexuality. It is the seat of joy, and the place where the 'inner child' resides. If the Sacral *chakra* is out of balance, sexual expression can either be overt and excessive, or repressed and hidden. This is the case with artistic expression too – either repressed or so fully expressed that the person has difficulty functioning.
  - Oils useful for the Sacral *chakra* are jasmine, ylang ylang, patchouli and sandalwood.

- The Solar Plexus *chakra* allows the personal will and mind to find expression. A link is established here between the mind and the lower emotions based on fear, such as anxiety, insecurity, jealousy and anger (Angelo 1997). In balance, growth and maturity flows easily; when stuck, the 'wounded child' can surface, negative energies are not processed properly and the emotions of fear surface. There may also be a lack of responsibility.

- Oils useful for the Solar Plexus *chakra* are lime, bitter orange, Roman chamomile and geranium.

- The Heart *chakra* is the place of soul or inner guidance, and the higher emotions such as love, trust, empathy and kinship. In balance, the individual is able to express true love for themselves and others, including all sentient beings. Out of balance, love is suppressed or overabundant – a constricting love. The person may find it difficult to feel good about themselves and others, and may have problems receiving and giving love.

  - Oils useful for the Heart *chakra* are rose, helichrysum and bergamot.

- The Throat *chakra* is involved with expression and communication of all kinds – dance, art, music, language, etc. From this free-flowing communication, truth and true expression of the soul is realised. In balance, the individual is able to express themselves, and is true to their word and actions. If the Throat *chakra* is 'stuck', then true expression is repressed, resulting in difficulty communicating with others.

  - Oils useful for the Throat *chakra* are clary sage, lavender and sweet basil.

- The Brow *chakra* (sometimes called the Third Eye) is responsible for intuition and soul knowledge. It has a governing role and oversees the *chakras* below it. When functioning well it allows the individual to trust their intuition in life, and to pursue their soul path with confidence. Out of balance, it leads to mistrust of this intuition, to overthinking and rationalising. This can block the soul's natural expression.

  - Oils useful for the Brow *chakra* are rosemary, tulsi and Douglas fir.

- The Crown *chakra* provides a direct link to 'Pure Consciousness' and deals with all matters of spirituality. Fully realised, it allows enlightenment or union with Spirit to take place, but for this to happen all the *chakras* below must be open and free. If the Crown *chakra* opens prematurely, it can lead to an individual being too 'spiritual' – a seemingly lost soul.

  - Oils useful for the Crown *chakra* are frankincense, frangipani and spikenard.

In this chapter we have just 'scraped the surface' of some of the ancient healing traditions, and given a short overview of how contemporary aromatherapy is being influenced by the psychosensory approach. Nevertheless, it is hoped that this will stimulate your appetite to explore and perhaps specialise in one of these. It is emphasised again that the molecular approach and the energetic approaches are by no means mutually exclusive, and in practice can work very well together.

In the next section we will focus on our aromatic materia medica.

The Essential Oils, Absolutes and Resinoids of Aromatherapy

CHAPTER 7

Botanical Principles in Aromatherapy

We will begin Part III by considering the aspects of botany that impact upon and influence contemporary aromatherapy practice. Then the essential oils will be presented according to their botanical sources, arranged by family. Perhaps the most important aspect is that of taxonomy, because essential oils are identified and traded under the Latinised names of their plant sources.

Taxonomy – the principles of classification

Taxonomy is the systematic study of the principles and practices of classification. The Swedish naturalist Carolus Linnaeus (to use his Latinised name) is considered to be the founder of the modern system of classification which is used in biology. There are many systems of classification of organisms, each with different merits. However, it is desirable that a system of plant classification should assist the rapid identification of a plant, based on features such as form, physiology and structure, and also indicate its natural interrelationships.

Over 1.2 million types of life exist on Earth. All have broadly similar requirements for life, and all living things are composed of cells. These are placed into three large, diverse groups called 'kingdoms' – see Table 7.1. Looking at the plant kingdom, we can see that two of the specific groups identified, the conifers and the flowering plants, are important in aromatherapy.

Table 7.1 Kingdoms

Kingdom	Characteristics	Examples
Protista	Single-celled (unicellular) organisms *or* Multicellular organisms lacking development of specialised tissues/organs	Protozoa, e.g. amoeba Algae, e.g. green algae, seaweed Blue-green algae Bacteria Viruses Fungi Yeasts Slime moulds
Plantae (plant)	Contain the green pigment chlorophyll Lack the power of motion by means of contracting fibres Have bodies made up of many cells specialised to form tissues and organs Have sex organs composed of many accessory cells Produce offspring that, as partially developed embryos, are protected and nourished for a time within the body of the parent plant	Primitive plants such as mosses and liverworts Ferns Conifers Flowering plants
Animalae (animal)	Do not possess chlorophyll Capable of movement by means of contracting fibres Are made up of many cells (multicellular animals)	Sponges Jellyfishes Worms Molluscs Spiders Insects Starfish Fish Amphibians Reptiles Birds Mammals

Taxonomy in the plant kingdom

The major taxonomic categories according to the International Code of Botanical Nomenclature are:

- phylum (or division); plural phyla – a group of similar classes

- subphylum

- class – a group of similar orders

- order – a group of similar families

- family – a group of similar genera

- genus; plural genera – a group of similar species

- species – a group of similar organisms that interbreed in their natural environment (and do not interbreed with other species)

- subspecies (or variety).

These categories are best illustrated by example, so see Table 7.2 for the classification of cornmint and its three varieties.

Mint is a familiar common culinary and medicinal herb, and there are many different types of mint – including peppermint and spearmint, whose essential oils are used in aromatherapy. These are distinct species – peppermint is the species *piperita* and spearmint is the species *spicata*. All of these are included in the genus called *Mentha*, and this genus belongs to a much larger family of related plants – the Lamiaceae. The Lamiaceae family contains many well-known herbs such as rosemary, marjoram, thyme and lavender. In turn, this family is placed in a larger group of families known as the order Tubiflorae, and the order is part of an even larger group – the subclass Dicotyledonae, which is one of only two subclasses within the vast class known as the Angiospermae.

There are more subdivisions within the orders and classes, but these are really only of concern to the plant taxonomist. For the aromatherapist it is sufficient to know the scientific name of a plant that denotes the genus and species, and in appropriate cases, the subspecies or variety. Staying with the genus *Mentha*, cornmint is known as *Mentha arvensis*, but there are three subspecies or varieties within this species. Varieties are indicated by the abbreviation 'var.' after the name of the species, followed by another Latinised name. The three varieties of cornmint are named *Mentha arvensis* var. *villosa*, *Mentha arvensis* var. *glabrata* and *Mentha arvensis* var. *piperascens*.

Table 7.2 Classification of cornmint, *Mentha arvensis*, and its varieties

Classification	Category	Comments
Kingdom	Plantae	The plant kingdom
Phylum	Tracheophyta	The presence of a water-conducting (vascular) system
Subphylum	Pteropsida	Plants with leaves
Class	Angiospermae	The flowering plants, including herbaceous perennials, annuals, biennials and many trees and shrubs
Subclass	Dicotyledonae	Plants with a two-part embryonic leaf (cotyledon)
Order	Tubiflorae	A group of families whose members are usually herbs with alternate or opposite simple leaves. The flower petals may be fused into a tube
Family	Lamiaceae	A large group of aromatic annual or perennial herbs or undershrubs, sharing specific characteristics such as stems that are square in cross-section, and five-petalled flowers fused into a tube that terminates in two distinct lips – hence the alternative family name, the Labiateae. The Lamiaceae is often called 'the mint family'
Genus	*Mentha*	A genus of some 25 aromatic perennials and a few annuals
Species	*arvensis*	Denotes cornmint, a mint that grows in a ploughed field
Subspecies	var. *villosa*	This has a shaggy appearance due to covering of soft glandular hairs
	var. *glabrata*	The leaves appear devoid of projections or glandular hairs
	var. *piperascens*	Known as Japanese mint

Hybrids are formed when two species interbreed, either in the wild or artificially. The Latin name will indicate this with the presence of a '×' between the genus and species. For example, *Mentha × piperita* is peppermint, a hybrid which is the result of a cross between *M. aquatica*, or watermint, and *M. spicata*, or spearmint. A cultivar is a variant, either natural or artificially produced, that is deliberately cultivated to maintain its characteristics. An example of this is *Mentha × piperita* 'Citrata' – the lemon-scented mint.

In aromatherapy and aromatic medicine there is another consideration – the concept of chemotypes. Sometimes the chemical composition of an essential oil from a named species can vary considerably – more than can be accounted for by minor, natural, normal variations. These variations can be due to external factors such as geography and climate, or to internal, genetic factors. For example, essential oil from rosemary – *Rosmarinus officinalis* – is available in three distinct chemotypes, designated *R. officinalis* CT camphor, *R. officinalis* CT 1,8-cineole and *R. officinalis* CT verbenone.

These scientific names are Latinised, and may be followed by the name, or an abbreviation of the name, of the taxonomist or botanist who originally identified and/or named the species. Here are some examples.

- Clove oil is obtained from *Syzigium aromaticum* L. (or Linn.). This means that the clove tree belongs to the genus *Syzigium* and the species is *aromaticum*, using the classification of Linnaeus.

- *Eucalyptus smithii* Baker is a species (*smithii*) belonging to the genus *Eucalyptus*. The plant is commonly known as gully-gum or Smith's gum, classified by Baker.

- The damask rose is known as *Rosa damascena* Mill., according to the taxonomist Miller.

When appropriate, it is important to use scientific names when referring to essential oil-bearing plants – it will accurately reflect the nature of the essential oil. In some instances the common name is insufficient. In aromatherapy literature it is not usual practice to include the name of the taxonomist. The scientific name should be italicised, the genus should have a capital letter, and the species should be lower case. Once a genus has been mentioned already in the literature, it is usual practice to abbreviate it by using only its first letter on subsequent occasions, for example *R. damascena*.

The gymnosperms and angiosperms

The aromatic plants all belong to the subphylum *Pteropsida*, which is composed of three classes:

- *Filicinae* – the ferns.

- *Gymnospermae* – the 'gymnosperms' are tree-like, seed-bearing plants, including conifers. They were dominant during the Devonian, Jurassic and early Cretaceous periods. Some essential oil-producing species belong to this class.

- *Angiospermae* – the 'angiosperms' are the flowering plants, now the dominant group, containing over 200,000 species. The rest of the plant kingdom comprises around 34,000 species. Many aromatic plants belong to this class.

Most gymnosperms are evergreen trees and shrubs. There are three orders within this class, namely the:

- *Cycadales* – the 'cycads', comprising tropical and subtropical plants resembling palms. Only one family exists, and this contains only around nine genera and about 100 species.

- *Ginkoales* – only one species has survived: *Ginko biloba*, a tall deciduous tree.

- *Coniferales* – in the gymnosperms, this order is the most common. The conifers are widely distributed, and are able to survive in cold climates. They are mostly evergreen trees, characterised by leaves in the form of needles, and their seeds are produced in cones. Within the order there are several families that contain essential oil-bearing species – notably the *Pinaceae* and the *Cupressaceae*. The sequoias (redwoods), spruces, pines, thuja, cypresses, *Chamaecyparis*, cedars and junipers are all in this order.

The largest class, the *Angiospermae*, is divided into two subclasses – the *Monocotyledonae* and the *Dicotyledonae*. The basis of the division is the form of the embryonic leaf within the seed, the cotyledon. The cotyledon also functions as the food-storing part of the endosperm within the seed.

- *Monocotyledonae* – the 'monocots' are flowering plants that have only a single cotyledon. As mature plants they may be distinguished by their narrow, parallel-veined leaves; their flower parts occur in multiples of three, they have a fibrous root system, and numerous, scattered vascular bundles (the water transport vessels). There are approximately 50,000 species. Monocots include the grasses – corn, wheat rice and cereals, and also aromatic grasses such as lemongrass, gingergrass, palmarosa and vetivert. Other examples are lilies, orchids, irises, tulips and food crops such as onions and asparagus. Monocots rarely possess a cambium (a tissue that lies between the bark and the wood) and secondary thickening; an exception is the family of palms.

- *Dicotyledonae* – the 'dicots' are flowering plants that have two cotyledons. As mature plants they are characterised by broader leaves with branching veins; their flower parts occur in fours or fives, they produce persistent, robust taproots and their vascular bundles are arranged in a ring. Unlike monocots, dicots usually possess a cambium; therefore they are often woody or herbaceous. This is a larger group of approximately 150,000 species and includes a wide variety of plants – deciduous trees, shrubs, herbs and cacti.

It is also useful to consider the basic principles of plant anatomy and physiology; this contributes to a deeper understanding of the biogenesis of plant volatile oils.

Plant anatomy

In this section we will consider the general structure of plants, from their cells and tissues to their gross anatomy.

Plant cells

Plant cells differ from animal cells in several ways. They have a cell wall, whereas animal cells have a cell membrane, and they contain organelles known as 'plastids'. A living plant cell consists of a 'protoplast' surrounded by an exterior cell wall. These cell walls are composed of cellulose, a rigid, porous material that provides strength to the entire plant. The cell wall also protects and supports the plant cell and provides routes for the passage of water and dissolved materials in and out of the cell. Some plant cells deposit a secondary cell wall between the protoplast and the primary wall. These additional layers of cellulose are impregnated with a cementing, woody material called lignin.

Within the cell are organelles, many of which have similar functions to their animal cell counterparts. The nucleus contains the chromosomes; it is enclosed by a nuclear membrane. *Rough* endoplasmic reticulum is an elaborate structure of membranes within the cytoplasm (the contents of the cell excluding the nucleus); sometimes small structures called ribosomes are located here – their main function is protein synthesis. *Smooth* endoplasmic reticulum does not have ribosomes adhering to it. It is active in the synthesis of plant materials such as polysaccharides and steroids.

The Golgi complex consists of stacks of membranes that sometimes connect to endoplasmic reticulum, allowing proteins to be transferred to the Golgi complex and assembled into granules before being secreted from the cell. Polysaccharides and mucus may also be assembled here before transport out of the cell. Mitochondria are the organelles where respiration occurs and energy in the form of 'adenosine triphosphate' (ATP) is produced.

The plastids mentioned above are in fact a group of organelles found in the cytoplasm of the majority of plant cells. They are surrounded by a double membrane and show a wide variety of sizes and structures. *Chromoplasts* contain pigment such as the red and yellow carotenoids – giving colour to the plant tissues. *Leucoplasts* are colourless, and are storage structures – for example, *elaioplasts* store oil (not essential oil). However, the most important plastid in the plant cell is the large, disc-shaped *chloroplast*, containing chlorophyll – the pigment essential for photosynthesis. Chlorophyll traps the energy of sunlight and enables it to be used for the manufacture of food.

Vacuoles are fluid-filled 'bubbles' in the cytoplasm, surrounded by a membrane. Vacuoles are numerous in young plant cells, but in mature cells they unite, forming a large central vacuole that contains dissolved nutrients, wastes and pigments. Crystals and oil droplets are sometimes found within a plant cell. Crystal deposits in the form of calcium salts are most common and are enclosed in a membrane. Oil droplets are not separated from the cytoplasm by a membrane – they serve as energy-rich cell fuel.

So there are considerable differences between animal and plant cells, giving rise to very different tissue types.

Plant tissues

Plant cells are organised into tissues; however, classification of these tissues is somewhat different to that of animal tissues, and is related to the function of the component cells.

Meristematic tissue is tissue where a high proportion of the cells are undergoing division. Its main function is the production of new cells, but meristematic tissue does not exhibit cell division all of the time – there will be dormant periods. 'Apical' (at the tip of roots or stems) meristems characterise the flowering plants, and occur in shoots and roots. Meristems that have differentiated tissues above and below are called 'intercalary' meristems. Cambium is a lateral meristem lying between the bark and the wood.

Epidermal tissues consist of cells in the outermost layer of plant structures – leaves, young stems and roots. Epidermis is permanent in some plant organs (such as leaves), but in some parts of mature plants (e.g. the bark of mature trees), other types of tissue may replace it. The main functions of epidermal tissue are protection and defence, strength and structure, flexibility (to allow growth), transparency (to allow the entry of light for photosynthesis), gas exchange via pores called stomata (see below), and finally the prevention of excessive water loss. A cuticle, a waterproof covering composed of cutin, may cover leaf epidermal tissue. 'Trichomes' are outgrowths of epidermal tissue: they can be simple hairs, or more complex multicellular structures. (Trichomes will be discussed in more detail when we examine plant volatile oils.) Outgrowths which arise from inner tissues, are called emergences – for example, thorns.

Photosynthetic tissue is found in the aerial (above ground) parts of plants, especially leaves, but also young stems, petioles (which join the leaf to the stem) and sepals (modified leaves which protect flowers). Photosynthetic tissue is located just beneath the epidermis in an area known as the mesophyll. Most photosynthetic tissue is classed as 'parenchyma'. Photosynthetic parenchyma consists of loosely packed cells with numerous chloroplasts and vacuoles; the cellulose cell walls are generally thin and the intercellular spaces allow for diffusion of gases.

Vascular tissue comprises the vascular system, which translocates materials around the plant. There are two distinct types of vascular tissue: *xylem* and *phloem*, which are closely associated, but quite different in both structure and function. Xylem transports water from the roots to the aerial parts in an upwards direction only. In addition to providing a means of transport, xylem also contributes support and strength to the plant, as the secondary cell walls of xylem tissue that form the outer walls of the vessels are lignified; lignin is a complex carbohydrate polymer that makes the xylem tissues more resistant to compression and tension. Phloem transports the products of photosynthesis and metabolism from the aerial parts downwards. It has two types of translocating cells – sieve tubes (found in angiosperms), and sieve cells (found in gymnosperms). Thickened cell walls may be found, but these are not lignified. Cells and fibres that are not involved in translocation are also found in phloem tissue. Phloem fibres may have very thick cell walls that may be lignified.

Strengthening tissues are necessary in all plants to help them withstand the elements and gravity. There are two main types: collenchyma and sclerenchyma. *Collenchyma* is living tissue which gives strength to the growing plant. It is often associated with parenchyma. The primary cell walls are thickened with cellulose and pectins, which are structural polysaccharides. Collenchyma is found in layers of strands underlying the epidermis in aerial parts such as petioles and stems. *Sclerenchyma* cells have thickened secondary walls – an addition to the primary wall, once the cell has stopped growing. The secondary wall is usually lignified, and the cells are frequently dead. Sclerenchyma fibres (cells) are often associated with vascular tissue, such as xylem and phloem. The fibres are arranged in bundles, which form strong and flexible strands; linen thread is made from the sclerenchyma fibres in the phloem of flax. *Sclereids* (also known as 'stone cells') are sclerenchyma cells that are not elongated in shape like the fibres, but are of irregular shapes; they may either occur singly or form accumulations and clusters. The hard shell of nuts consists of a dense sclereid coating; the granular texture of the flesh of a pear is caused by clusters of sclereids, and solitary, branched sclereids are found in the mesophyll of tea leaves.

Finally, *storage tissues* store surplus products of metabolism until these are required for growth or further metabolism. Like photosynthetic tissue, storage tissue is also classed as parenchyma, where the cells are relatively large and located close to other metabolising tissues. Sometimes mesophyll acts as a temporary storage tissue for the products of photosynthesis, but in most plants there are specialised areas for storage. For example, starch (the common storage carbohydrate in plants) is stored in insoluble grains in the cytoplasm of the cells in specialised organs such as stem and root tubers. Protein reserves may be stored as amorphous substances or crystals in the cells of seeds and tubers. Fats and oils may be stored in fruits and seeds.

The gross structure of angiosperms

Having outlined the different types of plant tissues and their functions, we can now look at how these tissues are organised into plant structures.

Roots and rhizomes

The root is the underground part of the plant. It is specialised for anchorage and absorption, and sometimes for food storage. In some cases – take, for example, the dandelion – there is a very obvious primary main root – often called the taproot. Roots may branch to form lateral roots, while in other plants the roots are very heavily branched and appear fibrous. There are also many root modifications – for example, aerial roots and climbing roots.

As anchorage and absorption are the main root functions, the vascular tissues normally form a solid, central cylinder known as a 'stele'. This is well able to withstand the tensions and pressures that roots are subject to. Root hairs are formed beyond the tip of the root. Root hairs are projections of the epidermal cells. They come into direct contact with the soil and increase the surface area available for absorption of water and dissolved nutrients from the soil.

Rhizomes are underground stems that grow horizontally. They form branches, and are a means of vegetative propagation. Some rhizomes are quite fibrous; others are fleshier. The fleshy types store reserves for the plant to over-winter and commence growth again in the spring. An example is the iris – orris root essential oil is obtained from the rhizome of the flag iris. Tubers are protuberances that form on roots or rhizomes. Their function is to carry reserve materials from the first season of growth to allow reproduction in the following season. Dahlias and potatoes are familiar examples of tubers (on roots and rhizomes, respectively).

Stems

Stems are the aerial parts of plants (often called shoots), which bear the leaves, flowers and buds. Stems contain the vascular structures that conduct water and dissolved nutrients from the roots to the aerial parts (xylem), and conduct products of photosynthesis, such as glucose, from the leaves to the areas that require them (phloem). The vascular system arrangement differs between the monocots and dicots. If seen in cross-section, the arrangement in dicots resembles a cylinder, while in monocots the vascular tissues are dispersed irregularly.

Stems are elongated and branched so that leaves can be displayed to the sunlight, and flowers are in suitable positions for pollination. There can be one main stem or trunk with side branches, or several equally prominent stems. Stem structure is complex. If observed in cross-section, a simple stem will consist of a central medulla, or pith, of inert parenchyma. This is surrounded by a starch sheath, which in turn is surrounded by vascular tissues and cambium. The outer layers comprise the cortex. The cortex consists of concentric layers of tissue – including photosynthetic tissue and collenchyma. The final layer of tissue is the epidermis and cuticle. Woody stems also have a concentric layer of phelloderm, a secondary cortex that produces a substance called phellem, or cork.

Bark is the tissue that arises to the outside of the phelloderm, and is the result of the epidermis being sloughed off. It can be fissured (for example, elm), and may be shed as scales (as in the plane tree) or as rings (typical of the birch tree). Any stem that forms continuous phellogen over its surface will also produce structures called lenticels, which allow communication, literally 'ventilation', between the internal and external environments of the plant.

Leaves

Leaves are the mains sites of photosynthesis, and their structure reflects this. The leaf is covered by epidermal tissue. A waxy layer called the cuticle (composed of a fatty substance called cutin and cellulose) protects the epidermis; this also helps reduce moisture loss via transpiration. The upper and lower epidermis is relatively impermeable; however, there are perforations called stomata (singular 'stoma') that permit interchange of gases with the atmosphere. Each stoma consists of two guard cells that lie side by side. Changes of pressure within the guard cells allow the pores to open and close.

Photosynthetic tissue is located just beneath the upper epidermis. The cells nearest the surface are elongated and appear to be closely packed, although they do have spaces between them, forming what is known as the 'palisade layer'. Palisade cells contain many chloroplasts, and being near the surface these cells receive the greatest light intensity. Just under the palisade layer is the area known as the mesophyll (literally meaning the middle of the leaf). The mesophyll is composed of the tissue known as parenchyma – the main photosynthetic tissue of the plant. Photosynthetic parenchyma consists of loosely packed cells with numerous chloroplasts and vacuoles; the cellulose cell walls are generally thin. The intercellular spaces allow for diffusion of gases; they form a continuous network that connects with the atmosphere through the stomata.

There is a wide variety of leaf forms. In a simple leaf, the lamina (the flattened blade-like part) is a single expanse, whereas in a compound leaf it is divided into several leaflets held together by stalks. Compound leaves may be *pinnate*, where the leaflets are arranged in two rows, one on each side of the midrib, or *palmate*, where four or more leaflets arise from a single point, as can be seen in the horse chestnut. There is also a vast variety of leaf shapes, such as *lanceolate* (narrow and tapering at both ends), *ovate* (egg-shaped), with the broadest part at the point of attachment, *acuminate* (gradually narrowing to a point) and *cordate* (heart-shaped, such as the violet leaf). Even the venation – the arrangement of the vascular strands – gives rise to a several possibilities. The veins may be open, where the veins branch but do not rejoin; reticulate, where the veins form a branched network; or parallel, linked by fine cross-connections.

Flowers

The flower is a reproductive organ, with seed production as is its main function. A flower is formed on the end of a stem known as a pedicel. The end of the pedicel is enlarged to form a portion called the receptacle, which contains the reproductive structures. The reproductive cells of plants are known as spores. There are two types, *microspores*, which germinate to form the male gametophytes (pollen) and *megaspores*, which develop into female gametophytes (ovules). In the angiosperms, both male and female spores are produced in flowers, and in most, both kinds are produced in the same flower. The microspores are produced in the male part of the flower – the stamen – and the megaspores in the female part – the carpel (or pistil). The stamen consists of a narrow stalk, the filament, which supports an anther. Yellow pollen grains (microspores) are formed in pollen-sacs in the anther. Most flowers contain several carpels, which are fused together. The carpel consists of a stigma, style and ovary. The stigma is adapted for the reception of pollen, and is usually carried on a stalk-like structure called the style. The ovules lie in a hollow structure called the ovary. For the production of seed, the pollen must travel from an anther to a stigma. This may happen in the same flower (self-pollination) or to a different flower (cross-pollination). Common pollinating agents are wind, insects and birds.

Pollination occurs at the stigma. Often the stigma is sticky – so that pollen will attach to it. A pollen tube grows down the style to the ovary, attracted by chemicals produced by the female sex cells in the ovary – the ovules. Fertilisation of the ovules occurs in the ovary. The fertilised ovule gives rise to the embryo, which is surrounded by nutritive tissue called the endosperm. These undergo mitotic cell division to form the seed.

Pollination, fertilisation and the development of the embryo and endosperm are all processes that involve plant hormones. In fleshy fruits, the outer and often edible layer is the 'pericarp', which is the tissue that develops from the ovary wall of the flower and surrounds the seeds.

In most cases, the organs of a flower are arranged in concentric circles, with the carpels at the centre, surrounded by the stamens. The part around this – the leaf-like structures – are known collectively as the perianth. The outer leaf-like structures are the sepals, which form the part known as the calyx, and the inner ones are the petals, which form the corolla.

As with leaves, there are many botanical terms used in flower description. The 'corolla' is the collective term for the petals. A corolla tube is formed when the margins of the individual petals are fused. A 'corona' is a crown-like outgrowth from the corolla tube; this is prominent in flowers such as daffodils.

An inflorescence is a flowering system consisting of more than one flower. It usually comprises individual flowers, bracts (modified leaves), peduncles (the main axis) and pedicels (the stalks). Inflorescences are either racemose, where the individual flowers are formed on individual pedicels on the main axis, for example lupins and broom; or cymose, where the apical tissues of the main stem and laterals lose their meristematic capacity, and differentiate into flowers. Older flowers may be found near the apex of the stem. A panicle describes a branching inflorescence, as in *Begonia* spp., and a spike is a racemose inflorescence on which the flowers are sessile (without stalks) and are borne on an elongated axis. This can be seen in *Lavandula* spp. In an umbel, the individual flower stalks arise from one point, at the tip of the stem, such as that of the African lily. The family Umbelliferae is named because of the appearance of the inflorescence typical of this family. The composite head, typical of the daisy family (the Asteraceae), and the sunflower family, consists of a cluster of many closely packed small flowers (central disc flowers surrounded by a ring of ray flowers).

Fruit

A fruit develops from the ovary wall as the seed or seeds enclosed in it mature; in other words, the ovary wall develops into the pericarp – which is familiar to us as the fleshy, edible layer of many fruits and berries. In some cases, the fruiting structure also involves parts of the perianth (the structure that protects the developing reproductive parts of the flower), the floral receptacle, bracts and bracteoles. In these cases a pseudocarp, or false fruit, is formed; examples are the strawberry and the rosehip.

Fruits are classed as succulent or dry. In succulent fruits, the mesocarp (the middle layer of the pericarp) develops into a fleshy covering. This serves as food for animals that are agents of seed dispersal. In dry fruits, this does not happen. Fruits may also be classed as 'dehiscent' or 'indehiscent'. Dehiscent fruits open in an organised manner to release the seeds; in indehiscent fruits the seeds are released only by accidental damage or decay, or the seeds germinate within the pericarp.

Seeds

The average seed is very small, although some are large – for example, the sunflower seed. Every seed contains an embryo, which develops into a seedling, and reserve substances that sustain the seedling in its early stages of growth. The reserves are located in the endosperm. Seed reserves vary – sometimes there is a high proportion of starch, for example in rice seeds, but proteins will also be present, and in some seeds, so will fats. Vitamins, minerals and hormones also form part of the reserve material. Both the embryo and the endosperm are enclosed and protected by a 'testa'. There is a distinction between seeds and one-seeded fruits, as in some of the grasses, which consist of a seed and its testa enclosed in a pericarp.

At this point it is appropriate to look at the basic principles of plant physiology.

Plant physiology
Metabolism

Metabolism can be defined as the exchange of matter and energy between an organism and its environment, and the transformation of matter and energy within the organism. The biochemical transformation of materials that occurs in the process is due to the presence of catalysts known as enzymes. A biological catalyst is a compound that enhances the rate of a biochemical reaction, without itself being used up in the process. Enzymes are protein molecules that are specialised to catalyse biological reactions. Their extremely high specificity and activity means that the living cell can function at physiological temperatures and various pH levels.

Metabolism is therefore the sum total of the enzymatic reactions that occur in a cell, organ or organism. In plants, two important processes are photosynthesis and respiration.

Anabolism and catabolism

Metabolism can be broadly divided into two processes, known as anabolism and catabolism. *Anabolism* is the phase in which small, simple molecules are built up into large, complex molecules. This process, known also as biosynthesis, is needed for growth, repair and reproduction. Anabolism requires energy. *Catabolism* is the breakdown of complex biological molecules such as sugars, amino acids, fatty acids and glycerol. These are broken down in stages, and the final stage is where simple molecules are broken down into carbon dioxide and water. Catabolism releases energy.

Specific metabolic processes are located in specific areas of the cell. For example, enzymes for the final stage of catabolism are found in the mitochondria, and protein synthesis, an anabolic process, occurs in the ribosomes. Photosynthesis occurs in the plastids called chloroplasts. There is a continuous turnover of the end products of cell metabolism.

The life of every living organism depends upon a steady supply of energy, derived from biological molecules that serve as fuel. For most living things, the primary fuel is glucose. A biological molecule, adenosine triphosphate (ATP), stores energy until it is required by the cell. Then energy may be released from the triple phosphate bonds in the molecule, leaving adenosine diphosphate (ADP).

Photosynthesis

Many metabolic processes are common to all living things. Animals depend for food on organic matter produced by other organisms: they are *heterotrophs*. Plants are *autotrophs*, which make their food or fuel from simple inorganic starting materials, using energy from sunlight. This process is known as photosynthesis. In very broad terms, photosynthesis is the process whereby energy from sunlight is converted into chemical energy. This is used to synthesise glucose, and ultimately all of the plant materials.

The process of photosynthesis occurs in plant cell organelles called chloroplasts. Chloroplasts are located in all green parts of a plant, but the main organ of photosynthesis is the leaf. A chloroplast consists of enclosures within an enclosure. Inside the outer membrane is a large space – the stroma – within which is found a membrane-bounded network of interconnected green, membranous flattened discs called thylakoids. Each has a liquid-filled centre called a lumen. Some of the thylakoids are organised into stacks called 'grana' (singular 'granum'). The thylakoids form the photosynthetic layers of the chloroplast.

Chlorophylls are photosynthetic pigments. They absorb red and blue-violet light and reflect green light, thus giving plants their characteristic green colour. They absorb light energy, and are involved in the light reactions of photosynthesis. Chlorophyll is located in the thylakoids, in the granal layers in the chloroplast.

Photosynthesis can be split into two types of biochemical reactions – light-dependent reactions and light-independent, or dark, reactions. The light reactions occur within the granal layers. The chlorophyll absorbs energy from sunlight, which initiates a chain of reactions. Water molecules are split, forming hydrogen atoms and molecular oxygen. This oxygen is given off into the atmosphere, and is the main source of atmospheric oxygen – essential for most life forms. The energy released in splitting the water molecules also forms ATP from ADP and inorganic phosphate. The ATP formed is then used in the dark reactions. The dark reactions occur in the stroma, via a cycle of reactions called the Calvin cycle. Here, carbon dioxide is 'fixed' into glucose – the primary fuel for the plant, and the starting point for synthesising more complex carbohydrates.

The photosynthetic reaction can be summarised in the following chemical equation.

$$6CO_2 + 6H_2O + \text{light energy} \rightarrow C_6H_{12}O_6 + 6O_2$$

Effectively, this means that six molecules of carbon dioxide plus six molecules of water in the presence of light energy, results in the formation of one molecule of glucose and six molecules of oxygen. The glucose formed by photosynthesis is subsequently converted into starch, cellulose and other polysaccharides.

Respiration

Cellular respiration is the oxidative breakdown of organic compounds within cells. It is a catabolic process, and occurs within the mitochondria. The process liberates energy for subsequent use in anabolic, biosynthetic reactions. Around 40 per cent of the energy liberated is stored in ATP. The process involves the absorption of molecular oxygen, with water and carbon dioxide as typical end products.

Respiration proceeds in two phases – first, glycolysis via the Embden-Myerhof-Parnas (EMP) pathway, where glucose is degraded to pyruvic acid, which then enters the tricarboxylic acid cycle (TCA cycle). The TCA cycle is found in all aerobic (oxygen-requiring) organisms. This cycle of biochemical reactions has both anabolic and catabolic functions.

Gaseous exchange

As already explained, the main function of the leaf is photosynthesis. Photosynthesis needs a substantial and steady supply of carbon dioxide, and produces an equivalent amount of oxygen. In the aerial parts of plants, gases pass through the stomata. When the internal pressure within the guard cells increases, the cells swell, blocking the stomata. Generally, stomata open when light strikes the leaf, and close at night.

Carbon dioxide diffuses through the stomata and into the air spaces in the spongy layer. It then dissolves in the film of moisture that surrounds the cells, bicarbonate ions are formed, and these diffuse into the cells where they are used in the dark reactions.

In contrast to the leaves, the gas exchange needs of roots and stems are not great. (Photosynthesis does not occur in the roots.) Oxygen enters the roots by dissolving in the film of moisture covering the root hairs, and then diffusing into the cells. Carbon dioxide produced by root cells leaves by the same route, in the reverse direction. Some older, thicker roots do not have the fine covering of root hairs. They are covered in a thickened layer of dead cells – cork. This may also be impregnated with a waxy water- and air-proof material. Here the tiny openings called lenticels allow gas exchange. In waterlogged soil there is no air between soil particles. This is why so few terrestrial plants can survive in such conditions.

Transport of water

Water enters the plant via the root hairs. It enters the xylem vessels in the vascular bundles, and moves upwards in these vessels (the tracheids), that run up through the root and stem. Water can pass laterally to supply the tissues, and continues upwards through the stems and petioles, finally reaching the leaves. At the end of the veins in the leaves, the water leaves the xylem, and enters the spongy and palisade layers. It is either used in photosynthesis, or exits the leaf in the process called transpiration. The degree of transpiration is also influenced by the degree of opening of the stomata. The surfaces of the cells in the spongy layer need to be covered in a film of water. When the stomata are open, water vapour diffuses out of the leaf. Therefore, fresh supplies must be drawn into the leaf to replace water lost by transpiration.

In dry conditions, transpiration can cause wilting. Some plants that flourish in dry conditions have developed features that will minimise water loss, such as waxy cuticles.

Transport of food substances

'Translocation' is the term used to describe the movement of food substances in the phloem tubes, the transfer of growth substances and the upward flow of dissolved salts in the transpiration stream.

Glucose is made in the leaves by photosynthesis. Much of this is converted into starch, which can be stored in the spongy layer. The starch is converted into soluble sugars, and these enter the phloem tubes. The sugars can be transported either upwards or downwards throughout the plant. Sugars ending up in the roots are reconverted into insoluble starch, and stored as a food reserve.

Excretion

Excretion is not a major problem for plants, because they have such slow rates of catabolism. Therefore metabolic wastes accumulate very slowly, and some are in fact recycled in plant metabolism. For example, water and carbon dioxide, the end products of respiration, are used in photosynthesis. In addition, plant metabolism is mainly carbohydrate metabolism – protein metabolism is less significant. The metabolic wastes produced are less toxic than the nitrogenous wastes of protein metabolism.

In terrestrial plants, wastes such as salts and organic acids are stored in the plant in the form of crystals, or in dissolved form in the central vacuoles of cells. Such wastes eventually leave the plant when the plant dies back, or the leaves are shed.

Responsiveness and coordination

In animals, the nervous and endocrine systems achieve homoeostasis – that is, maintain internal equilibrium by means of adjustments in their psychological processes, in response to changes in their internal or external environment. In the absence of nervous and endocrine systems, plants achieve their responsiveness and coordination with internal and external environments through a system of chemicals known as plant hormones.

Changes, whether from the external environment, or internal changes, act as stimuli that trigger responses. In plants, the response is usually growth of some kind. Two types of growth movements are known: nastic movements and tropisms. *Nastic* movements include the response to the stimulus of sunlight, causing certain flowers to open at sunrise. *Tropisms* include the phenomenon of plants growing in the direction of a light source; this is positive tropism. Responses to light are called 'phototropisms'. Responses to gravity are 'geotropisms'.

As well as growth movements, several developmental changes to stimuli can be observed. These include germination of seeds, stimulation of new growth, development of fruit and flowering.

Plants respond to light – its wavelength, direction and duration, gravity and temperature. These are all stimuli, and they require appropriate detectors, the plant pigments, in order that the plant can respond. Plant hormones act as chemical coordinators by initiating responses. Examples of plant hormones are *auxins*, which are substances responsible for growth, fruit development and root initiation, *cytokinins*, which regulate growth, and *dormins*, which repress gene activity and promote conditions for dormancy.

Duration

Duration relates to the pattern of growth of a plant and its lifespan. There are four categories: annuals, ephemerals, biennials and perennials.

Annuals die after less than one year. The normal life cycle is germination from seed, followed by a period of vegetative growth, flower production, seed is set, and then the whole plant enters the phase of senescence and dies. A few essential oils are produced from annuals, such as basil.

Ephemerals are annuals with a very short life, usually 6–8 weeks from germination to seed production and death. Generally, these are not aromatic plants, and are often weeds.

Biennials are plants such as (for example) carrots and parsnips, and some aromatic members of the Umbelliferae family, where the first year is devoted to the development of a body and food reserves; the plant flowers and produces seed in the second year, and then it dies.

Perennials are plants that flower every year once they have reached maturity, and their growth continues every year. Many of the aromatic plants are perennials.

The lifespan of plants varies widely – ephemerals complete their life cycle from seed to seed in months. At the other end of the scale, some of the conifers have lifespans in excess of 1000 years. The maximum recorded ages of many trees, such as *Pinus* (pine) and *Salix* (willow) species are between 100 and 500 years.

Some plants will succumb to extreme environmental conditions – frost, drought, severe competition for light, mechanical damage (e.g. from high winds), or as a consequence of insect attack or fungal or viral invasion. If death is not due to any of these factors, some internal factor will be the cause. The usual cause is the onset of senescence – the ageing process.

Woody and herbaceous plants

In woody plants the upright stem arises well above the soil and persists for many years. All woody plants are perennial and they may be trees, with one single, woody stem, or shrubs, which characteristically have several woody stems. The stems become thicker every growing season, and associated changes in the surface tissues may be seen. These include colour and texture changes resulting from cell death. Lenticels, which look like warts or pustules and are channels for the movement of gases, are formed. Bark is also formed; this increases in thickness and the texture becomes coarser over time – eventually becoming fissured, scaly or fibrous. In deciduous plants, the leaves are shed (by the process of abscission) at the end of the growing season; in evergreens they are shed after several seasons. The leaf positions will be marked by leaf scars.

Trees may take many forms, determined by the position of the branches on the main stem. The fastigiate habit is one in which the branches are almost upright and the crown of the tree is tall and narrow. The weeping habit is the opposite, where widely spread branches hang down.

In herbaceous plants the upright stem does not rise far above the soil, and it dies back after the first season. All annuals, ephemerals and biennials are herbaceous. Biennials may form tubers that act as reservoirs of foods produced in the first growing season, and be required for growth and reproduction in the second season – for example, the tubers we know as potatoes. However, most herbaceous plants are perennials. They survive winter by means of underground storage organs such as bulbs, corms, rhizomes and stem and root tubers. The foliage leaves and flowers die back in winter.

Plants and environmental stress

Many environmental factors pose threats to plant growth and development, and plants have evolved coping mechanisms to combat many of these. Stressors include heat, drought, freezing, excessive salt, predators, fungal invasion, competition for space and injury.

Overheating of leaves on a sunny day can threaten photosynthesis. Plants can stay cool by increasing their rate of transpiration, the process of losing water via the leaves. Transpiration can cool leaves to 3–5°C below the ambient temperature, thus protecting the leaf tissues from cell damage. Different plants function well in vastly different temperature ranges. For example, mid-latitude plants need moderate amounts of water and moderate temperatures of 30–40°C; xerophytes, or desert plants, require higher than normal temperatures, and are adapted for living in dry conditions; and there are also alpine, cold-loving plants.

At temperatures below zero, ice crystals can form inside the plant. This can rupture cell membranes and damage tissues. Some plants, such as the strawberry, have leaves that are colonised by bacteria (*Pseudomonas* species) containing a protein. The protein serves as a 'nucleation centre' around which the ice crystals form, leaving the leaves undamaged.

Salinity damages plants by interfering with water uptake, and sodium ions are toxic to plant cells. Some plants are more tolerant to salt – these are known as halophytes. It appears that these plants are able to exclude sodium ions at the cell membrane, while others have evolved a system of excreting salt. Examples of halophytes are the desert plant called the salt-bush, and the Mediterranean tamarisk shrub.

Most plants can suffer the loss of a few leaves and survive. Some have developed measures to deter predators, including physical deterrents such as thorns, thick cuticles, and hairy, or shiny, slippery leaves. Others produce astringent chemicals that repel insects; for example, stinging nettles squirt noxious substances directly into the cells of an invader.

The group of microorganisms known as the fungi can cause serious plant health problems. As essential oil-bearing crops are often grown in the system of monoculture (where only one species is grown in a dedicated area), fungal infection can cause serious damage to an entire crop. Some fungi are parasitic – they obtain their food from another living organism. Parasitic fungi invade a plant through open stomata, root hairs, and wounds or weak cells. The fungal spore (the reproductive structure) germinates, and mycelium (threadlike vegetative growth) penetrates the living cells. This can, if unchecked, kill the entire plant. Some plants can produce compounds in response to fungal invasion – phytoalexins that limit the spread of the fungus and protect the plant.

In the wild, plants compete for space. Many 'anti-plant' chemicals are produced by plants, which inhibit the growth of nearby plants, so that competition for nutrients and light is minimised. For example, the fruits of the black walnut tree produce juglone. This prevents the growth of any grass or herb on the ground around the tree – preserving water and minerals for the exclusive use of the tree.

Although plants can repair small wounds, massive damage can kill a plant. In cases of major injury, the plant can 'shut down'. Usually a plant will release ethylene gas in response to injury – this activates cell division at the site of the wound, accelerating tissue repair. Other substances, such as a group of chemicals known as jasmonates, can shut down active growth processes, thus conserving energy for repair processes.

Now, having looked at the basics of plant anatomy and physiology, we are in a good position to explore the subject of plant volatile oil biogenesis.

Volatile oil origins

Plant volatile oils are found in specialised cells which are located in various anatomical parts of plants. Frequently volatile oils are located in flowers, but they may also be found in leaves, bark, fruit and seeds, and also in woody parts such as stems and roots (Williams 1996).

Volatile oils are synthesised and stored in a variety of specialised glandular cells. Generally, these cells have a dense cytoplasm and a large nucleus. Their mitochondria are numerous and the endoplasmic reticulum is well developed. The large central vacuole found in many plant cells is absent. Each genotype (the genetic constitution of the plant) will determine the enzymes that catalyse the biosynthesis of the many chemicals that constitute its volatile oil. These specialised structures may be located on the surface of the plant, or within plant tissues. The secretory structures are usually family- or species-specific (Svoboda *et al.* 1996, 1999).

Single secretory cells

This is the simplest form of secretory structure – a single cell that contains the volatile oil. These single secretory cells are found in a variety of plant tissues, such as:

- leaf parenchyma, as in the scented grasses of the Poaceae family, such as lemongrass and citronella, in patchouli (of the Lamiaceae family) and bay laurel (of the Lauraceae family)
- seed coats, for example cardamom
- rhizomes, as in some members of the Zingiberaceae, such as ginger and turmeric
- roots, such as valerian and spikenard

- walls of fruits, such as pepper

- barks, including cinnamon and cassia.

Osmophores

Osmophores are found in flower tissues, their structure is distinct from adjacent cells. The osmophores found in some orchids are known as *isodiametric* cells.

Secretory cavities

These may be formed in two ways:

1. *Lysigenous glands* are formed from the breakdown of groups of cells, and each cavity is surrounded by the remnants of these cells – for example, the oil cavities in the leaves of citrus fruits, and in the leaves of the genus *Eucalyptus*. Several species of *Copaifera* (Leguminosae family) yield an oleoresin, a 'balsam' that is produced in lysigenous cavities.

2. *Schizolysigenous glands* originate from separation of intact cells, and by further enlargement due to cell breakdown. Examples are the oil cavities in the epicarp (the peel) of citrus fruits. Secretory cavities continue to increase in size; they may fill with cells, which not only synthesise, but also store the volatile oil.

Vittae

Vittae are resin canals (or ducts) or oil cavities. These form in a variety of ways and occur in fruits, seeds, and throughout the Umbelliferae, Pinaceae, Asteraceae and Cupressaceae families. In the Pinaceae and Cupressaceae they are known as resin ducts. Myrrh, benzoin and frankincense resins are formed in elongated secretory cavities or ducts located in the bark of small shrubby trees.

Schizogenous glands are enlarged intercellular spaces known as lumina and lacuna, enclosed by intact cells which have separated during development, and are lined with specialised secretory cells. These cavities join up to form ducts, such as the resin canals found in conifers. The vittae in the xylem can reach 10 cm in length and each needle-like leaf can have up to seven ducts.

All members of the Umbelliferae family have secretory ducts – these can be found in the fruits of caraway, aniseed, fennel, dill and coriander. In the case of parsley and coriander, the ducts extend from the roots, stems and leaves. This is why, for example, in the preparation of some recipes, finely chopped coriander stems are added during the cooking process and the more delicate leaves at the very end in order to retain their attractive appearance and fresh aroma.

Glandular trichomes

A trichome is an outgrowth of an epidermal cell. Trichomes vary in form and function – for example, root hairs increase the surface area of the root for water absorption. Glandular trichomes are modifications of epidermal hairs located in leaves, stems and calyces. They are multicellular structures where volatile oils are synthesised and accumulate. Glandular trichomes are widespread in the Lamiaceae family.

The secretory cells are either attached to a basal cell of the epidermis, or to a short 'stem' arising from the epidermis, and a cuticle encloses them. This effectively protects the trichome, and allows the volatile oil to accumulate within the structure before diffusing through the cuticle. There are genetic differences, and every species will have characteristic differences in the structure of their trichomes and in the number of the trichomes per leaf.

For example, both peltate and capitate glands can be found in clary sage. *Peltate* glandular hairs consist of one basal cell, a stalk and a multicellular head of secretory cells. *Capitate* glandular hairs consist of one basal cell, a stalk and one or two secretory head cells. There is chemical variation in the volatile oils found in these glands, even on the same plant and part (corolla, calyx and leaves), giving rise to the chemical variation in, for example, clary sage oils (Schmiderer *et al.* 2008).

Epidermal cells

Secretory cells also occur in flower petals – for example in rose and jasmine. As in these cases glandular hairs and trichomes are not present, the volatile oil diffuses through the epidermal cells and the cuticle to reach the atmosphere (Svoboda, Svoboda and Syred 2000).

The biosynthesis of plant volatile oils

A 'biosynthetic pathway' is a series of enzymatic reactions in which more complex molecules are built from simpler ones (anabolism). Plant volatile oils are composed of some of these complex molecules, and three main stages of their biosynthesis can be identified:

1. The first stage is the manufacture of simple organic molecules from inorganic molecules, as in the formation of glucose from carbon dioxide and water during photosynthesis. Glucose is a hexose – a sugar molecule that consists of six carbon atoms.

2. The second stage is where these simple molecules are converted to molecules that could be likened to building blocks – for example, the conversion

of hexoses (six-carbon sugars) to an intermediate compound known as pyruvate.

3. The third stage is the synthesis of macromolecules from the intermediate building blocks. In this stage we have the formation of aromatic molecules, fatty acids, amino acids (which are the subunits of proteins), nucleic acids and alkaloids, terpenoids and steroids.

The most important biosynthetic pathways in plants are:

- the *Calvin cycle* – formation of hexoses

- the *shikimic acid pathway (phenyl propanoic pathway)* – formation of aromatic compounds (here we mean compounds that contain a benzene ring structure, rather than just scented compounds)

- the *Kreb's cycle* (TCA cycle, citric acid cycle) – formation of amino acids

- the *acetate–malonate pathway* – formation of fatty acids

- the *acetate–mevalonate pathway* – formation of terpenoids and steroids.

Volatile oils are chemically complex; however, the constituents generally fall into two categories – the terpenoids and the phenyl propanoids that are formed in the acetate–mevalonate pathway and the shikimic acid pathway, respectively (Evans 1989).

Terpenes and their derivatives, the terpenoids

The name of this group of compounds comes from the word 'turpentine'. The terpenes, and their oxygenated derivatives, the terpenoids, are all based on the isoprene unit. This is a molecular subunit that consists of five carbon atoms, and molecules that are built from this are known as isoprenoids. Their carbon frameworks are combinations of short chains of carbon atoms attached to *cyclic, acyclic* and *bicyclic* carbon structures. Most of the terpenes and terpenoids found in essential oils are either *monoterpenes*, with ten carbon atoms in each molecule (e.g. the pinenes in pine oils and limonene in many citrus oils), or *sesquiterpenes*, with fifteen carbon atoms in each molecule (e.g. zingiberene in ginger oil).

The terpenoids are the oxygenated derivatives of both monoterpenes and sesquiterpenes, where the molecules have oxygen-containing functional groupings. This large group of essential oil constituents includes:

- monoterpene alcohols (such as linalool, found in lavender essential oil) and sesquiterpene alcohols (such as the santalols found in sandalwood oils)

- aldehydes (such as neral and geranial, found in neroli and geranium essential oils)

- ketones (such as menthone in peppermint oil)

- esters (such as linalyl acetate in lavender, clary sage and bergamot oils)

- oxides (such as 1,8-cineole in many *Eucalyptus* oils).

The terpenes and their derivatives are widely distributed in nature, and they dominate essential oil chemistry. The majority of essential oils contain a mixture of related constituents from this group.

Phenylpropanoids

The phenylpropanoids are formed via a distinct pathway called the *shikimic acid* or *phenyl propanoic acid pathway*. They are distinguished by the presence of a phenyl (aromatic) ring in their molecular structure. They are often called 'phenolics'. Although they are less common than the terpenes, they are also significant components of essential oils (Evans 1989). As with the terpenes, we also find oxygenated derivatives, the functional groups giving rise to classes of constituents such as:

- phenols (such as eugenol in clove bud oil)

- aromatic alcohols (such as phenylethanol in rose absolute)

- aromatic aldehydes (such as cinnamaldehyde in cinnamon leaf oil)

- ethers (such as *trans*-anethole in sweet fennel oil).

A comprehensive summary of essential oil constituents can be found in Appendix A.

However, essential oil biosynthesis is influenced by internal factors such as genetics, growth hormones and growth regulators, which influence plant development, including the development of secretory structures (Sharafzadeh and Zare 2011). External factors also have an impact on biosynthesis, including environmental, geographical and cultivation factors, but also less obvious influences such as soil microbial ecology, which has been shown to play a role in the formation of essential oils in roots and rhizomes (Alifono *et al.* 2010).

Only a relatively small proportion of plants produce volatile oils. These oils are produced for sound biological reasons, because in nature, energy-requiring processes are never wasted. So why do some plants produce volatile oils?

The biological role of plant volatile oils

First, we must explore the basic concepts of primary and secondary metabolism. *Primary metabolites* are so called because they are required for plant growth and development. They are formed from the first product of photosynthesis, glucose. Glucose is used in respiration and for energy-requiring activities. Glucose polymerises to form cellulose, required to form cell walls. Glucose can combine with minerals that have been absorbed via the water uptake by the roots, to form amino acids, which in turn polymerise to form proteins. Any excess glucose is stored as starch. Other examples of primary metabolites are glycerol, fatty acids (which form lipids) and nucleotides.

Secondary metabolites, by contrast, are not involved in growth and development. They are costly to produce in terms of resources and energy. Therefore, secondary metabolites should play an important biological role. However, sometimes the exact role is not known. Examples of plant secondary metabolites include the terpenes and phenylpropanoids – the common volatile oil constituents. Other examples are phenolics (such as tannins) and alkaloids (such as atropine, cocaine, nicotine, strychnine and morphine) (Evans 1989).

There is little doubt that plant volatile oils play important roles in the interactions between some plants and the environment.

Some essential oil components are the same as insect pheromones. Examples include verbenol and verbenone, which are aggregation (trail) signals for the bark beetle; β-farnesene, which is an alarm signal for aphids; while nepetalactol and nepetalactone (catmint) are sex pheromones that elicit mating in aphids; and citral and β-ocimene are sex pheromones for butterflies (Müller and Buchbauer 2011).

However, the main biological reasons for plant volatile oil production are defence and survival. Some of the possibilities are:

- Prevention of damage by herbivores; for example, snails have a marked distaste for phenolic compounds (Shawe 1996).

- Prevention of growth of plant pathogens. Phytoalexins are antifungal chemicals produced in response to the presence of pathogenic fungi. For example, the phenolic compound pisatin accumulates in the tissues of the pea plant, and the sweet potato resists attack by a fungus by producing the terpenoid compound ipomeamarone. It is possible that some microbial pathogens, including fungi, bacteria and viruses, may be inhibited by the presence of volatile plant oils. *In vitro*, many volatile oils exhibit antimicrobial activity – there is speculation as to whether this is a major function *in vivo* (Shawe 1996).

- Prevention of damage by insect pests. Some plants produce volatile oils that appear to repel insects. For example, pulegone, a constituent of some *Mentha* species, is repellent, as are several other widely distributed essential oil constituents. *Beta*-pinene and bornyl acetate are two terpenoids found in the Douglas fir; they are thought to impart resistance to attack by the larvae of the western spruce budworm. Limonene, a monoterpene abundant in the volatile oil in the oil glands in *Citrus* species may deter leaf-cutting ants. Pests such as aphids can cause a lot of damage; however, some plants produce an odour that is either repulsive to the pest, or attractive to another insect that will prey on the pest. Methyl salicylate, a phenylpropanoid found in wintergreen essential oil, may do this. This has been termed the 'SOS signal' (Day 1996).

- Chemical signals. When a plant is under attack, volatile oil production and its subsequent release into the environment increase. For example, if a caterpillar starts to eat a leaf, the plant responds to the crushing and tearing by releasing volatile chemicals. In such cases these are called 'semiochemicals' (sign chemicals), which will either attract more predators ('lunch is here'), or attract parasites that inadvertently come to the plant's defence ('SOS'), as they are in pursuit of their own menu – caterpillar... (Goode 2000).

- Reproduction, which ensures survival of a species. Pollination is the method of reproduction in plants and often relies on insects or animals. Volatile oils may be produced in flowers to attract insect pollinators, such as bees, beetles and moths. Usually the volatile oils are released at a time when their natural pollinator will detect them. This will vary in terms of the time of day and the season, according to the natural cycles of the pollinator, which could be night flying insects, or insects that are abundant on warm days. Animals that serve pollination, or as vectors for seed dispersal, will also be attracted. Birds are attracted by colour rather than odour (Shawe 1996).

- Allelopathy, a type of competition between plants. Plants must compete with each other in the environment for resources such as light, nutrients, water and space. Many of the secondary metabolites, including some terpenes, can inhibit the growth of other species in the immediate vicinity. For example, some species of thyme produce phenolic compounds that inhibit the germination of some species of grass. In some *Pinus* species, volatile compounds are produced which inhibit the development of their own seedlings. This is called 'autoallelopathy'. Another example of allelopathy can be seen in arid or semi-arid habitats, where aromatic plants release terpene-containing volatile oils from their leaves. For example, *Artemisia* species and *Salvia* species release substances such as camphor, which inhibit the germination of other herbaceous plants (Evans 1989).

- Reduction of transpiration. A film of volatile oil on a leaf surface may reduce water loss through transpiration; either by blocking the stomata or by increasing the density of the boundary layer at the leaf surface. This helps the plant survive in hot, dry conditions by conserving water (Shawe 1996).

In this chapter we looked at the plant kingdom – focusing on taxonomy, plant anatomy and physiology, and how and why volatile oils are formed in aromatic plants. These are useful underpinnings that help us to understand the nature of essential oils. In the following chapters, essential oils will be explored in the context of their botanical families and introduced by their botanical names. As will already have become apparent, this is the natural way to do this, as essential oils derived from particular botanical families often share characteristics, as do their plant counterparts.

Significant aromatic plant families and their essential oil and absolute products are summarised in Table 7.3.

Chapter 8 will explore essential oils from the Angiospermae in the alphabetical order of their botanical families, and in Chapter 9 the oils of the Gymnospermae will be addressed. Absolutes and resinoids can be found in Chapter 10. The botanical names are used throughout, but a quick reference to the essential oils according to their common names is supplied in Appendix E.

Table 7.3 Plant families and their essential oils

Family	Essential oils, absolutes and resinoids
Angiospermae	
Amaryllidaceae	Narcissus abs., tuberose abs.
Apocynaceae	Frangipani abs.
Annonaceae	Cananga, ylang ylang
Asteraceae	Chamomile (Roman, German, Moroccan), helichrysum (immortelle), mugwort, sweet inula, tagetes, tarragon, wormwood, yarrow
Burseraceae	Elemi, frankincense, myrrh, oponapax
Cannabaceae	Cannabis e.o.
Caryophyllaceae	Carnation abs.
Ericaceae	Wintergreen
Fabaceae	Genet abs.
Geraniaceae	Geranium (*Pelargonium* spp.), zdravetz
Illiciaceae, aka Magnoliaceae	Star anise, champaca abs.
Lamiaceae	Basil, clary sage, hyssop, lavender (true and spike), lavandin, melissa, oregano, patchouli, pennyroyal, peppermint, rosemary, sage spp., spearmint, sweet marjoram, thyme spp.

cont.

Family	Essential oils, absolutes and resinoids
Lauraceae	Camphor, cassia, cinnamon (bark and leaf), laurel (bay laurel), may chang, ravintsara, rosewood
Liliaceae	Hyacinth abs.
Magnoliaceae, aka Illiaceaea	Champaca abs., star anise
Mimosaceae	Cassie abs., mimosa abs.
Myristicaceae	Nutmeg
Myrtaceae	Clove bud, cajuput, *Eucalyptus* spp., lemon-scented tea tree, manuka, myrtle, niaouli, pimento (West Indian bay), tea tree
Nelumbonaceae	Pink and white lotus abs.
Oleaceae	Jasmine abs., osmanthus abs.
Orchidaceae	Vanilla abs.
Pandanaceae	Kewda abs.
Piperaceae	Black pepper
Poaceae	Citronella, lemongrass, palmarosa, vetivert
Rosaceae	Rose abs., rose e.o.
Rutaceae	Bergamot, bitter orange, lemon, grapefruit, lime, mandarin, neroli, orange blossom abs., petitgrain, sweet orange
Salicaceae	Poplar bud abs.
Santalaceae	Sandalwood spp.
Styraceae	Benzoin resinoid
Tiliaceae	Linden blossom abs.
Umbelliferae	Angelica, aniseed, caraway, coriander, cumin, dill, galbanum, lovage, parsley seed, sweet fennel
Valerianaceae	Spikenard
Violaceae	Violet leaf and flower abs.
Zingiberaceae	Cardamom, ginger, plai, white ginger lily abs.
Gymnospermae	**Order Coniferales**
Cupressaceae (dicots)	Cedar (Mexican, Virginian), cypress, juniper, thuja
Pinaceae (dicots)	Cedar (Atlas, Himalayan), pine spp., spruce spp., Douglas fir

Essential Oils of the Angiospermae

FAMILY ANNONACEAE

The Annonaceae family comprises tropical species and belongs to the order Magnoliales. The Annonaceae has around 120 genera, but only one genus, *Cananga*, is of significance from the essential oil perspective. *Cananga* probably originated in Southeast Asia, although now it has become naturalised in many other parts of the Pacific basin. It is particularly common in the Philippines, but it has been introduced into many other parts of the world as an essential oil-producing plant – with oil production commencing in the mid-nineteenth century. The main oil producing areas are now Indonesia and Madagascar, and the producers are often small companies. There are two distinct types of essential oil, known as cananga and ylang ylang, and both of these are now produced in Java. However, prior to this, when *Cananga* was introduced to the Comoro Islands, Réunion was renowned for its ylang ylang (Weiss 1997).

GENUS CANANGA

CANANGA ODORATA VAR. GENUINA – YLANG YLANG

C. odorata var. *genuina* is a tall tropical tree that produces numerous yellow-green, highly scented flowers. The name 'ylang ylang' means 'flower of flowers', although the words are derived from a Philippine phrase that describes how the flowers flutter in the breeze. The intense floral, narcotic, sensual fragrance of the flowers was used to perfume the bedlinen of newly married couples in traditional Indonesian culture. Ylang ylang has long been considered an aphrodisiac – its scent is considered to be very relaxing yet highly euphoric. The fresh flowers also have value, and are sold for personal and domestic adornment and to scent fabrics (Weiss 1997).

Fractional steam distillation of the flowers produces four or five grades of essential oil; each fraction has a different chemical composition and odour. For more detail, see Weiss (1997). Sometimes suppliers may offer 'complete' oil, but according to Weiss (1997), this may well be cananga or adulterated third grade oil. An absolute is also produced; this is intensely sweet and floral and is used in high-class perfumes and toiletries.

In aromatherapy, it is the fraction known as 'extra' that is most commonly used. However, this is not to say that the other fractions do not have therapeutic applications – they simply have not been investigated to the same extent. Ylang ylang extra is a pale yellow mobile liquid, with a sweet, persistent, floral odour that has a 'creamy' top note. Its chemical composition is very variable; however it will contain linalool (19%), terpenoid and aromatic esters, including geranyl acetate, benzyl acetate and methyl salicylate (giving a slightly medicinal note), which collectively will account for up to 64 per cent, phenyl methyl ethers (15%), sesquiterpenes such as farnesene and caryophyllene, and phenols, including eugenol. The extra has higher levels of p-cresyl methyl ether, methyl benzoate, linalool, methyl acetate and geranyl acetate than the other grades (Weiss 1997). Some major components of the various oils are shown in Table 8.1.

Table 8.1 Comparison of major components (%w/v) of ylang ylang and cananga oils (adapted from Weiss 1997)

Component	Extra	Grade 1	Grade 2	Grade 3	Cananga
Linalool	10.3	5.5	3.2	2.0	1.7
Benzyl acetate	12.6	4.2	1.2	0.5	Negligible
β-caryophyllene	6.8	11.5	12.8	16.3	37.0
Farnesene	18.0	16.8	17.0	21.0	12.2
δ-cadinene	8.9	15.1	20.4	16.3	5.4
Benzyl benzoate	4.3	8.5	9.7	5.3	2.9
α-caryophyllene	3.1	4.2	4.1	8.8	10.5

In indigenous medicine, the ylang ylang is mixed with coconut oil for the treatment of skin problems and in skin care products (Weiss 1997). In aromatherapy its scent is used to relax and uplift, and help the individual to connect with their senses and the physical realm.

Ylang ylang is often credited with 'balancing', sedative and calming properties – possibly due to the ester and linalool content (Bowles 2003), and is widely used to combat stress, tension, anxiety, tachycardia and insomnia (Price and Price 2007). A study conducted by Hongratanaworakit and Buchbauer (2004) that focused on the physiological effects and subjective feelings following exposure to the aroma, revealed a 'harmonising' effect, where blood pressure and heart rate decreased whilst attentiveness and alertness were increased. However, Moss et al. (2006), in a study that focused on the cognitive effects of aroma, demonstrated that ylang ylang could significantly increase calmness, but decrease alertness, reaction times, and impair memory and processing speed. A further study conducted by Hongratanaworakit and Buchbauer (2006) investigated the effects of ylang ylang via transdermal absorption, and again it was demonstrated that there was a significant decrease of blood pressure and increase in skin temperature in the ylang ylang group compared with the placebo. The ylang ylang group also reported feeling more calm and relaxed than the control group.

The essential oil also has antispasmodic properties, which may help with cramp and colic (Price and Price 2007) and muscular tension. Echoing its traditional uses, it is also of use in skin care – especially helping with oily skin/acne. For some uses in aromatherapy, please see Table 8.2.

Table 8.2 Ylang ylang essential oil in aromatherapy

System	Ylang ylang with
Nervous (anxiety, stress, tension, frustration, insomnia)	Frankincense, lavender, sandalwood, bergamot
Musculoskeletal and digestive (cramp)	Juniperberry, grapefruit, black pepper, ginger, clove bud, cinnamon leaf, West Indian bay
Integumentary	Sandalwood, palmarosa, lavender, bergamot

Cananga odorata var. *macrophylla* produces cananga oil. The cananga tree is a fast-growing, medium to tall evergreen tree with a single trunk. The wood has no commercial value. Its numerous leaves are thin, oblong and alternate, and its clusters of flowers are large, yellow-green and heavily scented. They consist of three sepals and six lanceolate petals about 4–8 cm in length. The flowers are often borne throughout the year.

The oil is steam distilled from the flowers, and contains over 30 per cent alcohols and esters at about 15 per cent (Price and Price 2007) – but there is wide variation and monoterpenes, sesquiterpenes, phenols, aldehydes and ketones are also present. The oil is a slightly viscous liquid that varies in colour from yellow to orange to greenish, darkening on exposure to light and oxygen. Its odour is reminiscent of ylang ylang, only heavier and more harsh, but with its sweet floral character and a woody/leathery note (Weiss 1997). However, Lawless (1996) describes cananga oil as a greenish-yellow viscous liquid with a sweet, floral and heavy scent, and classifies it as a base note.

C. latifolia also produces an essential oil; however, this has no commercial importance, and as a consequence it is generally not available for aromatherapeutic use.

FAMILY ASTERACEAE

This family is also called the Compositae, and is often referred to as the 'daisy' family. Essential oils obtained from this family are quite diverse; however, many contain fairly large amounts of a group of chemicals known as sesquiterpenoid lactones. Lactones are frequently implicated in allergic skin reactions – Bowles (2003) comments that plants from this family, such as chrysanthemums, are frequently responsible for allergic contact dermatitis in the floristry profession. However, members of this family produce several important essential oils.

GENUS ACHILLEA

ACHILLEA MILLEFOLIUM – YARROW

Yarrow is a large perennial herb with numerous aromatic, dark green, finely dissected leaves, giving a lacy, feathery appearance – the species name *millefolium* means 'a thousand leaves'. The flowers are small and white, tinged with pink or purple, and are borne on numerous flower heads. The essential oil is obtained from the dried flowering herb, and is a dark blue or greenish olive, mobile liquid (Lawless 1992). There are several chemotypes (Tisserand and Balacs 1995), the camphor and chamazulene types being the most commonly available. Its odour is herbaceous with a camphoraceous note – but this depends on the chemical composition.

According to Tisserand and Balacs (1995), notable constituents are camphor (a neurotoxic ketone) at 10–20 per cent, 1,8-cineole at 14 per cent and borneol at 9 per cent. However, Lawless states that the dominant constituent is 'azulene' at up to 51 per cent. This is presumably chamazulene, the inky-blue sesquiterpene with powerful anti-inflammatory properties (see also German chamomile). The sabinene, 1,8-cineole and chamazulene chemotypes do not present a hazard, but the camphor chemotype should be used with caution and is contraindicated via the oral route in pregnancy, epilepsy and fever (Tisserand and Balacs 1995).

The genus *Achillea* is named after the Greek Achilles, who is said to have been the first to use yarrow as an herb for healing wounds. This gives an insight into the aromatherapeutic uses of the essential oil. Yarrow is noted for its anti-inflammatory, anticatarrhal, decongestant, vasodilatory and cicatrisant qualities (Price and Price 2007). Tisserand and Balacs (1995) suggest that it can be used as a substitute for German chamomile. See Table 8.3 for some aromatherapeutic uses of yarrow.

Table 8.3 Yarrow essential oil in aromatherapy

System	Yarrow with
Musculoskeletal (pain, inflammation)	Lavender, spike lavender, Scots pine, juniperberry, sweet marjoram, grapefruit, black pepper
Cardiovascular (varicose veins and ulcers)	Lavender, cypress, patchouli, lemon, geranium

Genus Anthemis

Anthemis nobilis (also known as Chaemamelum nobile) – Roman chamomile

Roman chamomile essential oil is obtained from the daisy-like flowers of this creeping perennial. Roman chamomile was a staple of English herb gardens, and was even planted as ground cover in the form of a chamomile lawn, before grass was used for this purpose. It is known to gardeners as a 'companion plant', and the 'plant's physician' because it is protective of the health of other plants, even helping to prevent the 'damping off' of seedlings in greenhouses (Gordon 1980).

Roman chamomile essential oil has a distinctive pale blue colour and a strong, fruity, apple-like, herbaceous odour. The scent is intense and diffusive, so it is best used in low concentrations. The main geographical sources for the oil are Hungary, France and Italy (Lawless 1992). According to Bowles (2003) a typical Japanese essential oil contains isobutyl angelate at 35.9 per cent, 2-methyl butyl angelate at 15.3 per cent and methallyl angelate at 8.7 per cent. Roman chamomile essential oil is usually dominated by such non-terpenoid esters derived from short chain parent alcohols. Bowles (2003) cites Pénoël and Franchomme (1990), who state that such esters are especially oriented towards the head and the psyche, with cephalic and psychotropic characteristics. Additionally, isobutyl angelate is hailed as 'one of the grand antispasmodics of the pharmacopoeia' (Pénoël and Franchomme 1990, cited in Bowles 2003).

In aromatherapy Roman chamomile is widely used as an anti-inflammatory, antispasmodic, calming essential oil (Price and Price 2007). Moss *et al.* (2006) investigated its effects on mood and cognition. Their study showed that the odour of Roman chamomile had a calming, sedating effect, and reduced subjective alertness. However, as could be expected, the effects were influenced by induced expectancy.

An animal study by Seol *et al.* (2010) did not suggest that Roman chamomile had antidepressant effects (for more information, see *Salvia sclarea*, clary sage). However, it is interesting to speculate that the mode of administration influenced the effects experienced and observed. The Seol *et al.* study involved injection of diluted oils, and also inhalation. For some uses of Roman chamomile, see Table 8.4.

Table 8.4 Roman chamomile essential oil in aromatherapy

System	Roman chamomile with
Musculoskeletal (tension, pain, inflammation)	Lavender, ginger, sweet marjoram, lemongrass, bergamot
Nervous (insomnia;* stress, tension; headache/migraine**)	Lavender,* neroli;* clary sage, geranium, jasmine, citrus oils. For headache, peppermint**
Integumentary (eczema, inflammation, wound healing)	Lavender, helichrysum, geranium, yarrow, vetivert, patchouli, sandalwood, bergamot, rose

*Asterisks indicate a particular relationship between the condition and the oil (or oils) thus identified.

GENUS ARTEMISIA

ARTEMISIA ABSINTHIUM – WORMWOOD

Absinthium oil is obtained from the leaves and flowering tops of this large, hardy perennial. Although the herb has a long tradition of medicinal use, its essential oil is highly toxic and neurotoxic, and it is not used in aromatherapy (Tisserand and Balacs 1995). It contains high levels of thujone, generally 34–71 per cent. The herb itself is bitter, and it was used in traditional herbal medicine as a vermifuge – giving rise to the name 'wormwood'.

It is perhaps best known as an ingredient, along with anise, in the highly intoxicating and ultimately health-damaging greenish liqueur known as absinthe. This reached its height of popularity with the artists, writers and actors (including Henri Toulouse Lautrec and Vincent van Gogh) who frequented Parisian cafés in the late nineteenth century. Absinthe was fondly referred to as *la fée verte*, 'the green fairy', and the cafés introduced the concept of *l'heure vert* – the green hour. A French doctor who was interested in the digestive properties of herbs invented absinthe. Some of its drinkers believed that it also aided sexual prowess and heightened artistic awareness, so its popularity grew, despite the potential effects of depression, psychosis and madness. It has been noticed that thujone shares structural similarities with tetrahydrocannabinol (THC), found in cannabis, so it may have the potential for psychotropic effects (Turner 1993). In the same vein Balacs (1998/1999) commented on a report in the *New England Journal of Medicine* concerning a case of wormwood poisoning. He suggested that α-thujone in the essential oil could interact with the same receptors in the brain as δ-9-tetrahydrocannabinol. However, a recent study of authentic pre-1915 absinthe, post-ban 1915–1988 absinthe and modern commercial absinthe, suggested that 'absinthism' was due to the excessive use of alcohol, not its thujone content, which was in this case reported as β-thujone (Lachenmeier 2008, cited in Dobetsberger and Buchbauer 2011).

Meanwhile, Lachenmeier's 2010 paper revealed current thinking about the dose-dependent neurotoxic properties of thujone/wormwood, suggesting that seizures were due to GABA type A receptor modulation. He notes that studies have revealed that wormwood may have potential medical uses, such as the treatment of Crohn's disease, and that it might even have neuroprotective effects that could be harnessed in the treatment of strokes. It is emphasised, however, that a thorough risk–benefit analysis should be conducted if the therapeutic dose were to exceed the current threshold dose set by the European Medicines Agency.

ARTEMISIA DRACUNCULUS — TARRAGON

The name of this perennial herb is derived from Latin *dracunculus*, meaning 'little dragon', possibly because its roots are coiled like little snakes. Although it remains a popular culinary herb for many meat and fish dishes, and has a long tradition as a 'cooling' medicinal herb, the essential oil of tarragon is not widely used in aromatherapy. This is due to the presence of large amounts of estragole (also known as methyl chavicol), leading Tisserand and Balacs (1995) to advise that it should not be used in aromatherapy. However, Schnaubelt (1995) suggests that is it one of the best antispasmodic essential oils, which may be used with caution. For more information about estragole, see the profile of basil essential oil. In the right circumstances, and if used with care, tarragon can be useful for pain, spasm, and as a respiratory decongestant– which is one of its uses in herbal medicine.

ARTEMISIA VULGARIS (MUGWORT) AND ARTEMISIA ARBORESCENS (GREAT MUGWORT)

Mugwort essential oils are obtained from the leaves and flowering tops of these large perennial herbs. Like *A. absinthium*, the mugworts do have a tradition of medicinal use, but contain large amounts of thujone, rendering their essential oils toxic and neurotoxic (Lawless 1992; Tisserand and Balacs 1995). There are many other species of *Artemisia* that yield essential oils, all containing high levels of thujone, some containing 'artemisia ketone', and most are deemed unsuitable for aromatherapeutic use.

GENUS HELICHRYSUM

HELICHRYSUM ANGUSTIFOLIUM (H. ITALICUM) AND H. ORIENTALE (ESSENTIAL OIL), H. STOECHAS (ABSOLUTE) – IMMORTELLE, EVERLASTING

The essential oil from *Helichrysum angustifolium* (*H. italicum*) is the one used in aromatherapy practice. It is obtained from flowering tops of this large aromatic herb, and is a pale yellow, mobile liquid with a powerful, rich, sweet, honey-like odour. Chemically, it is dominated by α-pinene (21.7%), γ-curcumene (10.4%) and italidiones (diketones) at 8 per cent.

Italidiones, especially those found in *H. italicum* ssp. *serotinum*, are reputed to have anti-haematomal properties (Bowles 2003), and so are often used for bruises and trauma to the superficial soft tissues. Pénoël (1991), cited in Price and Price (2007), states that helichrysum is sometimes called the 'super arnica of aromatherapy'. Homoeopathic arnica is widely used for the healing of trauma.

Voinchet and Giraud-Robert (2007) investigated the therapeutic effects and potential clinical applications of *Helichrysum italicum* var. *serotinum* and a macerated oil of musk rose (*Rosa rubiginosa*) after cosmetic and reconstructive surgery. The objectives of reducing inflammation, oedema and bruising were all achieved, and more than half of the participants were able to go home in five rather than the usual 12 days. They attribute many of these effects to the italidiones, and commented that neryl acetate, a principal constituent, contributed to a pain-relieving effect. They commented on the 'particularly interesting' antistaphylococcal and antistreptococcal activity of the oil, which reduced infection by these commensal micro-organisms. Cicatrisant effects were also observed, the post-operative scarring was diminished, and it was thought that the musk rose oil helped to prevent keloid scar formation.

Helichrysum was also included in a study investigating the antimicrobial activities of essential oils whose principal constituents have floral-rosy aromas (Jirovetz *et al.* 2006). All of the oils and most of the principal aroma compounds showed medium to high antimicrobial activities against both Gram-positive (including *Staphylococcus aureus* and *Enterococcus faecalis*) and Gram-negative (including *Escherichia coli* and *Salmonella* spp.) bacteria and also the yeast *Candida albicans*.

Therefore helichrysum does indeed have some fairly unusual and very useful therapeutic properties. It is also thought to be anti-allergenic – so could be of help in cases of asthma, hay fever or eczema. Its cicatrisant properties suggest that it can be used to aid skin regeneration and help with wound healing. Finally, it is a useful phlebotonic – Price and Price (2007) claim that it is indicated for couperose skin (red veins), haematoma (even old haematomas), thrombosis and the prevention of bruises. Please refer to Table 8.5 for some aromatherapeutic prescriptions.

Table 8.5 Helichrysum essential oil in aromatherapy

System	Helichrysum with
Integumentary (eczema, inflammation, wound healing) Trauma	Lavender, Roman chamomile, geranium, yarrow, vetivert, patchouli, sandalwood, cypress, rose Can be used neat or diluted at 10–50% (Price and Price 2007)
Immune (allergic responses)	Rose, sandalwood, German chamomile
Musculoskeletal (arthritic conditions)	Wintergreen, sweet birch

Genus Inula

Inula graveolens – sweet inula

Sweet inula essential oil is obtained from *I. graveolens*, elecampane essential oil is obtained from *I. helenium*. Both essential oils are obtained from the dried roots and rhizomes of the perennial daisy-like plants, and both are characterised by the presence of chemicals known as lactones.

Elecampane has a long tradition of use as a medicinal and a cosmetic herb. It is named after the renowned beauty Helen of Troy who, according to legend, was in possession of the herb when Paris separated her from her husband Menelaus. However, elecampane essential oil is not used in aromatherapy because of the high risk of causing severe sensitisation (Lawless 1992; Tisserand and Balacs 1995) due to the large amounts of a sesquiterpenoid lactone known as alantolactone (52%) and *iso*-alantolactone (33%).

Sweet inula essential oil is a deep green essential oil (Lawless 1992) that does not have the sensitisation capacity of elecampane. Schnaubelt (1995) writes that it contains 50 per cent bornyl acetate as well as traces of the sesquiterpene lactones; while Tisserand and Balacs (1995) state that it contains mainly bornyl acetate and camphene. Sweet inula is mainly used in French aromatherapy, probably due to the influence of Franchomme, cited in Lawless (1992) and Schnaubelt (1995), who states that it is the strongest mucolytic to be found in aromatherapy. This effect can be found even below the odour threshold. Schnaubelt (1995) recommends that it is administered by diffusion, and is invaluable for all bronchitis and catarrhal conditions of the throat/nose, and also spasmodic conditions affecting the respiratory tract.

GENUS MATRICARIA

MATRICARIA RECUTITA – GERMAN CHAMOMILE

German chamomile is an annual herb, and like its Roman relative, it too has an herbal tradition. The herb is also known as 'scented mayweed', and its generic name *Matricaria* comes from the Latin '*matrix*' (womb) or '*mater*' (mother), because of its tradition of use as a uterine tonic.

The essential oil is obtained from its daisy-like flowers. It is a deep, inky-blue liquid – the colour is due to a constituent called chamazulene, formed during the distillation process from the parent chemical, matricine, which is found in the flowers. German chamomile oil is characterised by the presence of chamazulene, farnesene (both sesquiterpenes) and α-bisabolol (a sesquiterpene alcohol). There are several chemotypes, so there is a wide variation in the proportions of these. Price and Price (2007) indicate that chamazulene ranges from 1–35 per cent; Bowles (2003) gives a chamazulene content of 17 per cent. The α-bisabolol content ranges from 2–67 per cent (Price and Price 2007), while the farnesene content (*trans*-α-farnesene) is in the region of 27 per cent. Bisabolol oxides (A and B) are also significant. Price and Price (2007) state that the dominant α-bisabolol oxide A content can range from 0–55 per cent. This is a case where many of the therapeutic properties ascribed to an essential oil can easily be related to its chemical constituents. Price and Price (2007) highlight its anti-inflammatory actions, and their observations include research that has been done investigating its anti-allergenic potential.

Chamazulene itself has interesting effects. Bowles (2003) states that it is anti-inflammatory *in vivo*, citing the work of Safayhi *et al.* (1994), who suggest that this effect is due to the blocking of formation of leukotriene B4, an inflammatory mediator produced by neutrophils at sites of inflammation. Mills (1991) cited in Price and Price (2007) also states that chamazulene (and α-bisabolol) are not only anti-inflammatory but also antispasmodic, and can reduce histamine-induced reactions. The cutaneous benefits of German chamomile were investigated by Baumann (2007a) and it was also shown to have antipruritic potential. This would suggest that German chamomile oil has applications in cases of allergic problems, including hay fever and some types of asthma and eczema. When referring to 'azulenes' Mills (1991), cited in Price and Price (2007) suggests that they can 'calm the nervous system both peripherally as in nervous tension and centrally as in anxiety, nervous tension and headaches'.

The other significant component in German chamomile is α-bisabolol. This is a sesquiterpene alcohol with considerable therapeutic potential. It is non-toxic and non-irritant, it is more anti-inflammatory than chamazulene (Bowles 2003), and research has also indicated that α-bisabolol has 'a strikingly efficient and potent cytotoxic effect on human and rat malignant glioma cell lines' (Cavalieri *et al.* 2004), leading to their conclusion that α-bisabolol may have a potential use in clinical treatment of glioma, a highly malignant brain tumour.

A study conducted by Pauli (2006) investigated the antifungal activity of α-bisabolol. This research revealed that α-bisabolol 'may play an extraordinary role among natural antimicrobials', suggesting that it is a potential selective, non-toxic inhibitor of ergosterol biosynthesis. Ergosterol synthesis is an important step in the formation of fungal cell walls. This is a different mode of action to that of existing antifungal drugs, and this is significant because of emerging problems with resistance – for example in the case of *Candida albicans*. For some uses of German chamomile, please see Table 8.6.

Table 8.6 German chamomile essential oil in aromatherapy

System	German chamomile with
Musculoskeletal (inflammation, spasm)	Lavender and others appropriate to circumstances
Integumentary (eczema, inflammation, allergy, irritation, wounds)	Lavender, helichrysum, vetivert, patchouli, peppermint, spearmint, rose
Immune (hay fever)	Peppermint, sandalwood, rose, lavender
Nervous (tension, headache)	Peppermint

GENUS ORMENIS

ORMENIS MULTICAULIS – MOROCCAN CHAMOMILE

An essential oil, 'chamomile maroc' is distilled from the flowers of this species (also known as *O. mixta*), which is common in the Mediterranean region. It belongs to the same botanical family as the German and Roman chamomiles, but this essential oil is very different and should not be considered as a 'substitute' (Lawless 1992). It does not have a tradition of use in aromatherapy practice, although it has been described as having calming effects. Its major components are the non-hazardous α-pinene and artemisia alcohol (Tisserand and Balacs 1995).

GENUS TAGETES

TAGETES MINUTA, T. GLANDULIFERA – TAGETES

This is also known as 'Mexican marigold'. An essential oil is distilled from the bright orange, daisy-like flowers and flowering tops of this annual herb. The fresh oil is a mobile liquid; however it thickens and becomes sticky with age and exposure to the air. The essential oil has a distinctive green, fruity, herbal odour, which is used in perfumery to impart apple notes (Williams 2000).

The main constituent of this essential oil is a ketone – tagetone – present at 50–60 per cent; however, the presence of a group of chemicals known as furanocoumarins means that tagetes oil is strongly phototoxic, and for this reason it is not widely used in aromatherapy. Perhaps this is compounded by Lawless' (1992) reference to Arctander (1960) – 'it is quite possible that "tagetone" [the main constituent] is harmful to the human organism.'

Family Burseraceae

This family includes some of the shrubs and trees that exude fragrant oleo-gum resins, which can be extracted to produce essential oils and absolutes. Many of these species, such as frankincense, myrrh and oponapax, have biblical or Middle Eastern connotations. Several essential oils from this family are used in aromatherapy practice, mainly to aid the respiratory system and the skin, although other uses are reported.

Genus Boswellia

Boswellia carteri – frankincense

Frankincense or olibanum essential oil is obtained from an oleo-gum resin formed in specialised resin ducts in the tissues of this small shrubby tree that grows in Northeast Africa. Incisions can be made in the bark, and in response a milky white resin exudes, and then solidifies in tear-shaped amber drops. These are harvested and usually exported to Europe for distillation of the essential oil (Lawless 1995). The essential oil is a pale yellow, mobile liquid that has a spicy, pine/resinous, woody odour, with lemony top notes and a balsamic dryout (Williams 2000). According to Bowles (2003) its dominant chemical constituent is α-pinene at 34.5 per cent, followed by α-phellandrene at 14.6 per cent and *para*-cymene at 14 per cent. These are all classed as monoterpenes, a large group of chemicals often attributed with stimulating, decongestant and analgesic qualities.

More recently, Mertens *et al.* (2009), in an extensive review of the volatile constituents, identified that the main constituents common in most species are α-thujene, α-pinene, myrcene, incensole acetate, (*E*)-β-ocimene, duva-3,9,13-triene-1,5a-diol-1-acetate (a complex multi-carbon ring structure with hydroxyl and ester functional groups), phyllocladene (which has a tricyclic carbon framework), limonene, octanol acetate and octyl acetate. They also comment that another compound has been found – another complex carbon structure named verticilla-4(20),7,11,triene – and so far this has not been found in any other naturally occurring resin, so it could be a 'marker' for frankincense products. Despite this, no compound has been found that is typical of frankincense odour.

Price and Price (2007) highlight frankincense essential oil's anticatarrhal, antidepressant and immunostimulant properties, therefore this oil is particularly useful for respiratory congestion associated with asthma and bronchitis, for those with compromised immune systems and for alleviating anxiety and depression. Please see Table 8.7 for the use of frankincense in aromatherapy.

Table 8.7 Frankincense essential oil in aromatherapy

System	Frankincense with
Respiratory (catarrh, asthma, bronchitis)	Pine, lemon, bergamot, ginger, lavender. Also with sandalwood, Atlas cedarwood
Nervous (anxiety, stress, tension, depression)	Lavender, neroli, geranium, jasmine, lime, mandarin, sandalwood
Immune (colds, flu, myalgic encephalomyselitis or ME, convalescence)	Lavender, rosewood, palmarosa

GENUS CANARIUM

CANARIUM LUZONICUM – ELEMI

Elemi essential oil is distilled from a gum-like pathological exudate from a large tropical tree; the main production is in the Philippines and the Moluccas. Although the gum has a long tradition of use, including its application as an embalming agent in ancient Egypt, and as a stimulant for the skin and the respiratory system (Lawless 1992), it is either not used, or used only with caution in aromatherapy, as the essential oil may be carcinogenic (Tisserand and Balacs 1995). This is due to the presence of a chemical known as elemicin, which is present at 3–12 per cent. However, the dominant constituent of elemi essential oil is the monoterpene d-limonene. This could counteract the potential for carcinogenesis, as d-limonene itself could well have cancer prevention properties (Tisserand and Balacs 1995; Bowles 2003), leading Tisserand and Balacs to state, 'the chances of elemi oil causing serious problems in aromatherapy seem remote'. If it is selected for aromatherapeutic use, it is usually to rejuvenate the skin, with other oils derived from resins such as frankincense and myrrh as an expectorant, or to alleviate stress (Lawless 1992).

Genus Commiphora

Commiphora erythraea — opopanax

Opopanax essential oil is obtained from the oleoresin of a tropical tree which is of the same genus as myrrh. The oil has a sweet, balsamic, spicy scent and it thickens into a sticky mass upon exposure to the air. The oil is phototoxic and is not produced in significant quantities. Information is limited; therefore opopanax is not widely used in aromatherapy.

Commiphora myrrha — myrrh

Myrrh essential oil is distilled from crude myrrh oleoresin. The *Commiphora* genus is composed of small trees and shrubs native to the Red Sea region. They have specialised resin ducts that exude an oleoresin – see frankincense and opopanax – the harvesting and processing is similar. Myrrh essential oil is a pale yellow, mobile liquid with a sweet, spicy medicinal odour. Like opopanax, it becomes sticky and resin-like upon exposure to air.

A detailed breakdown of this chemically complex oil may be found in Price and Price (2007). Suffice it to say that it is dominated by sesquiterpenols – a group of constituents associated with some interesting therapeutic actions, including anti-inflammatory effects, and a ketone known as curzerenone. Myrrh essential oil does indeed have an anti-inflammatory effect (Bowles 2003). Price and Price (2007) emphasise its antiseptic qualities, its indications for the urinary tract and for cleansing sores and ulcers. They cite Bartram (1995), who wrote that myrrh was a leucocytogenic agent which is bacteriostatic against *Staphylococcus aureus* and other Gram-positive bacteria, and also commented that it is perhaps the most widely used herbal antiseptic. Lawless (1992, 1995) and Price and Price (2007) concur that myrrh is also indicated for healing the skin (it is cicatrisant) and for the respiratory system, where it can act as an expectorant. Please refer to Table 8.8.

Table 8.8 Myrrh essential oil in aromatherapy

System	Myrrh with
Respiratory (congestion, bronchitis, laryngitis)	Frankincense, thyme, sandalwood, benzoin
Integumentary (skin and wound healing)	Lavender, patchouli, helichrysum, geranium
Genito-urinary (urinary tract infections, cystitis, pruritus, thrush)	Lavender, juniperberry, bergamot, sandalwood

FAMILY CANNABACEAE

GENUS CANNABIS

CANNABIS SATIVA — CANNABIS

C. sativa yields an essential oil from its flower buds and flowers. Cannabis is probably best known as a recreational drug whose psychotropic effects are due to constituents known as THCs, but it also yields a fixed oil from its seeds that has skin healing properties and is used in massage practice as well as in phytocosmeceuticals.

The essential oil has a characteristic 'cannabis' odour. This varies according to its composition, which is related to many factors such as the time of harvesting, the maturity of the flowers and the seed ripeness. Consequently, there are some oils dominated by sesquiterpenes and some by monoterpenes; and the oils with a predominance of monoterpenes are usually regarded as having more pleasant odours. Even though it is present in small amounts, caryophyllene oxide is important in the aroma – this is one of the components that is detectable by sniffer dogs. The THC component is non-volatile, therefore does not come over in the distillation process into the essential oil (Mediavilla and Steinemann 1997).

Hadji-Mingalou and Bolcato (2005) investigated its use in a formulation for the replacement of dermacorticoid drugs, and give its components as myrcene (33%), trans-β-ocimene (15%), terpinolene, β-caryophyllene and caryophyllene oxide (1.4%). They state that the oil is obtained from the whole fresh plant, not just the flowering tops. This profile of constituents would certainly suggest that cannabis essential oil has analgesic potential. It has anti-inflammatory potential too; Baylac and Racine (2004) demonstrated that, *in vitro*, it was one of the oils that could inhibit the enzyme 5-lipoxygenase, which is involved in a cascade of reactions in the formation of pro-inflammatory leukotrienes.

Tubaro *et al.* (2010) investigated the anti-inflammatory activity of isolated cannabinoids and cannabivarins, from the flowers of non-psychotropic plants, confirming their anti-inflammatory activity but raising more questions about the cannabinoid receptors. Essential oils obtained from industrial hemp (non-psychotropic, legal) varieties of *C. sativa* also have considerable potential as antimicrobials in human and animal health, particularly in cases of antibiotic resistance. Therefore, it could be argued that cannabis/hemp essential oil should have a more prominent role in aromatic medicine and aromatherapy.

Family Ericaceae

Genus Gaultheria

Gaultheria procumbens – wintergreen

Wintergreen is an aromatic perennial herb that is native to North America and Canada, where it is found in pine forests, woodlands and clearings. Its leaves are spicy and aromatic; it produces white flowers followed by red, berry-like capsules, and is known as the Canada teaberry. Traditionally it was a remedy for rheumatism, sciatica, bladder disorders and skin diseases, also used in gargles, poultices and antiseptic washes. It is still used in some dental products (Gordon 1980).

The essential oil is steam distilled from the leaves, which first need to be soaked overnight in warm water at 49°C; this induces hydrolysis of a glucoside called gaultherin (Jouhar 1991) and promotes the production of the volatile oil. Wintergreen oil is a pale yellow, mobile liquid with a strong, medicinal, ethereal-fruity, sweet, woody odour (Lawless 1992). It contains a great deal of methyl salicylate, around 98 per cent, an aromatic ester which is toxic if taken internally. Lawless (1992) suggests that it should not be used in aromatherapy; however, it is a useful counter-irritant and anti-inflammatory, and can be used with caution in prescriptions for muscular aches and pains and sciatica. The genuine oil can be difficult to obtain; often synthetic methyl salicylate or the similar oil distilled from the bark of *Betula lenta* (sweet birch) is sold as wintergreen oil.

Family Geraniaceae

There are five genera in the Geraniaceae family. Of these, only the genus *Pelargonium* ('stork's bill') and the genus *Geranium* ('crane's bill') are essential oil producers. The term 'geranium' is commonly used to refer to both *Pelargonium* and *Geranium*, and it is in fact the *Pelargonium* species that are cultivated to produce 'geranium' essential oil. The only species of the genus *Geranium* that is grown for essential oil production is *Geranium macrorrhizum*, the essential oil from which is known as *zdravetz* oil (Brud and Ogyanov 1995).

Geranium oils require close attention to taxonomy. Consideration must also be given to the influences of ecological factors, such as geography and growth conditions, on essential oil quality and odour.

Genus Geranium

Geranium macrorrhizum – zdravetz

This species is known in Bulgaria as the big-root geranium, or long-rooted cranesbill, as its species name would suggest. It is an herbaceous perennial with large brown rhizomes, and all parts of the plant have a role in indigenous medicine, where it is used for stomach disorders and as a general tonic. The foliage is strongly aromatic, and it produces magenta-pink or red flowers. Its essential oil is known as *zdravetz* (from the Bulgarian word meaning 'health') and may be obtained from both the foliage and the rhizomes. All oil is distilled from wild plants in Bulgaria, Russia and the former Yugoslavia.

Zdravetz oil is a pale green or pale yellow, slightly viscous liquid, due to crystals that form at below 32°C. The scent is 'warm-fresh, sweetly herbaceous, rosy woody and tenacious' (Brud and Ogyanov 1995). It is mainly composed of sesquiterpenes, present in the region of 90 per cent, and around half of these are germacrone (Weiss 1997). It is used occasionally in perfumery, but rarely in aromatherapy. The aromatherapeutic properties have not been investigated, but it has a low toxicity, and Brud and Ogyanov (1995) suggested that it probably has strong antimicrobial activity, which could be harnessed as an antiseptic in skin care, and that it could have hypotensive effects.

GENUS PELARGONIUM

In contrast, *Pelargonium* species essential oils are some of the most widely used oils in aromatherapy practice. The genus consists of aromatic, hairy, perennial shrubs that thrive best in warm temperate climates. The *Pelargonium* genus was first named in South Africa, when *P. cucullatum* was collected from Table Mountain in 1672. There are many microhabitats in the South Western Cape region, allowing up to 70 species to flourish. *P. graveolens* was introduced to Britain in the early 1700s and was cultivated for essential oil for the first time in the early nineteenth century around Grasse in France. The main area of cultivation then moved to Réunion, where 'Bourbon' or rose geranium is produced (*P. capitatum* × *P. radens*), and now oils are produced in Algeria, Morocco and Egypt (Weiss 1997), and also India (with plants that originated in Réunion) and China (*P. roseum*).

The genus contains about 250 species; however, only a few species are used for essential oil production. These are *P. graveolens*, *P. odoratissimum*, *P. capitatum* and *P. radens*, and also *P. roseum*, a hybrid of *P. capitatum* × *P. radens*. The oil is found in glands throughout the green parts of the plant. Geranium oil is steam- or hydro-distilled from the fresh herbage. The oil is usually designated by country of origin. Adulteration is common, but oils from France, Egypt and Réunion are usually good quality (Weiss 1997).

The aroma of the oil will vary according to the geographical origin, but other factors will affect odour, such as the age of the plants, and time of harvesting. The main constituents are citronellol, geraniol, linalool and *iso*-menthone, and it is their relative proportions that influence the odour of the oil. Geranium oil from Grasse has a fine, rose-like scent, but it is the oil from Réunion that sets the standard for perfumery. This may have a fresh, mint-like note due to the *iso*-menthone, and also rosy, sweet and fruity notes. The Moroccan oil is dark to mid-yellow with a sweet, rosy and herbaceous aroma; Egyptian oil is yellowish-green with a similar aroma to that from Morocco. Oil from China is more variable in quality because of the differences in distillation methods and also the number of variants under cultivation. Generally, Chinese oil is a darker olive green with a harsher odour than Réunion, but more lemony and rosy, sweet and herbaceous; it is not considered a substitute for the others in perfumery (Weiss 1997).

Geranium oil will contain, as major constituents, the alcohols citronellol, geraniol and linalool (55–65%), esters (15%) and ketones such as *iso*-menthone (1–8%) (Price and Price 2007) and because of variability, the proportions of each of these affect the aroma (Weiss 1997). Aldehydes (neral, geranial and citronellal) up to 10 per cent are found in the Bourbon variety (Price and Price 2007). Price and Price (2007) also state that oxides are only found in the Chinese variety. A comparison is shown in Table 8.9.

Table 8.9 Comparison of the main chemical constituents (%w/v) of geranium oils (adapted from Weiss 1997)

Component	Algeria	China	Egypt	Morocco	Réunion
Iso-menthone	5.38	5.70	5.39	5.20	7.20
Linalool	5.26	3.96	9.47	6.80	12.90
Citronellyl formate	7.57	11.35	6.74	6.02	8.37
Geranyl formate	5.90	1.92	4.75	6.55	7.55
Citronellol	22.90	40.23	27.40	19.28	21.28
Geraniol	17.07	6.45	18.00	18.40	17.45
10-Epi-gamma eudesmol	4.20	–	4.00	5.10	–

Geranium oil is used in traditional medicine as an insecticide, nematicide and antifungal (Weiss 1997). Lawless (1996) suggests that it can be used for skin care (including alleviating problems associated with acne and oily skin), oedema, poor circulation and cellulitis, sore throats, premenstrual syndrome and menopause, to stimulate the adrenocortical glands, as well as for nervous tension and stress. It is potentially fungicidal, probably due to geraniol and aldehydes, and contains anti-inflammatory esters. For information on its aromatherapeutic uses, please see Table 8.10.

It is thought that cutaneous application of geranium can suppress inflammation by suppressing neutrophil accumulation, and consequently Maruyama *et al.* (2006) investigated its effects, via injection, on induced oedema and arthritis in mice. The study revealed that geranium could reduce swelling and inflammation in both the early and later phases of the inflammatory response, and that neutrophil accumulation was also decreased – however, the intraperitoneal injections had toxic effects. They suggested that geranium might be used in the treatment of rheumatoid arthritis, as this has several features in common with the collagen-induced arthritis in mice. Cutaneous application should be used to avoid potential toxicity.

Geranium has also been shown to provide temporary relief in postherpetic neuralgia – a condition that can be severe and disabling, and difficult to treat. A multi-centre, double-blind crossover study (Greenway *et al.* 2003) showed that geranium (at various concentrations from 100% to 10% in mineral oil) could relieve pain in 'minutes' and that 25 per cent of the patients had 'dramatic relief of spontaneous pain'. The oil was well tolerated, with only a few cases of minor skin irritation, even at 100 per cent.

Some have suggested that it is a 'balancer' of mood swings related to hormone activity (Bowles 2003), possibly by influencing the adrenocortical glands. Bowles states that this may be due chemical similarities in the pathway that produces geraniol and that which produces steroid hormones, reasoning therefore that geraniol may increase oestrogen levels. However, this balancing effect could also occur via olfactory stimulus. Regardless of the mechanism of action, geranium has certainly been shown to reduce anxiety when inhaled (Morris *et al.* 1995).

Table 8.10 Geranium essential oil in aromatherapy

System	Geranium with
Integumentary (including inflammation)	Lavender, bergamot, helichrysum, palmarosa, sandalwood, German chamomile, tea tree, manuka
Musculoskeletal (spasm, pain, inflammation)	Lavender, clary sage, rosemary, marjoram, black pepper
Nervous (stress, anxiety, premenstrual syndrome or PMS, mood swings, postnatal depression)	Lavender, bergamot, clary sage, lemon, grapefruit, mandarin, rose

Family Illiciaceae

In this family (also referred to as the Magnoliaceae), the genus *Illicium* comprises around 40 species of trees and shrubs. Of these only one species, *Illicium verum*, is of importance in aromatherapy, and this yields star anise essential oil. This essential oil should not be confused with that of aniseed (*Pimpinella anisum*), which it resembles in terms of scent.

Genus Illicium

Illicium verum – star anise, Chinese star anise

Star anise essential oil is distilled from the fully ripe, star-shaped fruits of this tall evergreen tree (Weiss 2002). The essential oil is a colourless or pale yellow, mobile liquid, with a sweet anise, liquorice-like odour (Lawless 1995). Star anise contains around 70 per cent *trans*-anethole (Bowles 2003), the phenolic ether also found in sweet fennel essential oil, which is thought to have 'oestrogenic' properties. *Trans*-anethole may also have antispasmodic and anaesthetic effects (Bowles 2003), hence its use in aromatherapy for muscular aches and pains, colic and cramp. Star anise is also used for the respiratory system because of its expectorant properties (Lawless 1995). See Table 8.11.

For reservations and cautions due to the *trans*-anethole content, refer to the sweet fennel profile, where hazards associated with this constituent are discussed.

Table 8.11 Star anise essential oil in aromatherapy

System	Star anise with
Female reproductive	Rose, geranium, juniperberry
Digestive	Black pepper, coriander seed, cardamom, sweet orange, mandarin
Respiratory	Lemon, Scots pine, sandalwood, Atlas cedarwood

Family Lamiaceae

This family is also known as the Labiateae, and it is often referred to as the mint family. Many essential oil-bearing plants are found in the Lamiaceae; it is one of the ten largest families, comprising some 3200 species of herbs and shrubs. Members of the Lamiaceae are distinguished by their flowers, which have discreet, gaping lips (hence the term 'labiate'), opposite leaves and angular petioles, and a four-part ovary. In many cases the leaves are highly aromatic. Typically, the volatile oil is found in glandular cells or glandular hairs (trichomes) mainly located on the leaves. The genera and species of most importance in aromatherapy are described below.

Genus Hyssopus

Hyssopus officinalis – Hyssop

Hyssop is a highly aromatic perennial, although it is not entirely hardy in cooler climates. The herb was used in ancient times in purification rituals and for 'cleansing' lepers, and it even played a role in the consecration of Westminster Abbey (Gordon 1980). Hyssop essential oil is obtained from the leaves and flowering tops of the herb. It is produced in Hungary and France, and is a colourless or pale yellow-green, mobile liquid (Lawless 1995) with a strong, camphoraceous, warm, spicy odour (Williams 2000). Hyssop essential oil is not widely used in aromatherapy because of its numerous contraindications, including epilepsy, fever, pregnancy, and on children aged less than two years. This is because the oil is moderately toxic, and neurotoxic, with the potential to cause convulsions. The components that are responsible for this hazard are ketones – pinocamphone and *iso*-pinocamphone. Despite this it is a very useful expectorant and mucolytic, best used with less toxic herbal essential oils such as lavender, rosemary CT 1,8-cineole, sweet marjoram, thyme CT linalool or *Thymus mastichina* (Spanish marjoram).

Genus Lavandula

The lavenders are aromatic, evergreen, woody shrubs, native to the Mediterranean coast. They were used by the Romans to scent bathing water, giving rise to the generic name *Lavandula*, from the Latin *lavare*, 'to wash'. Over the years, lavender has acquired many associations within folk tradition and medicine. These included a dedication to Hecate, the goddess of witches and sorcery, and as a means to avert 'the evil eye' (Gordon 1980).

Lavender is now cultivated in many countries for its essential oil (Lawless 1992). Lavender essential oils are obtained by steam distillation of the flowering tops. The essential oils were originally produced for the perfumery industry, but in recent years lavender essential oil has become one of the best known (and investigated) and most popular essential oils. It is probably the most useful and versatile of the therapeutic essential oils.

Lavandula angustifolia, *L. vera* and *L. officinalis* are the true lavenders; they hybridise easily, therefore many subspecies (ssp.), for example *delphinensis*, and many cultivars are in existence. Other species in this genus include *L. latifolia* (also known as *L. spica* and its subspecies *fragrans*), which yields spike lavender essential oil, and *L. stoechas*, which yields an essential oil known as French lavender. The hybrid *Lavandula* × *intermedia* is a cross between true lavender and spike lavender; it yields an essential oil called lavandin.

LAVANDULA ANGUSTIFOLIA — TRUE LAVENDER

Lavender essential oil is produced in several countries including France, Spain, Bulgaria, Tasmania and the UK (in Norfolk, Suffolk and Kent). It is a pale yellow or colourless, mobile liquid and its odour will vary according to its geographical source. Lavender has an herbal, fruity, floral, woody aroma, with a nondescript dryout (Williams 2000); French lavender 40/42 is typical. The '40/42' refers to its linalyl acetate (an ester) content. Linalyl acetate can be present at anywhere between 36 per cent and 53 per cent (Price and Price 2007). High altitude French lavender, sold as '50/52' is also available, and in this a distinctive 'pear drops' ester note is detectable. This component, along with *l*-linalool (a monoterpene alcohol) present at 26–49 per cent, may contribute to lavender's sedative effect on mice (Buchbauer *et al.* 1991a, cited in Bowles 2003) and in humans (Buchbauer *et al.* 1993).

Lavender has been shown to reduce sympathetic nervous system activity and stimulate parasympathetic nervous system activity. Essential oil of lavender is perhaps best known for its sedative, calming and mood-enhancing effects, evidenced in several studies on humans (Ludvigson and Rottmann 1989; Diego *et al.* 1998; Moss *et al.* 2003; Lehrner *et al.* 2005).

An animal study conducted by Shen *et al.* (2005) explored the effects of inhalation of lavender essential oil and isolated linalool on lipolysis, heat production and appetite in rats. It was found that sympathetic nervous activity was supressed, so metabolism in white adipose tissue was reduced, indicating an anti-lipolytic effect. The reduced nervous activity in the brown adipose tissue appeared to reduce heat production and thus energy consumption. Sympathetic nervous system activity is also related to appetite, and the food uptake of the rats increased. It was concluded that lavender, by virtue of its relaxing, stress-reducing actions, also could result in decreased lipolysis, increased appetite, and consequently weight gain. Given the increasing problems with weight and obesity in humans in affluent countries, this may not be seen as desirable. However, it would indicate that inhalation of lavender and similar sedative oils may have uses in helping those with poor appetite and related problems. (Those with over-weight issues might consider using grapefruit instead – see page 214.)

In addition to its sedative and calming effects, lavender has many other useful therapeutic properties. It is a useful analgesic agent in the context of aromatherapy. Brownfield (1998) demonstrated that massage with lavender was a more effective analgesic than massage alone in chronic rheumatoid arthritis. Its anti-inflammatory potential has also been investigated. Kim and Cho (1999) conducted *in vitro* and *in vivo* animal experiments which indicated that lavender oil had concentration-dependent anti-inflammatory effects; it could inhibit immediate allergic type responses by inhibiting mast cell degranulation and the secretion of histamine.

However, it is worth noting that there is one reservation to the use of lavender, and that, somewhat surprisingly, is in relation to the skin. Baumann (2007b) suggests that lavender has a 'dark side', citing a study conducted by Prashar *et al.* (2004). It was found that lavender had a cytotoxic effect on endothelial cells and fibroblasts, possibly due to cell membrane damage, leading Baumann to comment that lavender is perhaps unsuitable in preparations specifically designed to have an anti-ageing effect.

Price and Price (2007) noted that lavender is analgesic, anti-inflammatory, antispasmodic and cicatrising. This broad spectrum of therapeutic actions allows many varied applications, some of which can be seen in Table 8.12.

Table 8.12 True lavender essential oil in aromatherapy

System	True lavender with
Nervous (pain,* migraine,* insomnia,** anxiety***)	Peppermint,* clove bud, marjoram, Roman chamomile,** neroli, Geranium,*** ylang, ylang, clary sage, frankincense, sandalwood, rose, bergamot and citrus oils
Musculoskeletal (aches and pains, tension)	Sweet marjoram, rosemary, geranium eucalyptus, clary sage, juniperberry, basil, lemon, lemongrass, black pepper, ginger

Integumentary:
  irritation, eczema
 	
  infection
  itching
 	
  healing
  phlebitis
	Geranium, rose, sandalwood, patchouli, vetivert, German chamomile
	Tea tree, manuka
	Tea tree, bergamot, peppermint, German chamomile
	Helichrysum, myrrh
	Patchouli, bergamot, cypress

*Asterisks indicate a particular relationship between the condition and the oil (or oils) thus identified.

LAVANDULA × INTERMEDIA — LAVANDIN

Lavandin is a cross between true and spike lavender; this is apparent in its scent, which is less 'fruity/pear drops' than lavender, but not as penetrating and camphoraceous as spike lavender. Depending on the source, the essential oil contains *l*-linalool (20–60%), linalyl acetate (15–50%), camphor (5–15%) and 1,8-cineole (5–25%). Again, this oil should be used with care, due to its camphor content (Tisserand and Balacs 1995). Like spike lavender, it is a useful mucolytic and expectorant and it has analgesic potential. It is perhaps best viewed as occupying the space between true and spike lavender.

L. latifolia (also known as L. spica) – spike lavender

This is quite different from true lavender in odour, chemistry, and consequently its therapeutic applications. It has a camphoraceous, herbal, woody odour (Williams 2000); it is sharper and fresher, lacking the softer, floral/fruity notes of true lavender. This is because it contains 1,8-cineole at 36.3 per cent, linalool at 30.3 per cent and camphor (the ketone) at 8 per cent (Bowles 2003).

1,8-cineole is an oxide found in many essential oils – and in high amounts in many *Eucalyptus* oils. At high doses, 1,8-cineole can have neurotropic effects (such as slurred speech, coma, even convulsions), and it can cause respiratory irritation, as it is a rubefacient and mucous membrane irritant. However, 1,8-cineole is an expectorant, an anti-inflammatory in cases of bronchial asthma, and it may also be a stimulant of the trigeminal nerve – hence its ability to increase alertness (Bowles 2003). Buchbauer (1996) states that 1,8-cineole can increase cerebral blood flow, and has also suggested that it has spasmolytic properties (Buchbauer 1993). Balacs (1997), in a comprehensive review of cineole-rich oils, explores the pharmacokinetics of 1,8-cineole, emphasising that this compound is absorbed very quickly from the air into the bloodstream.

The camphor (a neurotoxic ketone) content is not high – even true lavender has a camphor content of <1 per cent (Tisserand and Balacs 1995) – but it is present in sufficient quantity to class it as an oil to be used with caution, and avoided in epilepsy, fever and pregnancy. Spike lavender is a stimulating essential oil, with mucolytic and expectorant properties. It can be useful for muscular aches and pains and respiratory congestion. Its odour is very compatible with that of rosemary, *Eucalyptus* spp., pine, clove bud, and also true lavender and lavandin – all of which would also be indicated for these complaints.

Lavandula stoechas – French lavender

The so-called 'French' lavender oil originating from *L. stoechas* is distinct from true lavender that originates in France. This oil has a fairly high camphor content at 15–30 per cent, and a fenchone content of 45–50 per cent. Fenchone is another ketone, and this one has the potential to irritate the skin. For these reasons, *L. stoechas* is usually avoided in aromatherapy. However, this does not mean that it does not have therapeutic potential. The herb is used in the Unani Tibb system of medicine (the forerunner of modern Western herbalism) to treat brain disorders, including epilepsy. Zaidia *et al.* (2009) conducted an animal study to investigate its anticonvulsant potential and neurotoxicity. This study indicated that *L. stoechas* essential oil does have anticonvulsant activity, which the authors attributed to linalool, pinene and linalyl acetate. They also identified that the LD_{50} (the dose required to kill 50% of the test animals) was 2.5 ml/kg in mice. So if an anticonvulsant action is required in the context of aromatherapy, it would be more advisable to consider using true lavender essential oil, where the LD_{50} is >5.0 g/kg (for rats).

GENUS MELISSA

MELISSA OFFICINALIS — LEMON BALM

This is a common cottage garden herb that is very attractive to bees. It is a perennial herb with a long tradition of use as a culinary herb, a 'strewing herb', for calming the nerves and the heart and perfuming the home (Gordon 1980).

Melissa essential oil is a pale yellow, mobile liquid that has a citrus/herbal odour (Williams 2000). Williams also indicates that it is little used. This could be due to the fact that melissa essential oil is frequently adulterated, or even synthetic, and in the past it has been difficult to purchase the genuine essential oil (Price and Price 2007). The yield is very low, and the essential oil commands a high price. Authentic, laboratory-distilled melissa contains around 80 per cent citral (Sorensen 2000). Citral is the name given to a naturally occurring mixture of two aldehydes – geranial and neral – chemicals that are isomers (same molecular formula, but minor differences in molecular structure). Another aldehyde, citronellal, is present, but a high level of this is an indicator of adulteration (Sorensen 2000).

Many writers of aromatherapy books that are aimed at both the general public and the professional ascribe therapeutic properties to melissa, notably that it is a calming, sedative essential oil (Price and Price 2007). Tisserand and Balacs (1995) suggest caution due to the citral content, as this may cause sensitisation, while Price and Price (2007) suggest that care should be exercised if using the oil on skin that is exposed to direct sunlight. Sorensen (2000) suggested that there was very little evidence to support melissa's therapeutic use, other than speculation about the effects that citral may impart.

However, following reports that melissa essential oil could reduce agitation in severe dementia, and extend the time spent on constructive activities while reducing the time of social withdrawal (Ballard *et al.* 2002), Elliot *et al.* (2007) conducted a preliminary investigation to determine the bioactivity of the oil, especially in relation to its ability to bind with the key neurotransmitter receptors that are important in the mediation of agitation. They found that melissa had a wide receptor binding profile (greater than that of lavender), which could explain its calming and cognition enhancing actions. They also suggested that the topical application or inhalation of melissa could be a better way of delivering a treatment for agitation than the usual intramuscular injections or tablets.

Genus Mentha

Mentha × piperita – peppermint

Botanically, peppermint is a cross between *M. viridis* (spearmint) and *M. aquatica* (watermint). It is a widely cultivated perennial herb whose essential oil is produced in many countries, including the USA, France and England (notably in Mitcham).

Peppermint oil is extensively used in the flavour and fragrance industry, and also in the pharmaceutical industry. It is a pale yellow or colourless, mobile liquid, with a strong, fresh, minty, green odour (Williams 2000). The odour is mainly due to menthol, a monoterpene alcohol present at around 42 per cent, and menthone, its corresponding ketone, at 20 per cent. Menthol produces a cooling sensation when applied to the skin and there is evidence to support its analgesic effects. Menthone is not a neurotoxic ketone. It may well have some of the properties attributed to ketones – notably their effects on mucosal secretions and their wound healing properties (Bowles 2003). These two constituents can at least partly account for the therapeutic properties associated with peppermint essential oil.

Price and Price (2007) give a long list of properties and indications, citing several research papers. In summary: the main uses for peppermint essential oil are for the respiratory system, especially bronchitis and asthma, as it is antispasmodic, expectorant and mucolytic; for the integumentary system, especially eczema, rashes and itching, as it is anti-inflammatory, antipruritic and analgesic; for the nervous system, pain, migraine, neuralgia and sciatica, as it is analgesic and cephalic; for the digestive system, especially indigestion, nausea, colic and digestive dysfunction such as irritable bowel syndrome, because of its antispasmodic properties; in addition, it is thought to reduce colonic motility.

Gobel *et al.* (1995) conducted a double-blind, placebo-controlled study to investigate the effects of peppermint and eucalyptus essential oils on headache mechanisms. It was found that a combination of these oils increased cognitive performance and had a physically and mentally relaxing effect, but did not affect sensitivity to pain. However, a 10 per cent preparation of peppermint applied to the forehead and temples had a marked analgesic effect in relation to headache.

Davies, Harding and Baranowski (2002) reported a case of a patient suffering from intractable pain, thought to be due to an 'irritable nociceptor' pathophysiology. Peppermint essential oil (applied neat) was a very successful and quick acting treatment for this type of neuropathic pain. This again demonstrates its analgesic potential.

In 2007 Cappello *et al.* conducted a double-blind, placebo-controlled study investigating the use of peppermint essential oil, this time in enteric coated capsules, as a treatment for the symptoms of irritable bowel syndrome (IBS). The study revealed that after four weeks there was a more than 50 per cent reduction in symptoms in 75 per cent of patients who had received the peppermint capsules, compared with 38 per cent of the placebo group. This would certainly support the use of peppermint oil in aromatherapy for clients with IBS, although it is not known if a topical application would have the same level of efficacy.

Peppermint oil is contraindicated for babies and young children as it can cause reflex apnoea, or laryngospasm (Tester-Dalderup 1980, cited in Price and Price 2007). Caution is also suggested with high doses, as this could cause sleep disturbance and skin irritation. A maximum of 3 per cent is recommended for application to mucous membranes, and it is contraindicated in cardiac fibrillation (Tisserand and Balacs 1995).

Table 8.13 Peppermint essential oil in aromatherapy

System	Peppermint with
Respiratory (congestion, bronchitis asthma)	Eucalyptus (1,8-cineole types), rosemary, sweet marjoram, clary sage, lavender, spike lavender, benzoin
Integumentary (eczema, itching, rashes, wound healing)	Lavender, bergamot, tea tree, patchouli, helichrysum, German chamomile, myrrh, geranium, rose
Digestive system	Lavender, cardamom, coriander seed, sweet marjoram, citrus oils, clove bud, black pepper
Nervous system (pain)	Lavender, ravintsara, geranium, nutmeg, clove bud

MENTHA PULEGIUM – PENNYROYAL

This contains 55–95 per cent of a ketone, *d*-pulegone. This is a very toxic ketone; it is hepatotoxic, and the high levels in pennyroyal oil render it unsafe for therapeutic use (Tisserand and Balacs 1995). The herb, however, had many uses. It was not valued as a culinary herb, but it was used to treat many pains and ills, including toothache, headache and colic.

MENTHA SPICATA – SPEARMINT

This has a sweeter, warmer, minty odour than peppermint (Williams 2000). The main chemical constituent is *l*-carvone at around 50–70 per cent (Lawless 1996). Carvone is a ketone that has two chiral forms, which are mirror images of each other. The *d*-carvone molecule has the odour of caraway, while the *l*-carvone molecule smells minty. Carvone is not toxic (Tisserand and Balacs 1995), and so spearmint is often thought to be a better option than peppermint for children (Lawless 1992). The indications are similar to peppermint; however there is less evidence to support its use. Traditionally, spearmint was used to scent bathwater and the herb was used as a digestive, especially if meat had been consumed. It is the only mint described by the herbalist Culpepper, who suggested that it should form part of a tonic for 'delicate and consumptive young women' (Gordon 1980).

GENUS OCIMUM

OCIMUM BASILICUM – BASIL

The herb is not hardy in cooler climates, where it is treated as an annual. The name comes from the Greek word for 'royal', indicating that it may have been used in royal medicines. It was and is a very popular herb in Greek, Italian and French cuisine. It was used in folk medicine as a digestive aid.

Essential oils may be obtained from several cultivars of basil, and different chemotypes are available. These are Comoran, or exotic basil, European basil, and methyl chavicol and linalool chemotypes. Basil essential oil is a colourless, mobile liquid with a sweet, warm herbal, anisic odour. It is distilled from the leaves of the herb in France, and also in the Comoro islands and Madagascar. The geographical influences and growing conditions give rise to significant differences in the chemical compositions of the essential oils, despite the fact that they are derived from the same botanical species.

A constituent called estragole, also known as methyl chavicol, dominates Comoran basil. This belongs to a group of chemicals known as phenolic ethers. Estragole itself is not toxic, but is converted during its metabolism into a chemical, 1'-hydroxyestragol, which is carcinogenic and hepatotoxic. This is rapidly detoxified in the body, and basil oils with lower estragole contents are not a cause for concern (Tisserand and Balacs 1995). Comoran basil may contain 40–87 per cent estragole, up to 4 per cent methyleugenol (which is thought to be genotoxic and carcinogenic) and the monoterpene alcohol, linalool, at up to 6 per cent.

European basil oil is usually the linalool chemotype, as the dominant constituent is linalool at up to 75 per cent, along with estragole at up to 16.5 per cent and methyleugenol in traces or up to 2 per cent (Tisserand and Balacs 1995). Therefore, for use in aromatherapy, it is strongly recommended that the low estragole (i.e. <5%) be used. Bowles (2003) suggests that methyl chavicol has antispasmodic qualities, and indeed this is one of the properties attributed to basil essential oil (Lawless 1992 and Price and Price 2007). These authors also state that basil is a 'tonic' for the nervous and digestive systems, and is a stimulating oil with cephalic qualities. Therefore it can be of use in a wide variety of stress-related symptoms such as muscular tension, headaches, poor concentration and nervous indigestion. For the uses of basil CT linalool in aromatherapy, please see Table 8.14.

Table 8.14 Basil essential oil in aromatherapy

System	Basil with
Musculoskeletal (muscle tension, pain, stress)	Lavender, rosemary, geranium, sweet marjoram, clary sage, black pepper
Nervous system (stress, headaches, poor concentration, fatigue)	Lavender, rosemary, lemon, eucalyptus, peppermint
Digestive system	Lavender, sweet marjoram, clary sage, citrus oils, sweet fennel, peppermint, spearmint, black pepper

OCIMUM GRATISSIMUM

This species of basil is indigenous to tropical regions, especially India and West Africa. It has been extensively used in traditional medicine, and as a culinary herb. The leaves and flowers are rich in volatile oil, and the herb has a myriad of uses, including the treatment of headaches, fever, respiratory problems, infections, fever and skin diseases.

Recently it has been used in topical preparations for its antiseptic properties and for the treatment of minor wounds, boils and pimples. A review of the research into 'ocimum' revealed that extracts and the essential oil have many biological actions, and considerable therapeutic potential. These included antibacterial, antifungal, antidiarrhoeal, anti-inflammatory, analgesic, immunostimulatory, hepatoprotective, antioxidant and anticonvulsant actions.

The essential oil is dominated by eugenol, at around 54 per cent, and 1,8-cineole at 21–22 per cent, a variety of mono- and sesquiterpenes, their oxygenated derivatives and 'gratissimol'. Some toxicology studies have revealed that persistent use of relatively large quantities can provoke an inflammatory response, that it can affect macrophage functioning, and has hepatocarcinogenic potential (Prabhu *et al.* 2009). However, the levels used in topical preparations are regarded as safe.

Ocimum's antimicrobial activity is regarded as 'potent'; therefore it has been investigated with regard to its potential use in wound healing (Orafidiya *et al.* 2006) and acne treatments (Orafidiya *et al.* 2004). Studies in these areas have revealed that it is more active in hydrophilic media than oil bases. It was found that a 2 per cent formulation of *O. gratissimum* in honey, which itself has antibacterial and wound healing properties, possibly due to its osmotic effects, had a 'remarkable' antibacterial effect. In this case, the authors suggest that this is partly due to its thymol content (Orafidiya *et al.* 2006), rather than eugenol. They concluded that this formulation could be invaluable as a topical antiseptic for wounds. Ocimum oil has also been used in conjunction with aloe vera gel in a study that looked at the treatment of acne vulgaris, demonstrating that aloe vera gel enhanced the effects of ocimum on inflammatory lesions, and that the combination of 2 per cent ocimum in 50 per cent aloe vera gel was more effective than a commercial synthetic anti-acne agent.

The wound healing study (Orafidya *et al.* 2003) investigated the effects of *O. gratissimum* essential oil on full thickness wounds in test animals. The study demonstrated that this essential oil enhances wound healing; it accelerated scab formation, wound contraction and the formation of granulation tissue, and significantly it was effective against both bacterial and fungal wound-infecting micro-organisms.

So although aromatherapists do not commonly use this oil, it certainly has potential for applications in wound healing and in anti-acne hydrophilic preparations.

OCIMUM SANCTUM – HOLY BASIL, TULSI

This species of basil is native to India and sacred to the Hindus; it is also known as *tulasi*. It is worshipped as the plant of Lakshmi, wife of Vishnu, and is planted near temples and in courtyards to purify the air and invite the gods to these areas. The herb is widely used in Ayurvedic medicine (Svoboda 2004).

O. sanctum yields an essential oil known as tulsi. This is not widely used in aromatherapy; however, a study investigating the *in vitro* activities of essential oils for acne control included holy basil, revealing that it was more effective against *Propionibacterium acnes* than sweet basil, and that its antioxidant activity suggested that it would be useful for the prevention of scar formation (Lertsatitthanakorn *et al.* 2006).

GENUS ORIGANUM

ORIGANUM MAJORANA – SWEET MARJORAM

Other species include *O. vulgare* or common oregano, which has many varieties such as *O. glandulosum, O. virens* and *O. heracleoticum*. In aromatherapy practice it is important to distinguish between sweet marjoram and some of the thyme species that are commonly known as marjoram – see *Thymus* genus on page 176.

Origanum species are native to Mediterranean regions; it is known that the ancient Greeks cultivated marjoram for its scent, as well as for culinary and medicinal purposes. In mediaeval Europe, marjoram was a valued strewing herb; it was used in brewing before the advent of hops, and was used medicinally too – to maintain good health and to relieve pain.

Sweet marjoram essential oil is distilled from the dried flowering herb – the geographical sources include France, Tunisia and Morocco (Lawless 1992). The essential oil has a warm, camphoraceous, herbal, spicy odour (Williams 2000). Chemically it is characterised by monoterpenes (40%) and their alcohols (50%), notably myrcene, *para*-cymene, terpinen-4-ol and α-terpineol (Price and Price 2007). Myrcene, *para*-cymene, linalool and α-terpineol have all been attributed with analgesic properties (Bowles 2003); terpinen-4-ol may have diuretic properties (Schilcher 1985, cited in Baerheim Svendsen and Scheffer 1985).

Marjoram is regarded as being of most use as an analgesic – especially for arthritic and muscular pain and rheumatism, and as a nervous sedative (Duraffourd 1982, cited in Price and Price 2007). For some uses in aromatherapy, please refer to Table 8.15.

Table 8.15 Sweet marjoram essential oil in aromatherapy

System	Sweet marjoram with
Muscular (muscle tension, pain, spasm, soft tissue trauma)	Lavender, rosemary, lemongrass, basil, clary sage, helichrysum, black pepper
Joint pain, arthritis	Lavender, juniperberry, Atlas cedarwood, plai, black pepper, grapefruit
Nervous system (stress, anxiety)	Lavender, geranium, sweet or bitter orange, tangerine, mandarin

GENUS POGOSTEMON

POGOSTEMON CABLIN – PATCHOULI

There are around 40 species in this genus that are native to Southeast Asia and India; however, only one species is of commercial importance – the botanical source of patchouli essential oil, *Pogostemon cablin*. Patchouli has a very long history of use in the East as an incense and personal and fabric perfume, as an insect repellent and for sacred use in temples. The scent was introduced to Europe via the scented fabrics that were imported from India, and in the nineteenth century, essential oil production commenced (Weiss 1997).

P. cablin is the only modern botanical source of patchouli essential oil. Patchouli is an aromatic, large, bushy, perennial herb with a hairy appearance. The volatile oil is contained in glands on the underside of the leaves. Patchouli essential oil is distilled from the leaves of the herb. Often harvesting is selective – only removing stems with three to five pairs of mature leaves. This allows rapid regrowth. The fresh leaves will not yield much oil, so they are left to dry and ferment slightly. This controlled process alters the cell wall structure, so that the cells are more permeable and the oil can be liberated (Weiss 1997). The scent of the fresh leaves is quite different from the essential oil; it is lighter and fresher in character.

Patchouli essential oil has a clear amber appearance; it is slightly viscous. The odour is quite distinctive; it is rich, sweet herbaceous, earthy, heavy and very persistent. The oil ages well, and the odour will improve rather than deteriorate. Patchouli oil is an important perfumery material, and it is also used to flavour tobacco. The aromatherapy trade supplies refined oil, rather than the crude, whole oil for therapeutic and perfumery purposes.

The chemistry of patchouli oil is very complex, with around 60 constituents identified (Weiss 1997). However, the dominant constituents are the sesquiterpene alcohols – especially patchoulol (40%) according to Bowles (2003), and sesquiterpenes at up to 50 per cent, including α- and β-bulnesene (Price and Price 2007).

Patchouli is particularly useful for the skin – as it is both anti-inflammatory and cicatrising, it may be of support to the immune system, and it is one of the few essential oils cited as a phlebotonic (Price and Price 2007). For some uses of patchouli in aromatherapy, please see Table 8.16.

Table 8.16 Patchouli essential oil in aromatherapy

System	Patchouli with
Integumentary (acne, inflammation, eczema*)	Lavender, sandalwood, vetivert,* rose, geranium, helichrysum, bergamot
Allergies	German chamomile, rose, helichrysum
Nervous system (stress, anxiety)	Lavender, rose, geranium, ylang ylang, jasmine, citrus oils (especially lime), sandalwood
Vascular	Lemon, bergamot, cypress, geranium, helichrysum

*Asterisks indicate a particular relationship between the condition and the corresponding oil.

GENUS ROSMARINUS

ROSMARINUS OFFICINALIS – ROSEMARY

There are many cultivars of rosemary, and several chemotypes of the essential oil are available. The ones that have applications in aromatic medicine and aromatherapy are CT 1,8-cineole (Tunisia), CT verbenone (France) and CT camphor (Spain). Rosemary is a strongly aromatic perennial shrub, and, like many of the Lamiaceae, is native to the Mediterranean coast. In fact, the name is derived from *ros marinos*, meaning 'dew of the sea'. Mankind has known rosemary for a long time – an early eleventh-century herbal mentions its use as a culinary herb, a medicine, a strewing herb, a perfume (it was an ingredient in 'Hungary water', the predecessor of 'eau de Cologne') and a bee plant. It was one of the first herbs to be distilled for its oil, around 1330, and by then it had been noted for its ability to clear the head (Gordon 1980).

The essential oil is distilled from the flowering tops and leaves. Rosemary essential oil has a strong, fresh, herbal, resinous, woody aroma (Williams 2000). Depending on the chemotype, it is dominated by 1,8-cineole or camphor (the verbenone type is rare). The other dominant constituent is α-pinene; minor constituents are mostly monoterpenes and their alcohols and esters (Bowles 2003).

The most commonly cited uses for rosemary oil are as an analgesic, mucolytic and cephalic; Price and Price (2007) also state that it has 'neuromuscular action'. It is almost always described as a stimulating essential oil. Some animal studies have indicated that rosemary has anti-inflammatory activity, probably by inhibiting leukocyte chemotaxis, and analgesic (antinociceptive) activity (Takakai *et al.* 2008).

There are a few authors who give conflicting information regarding the safety of this oil – especially with regard to its uses in pregnancy and epilepsy (Price and Price 2007). Tisserand and Balacs (1995) suggest that oral doses are contraindicated in pregnancy, epilepsy and fever, and that the Tunisian 1,8-cineole CT should be used in aromatherapy practice, as it has a lower camphor content (10–13% compared with 17–25% in the Spanish oil). For some uses of the 1,8-cineole type, please see Table 8.17, and for more detail about the chemotypes, see Soulier (1996) and Mailhebiau, Goëb and Azémar (1996).

Table 8.17 Rosemary CT 1,8-cineole essential oil in aromatherapy

System	Rosemary with
Musculoskeletal (pain)	Lavender, lavandin, marjoram, basil, clary sage, juniperberry, lemongrass, black pepper
Nervous system (pain, e.g. migraine or headaches, neuralgia)	Lavender, peppermint, German chamomile, geranium, clove bud
Debility, fatigue	Lavender, thyme CT linalool, *Thymus saturoides*, pine, basil
Respiratory (catarrh, congestion, bronchitis, coughs)	*Thymus mastichina*, eucalyptus (1,8-cineole types), peppermint, Atlas cedarwood

Genus Salvia

There are four essential oil-bearing plants that belong to this genus. These are Spanish sage, common sage, Greek sage and clary sage.

Salvia lavandulaefolia — lavender-leaved sage, or Spanish sage

In Spain this plant is used to treat a myriad of ills, but is noted for helping maintain and restore health, protect against infection, relieve pain, aid digestion and treat menstrual problems and infertility. The essential oil is dominated by camphor and 1,8-cineole, but some oils also contain significant amounts of limonene and pinene (Lawless 1992). This would indicate applications for the respiratory system and as a general stimulant, but with caution with regard to the camphor content.

Kennedy *et al.* (2010) noted that sage extracts, including that of *S. lavandulaefolia*, have been used for over 2000 years to improve cognition and protect against cognitive decline. An *in vitro* study had already revealed that these extracts inhibit cholinesterase; several current treatments for Alzheimer's disease are plant-derived alkaloids that inhibit cholinesterase, but have side effects. Their 2010 study followed a preliminary *in vitro* investigation, and was a double-blind, placebo-controlled, balanced cross-over study that examined the cognitive/mood effects of a single oral dose of the extract in the essential oil. It was demonstrated that the extract was a cholinesterase inhibitor that improved both mood and cognitive performance in healthy young adults, and suggested that this could be a potential treatment for dementia and the elderly. However, this study involved a single oral dose, and the effects may be different with inhalation or skin absorption. The study by Robbins and Broughan (2007) showed that with inhalation, the effects of *S. lavandulaefolia* on memory are influenced by expectation.

Salvia officinalis — common or 'Dalmatian' sage

Sage was one of the most important herbs of antiquity, and has retained an important place in modern herbalism. Dalmatian sage essential oil is distilled from the leaves of the perennial herb, and has a strong, sweet, herbal, camphoraceous odour (Williams 2000). The essential oil contains α-thujone and β-thujone, neurotoxic ketones, at up to 50 per cent, and camphor, another neurotoxic ketone, at around 26 per cent — not surprisingly, Tisserand and Balacs (1995) state: 'the usual thujone content is sufficiently high to warrant its exclusion from aromatherapy'. Despite this, it is available to aromatherapists, and is used occasionally for its possible action as an emmenagogue.

Salvia sclarea — clary sage

Closely related species are *S. verbenaca* (wild English clary) and *S. praetensis* (meadow sage) — both widely used in past times for diseases of the eyes, as digestives, and in brewing beers and flavouring muscatel-type wines.

Clary sage is sometimes classed as a biennial herb, sometimes as a perennial. The essential oil is extracted from the flowering tops and leaves (Lawless 1995). It has very distinctive odour – sweet, warm, herbal and tea-like (Williams 2000).

Chemically, it is complex, containing over 250 constituents. The dominant constituents are monoterpene alcohols, notably linalool at up to 26 per cent, and esters, especially linalyl acetate, at up to 75 per cent (Price and Price 2007). These are also the dominant constituents of true lavender essential oil. However, clary sage also contains an unusual constituent – sclareol, a diterpene alcohol – a larger molecule with 20 carbon atoms and two hydroxyl functional groups. Molecules of this size are not common in essential oils as they are often too big, and insufficiently volatile, to distil over in the essential oil. Sclareol is present at up to 7 per cent (Price and Price 2007). Its molecular structure resembles oestradiol, and it has been suggested that this is responsible for its 'oestrogenic' effects, although there is no evidence for this (Bowles 2003). It could also be possible that these effects are brought about via the limbic system.

Clary sage is an exceptionally useful essential oil. In addition to its potential therapeutic benefits to the female reproductive system, possibly helping with irregular menstruation, painful menstruation, menopausal symptoms, perimenopause and PMS, it has antispasmodic, neurotonic, analgesic and antidepressant actions, coupled with the ability to bring about a state of euphoria.

In 2010 Seol *et al.* conducted an animal study to examine the antidepressant effects of several essential oils, and demonstrated that of all the oils tested, clary sage (at a 5% concentration) has the strongest anti-stressor effect, probably by modulating dopamine activities. They suggest that clary sage could be developed as a therapeutic medication for depression.

It is not toxic, although some writers indicate that it is contraindicated in pregnancy. It is also often said that it is not advisable to either consume alcohol or even drive if clary has been used; however, there is absolutely no evidence to support these cautions. For the use of clary sage in aromatherapy, please see Table 8.18.

Table 8.18 Clary sage essential oil in aromatherapy

System	Clary sage with
Musculoskeletal (pain, spasm)	Lavender, Roman chamomile, basil, geranium, juniperberry, lemongrass, black pepper
Female reproductive	Geranium, rose, jasmine, sweet fennel
Nervous system (debility, depression)	Lavender, geranium, jasmine, rose, citrus oils, especially bergamot, mandarin, sweet orange, bitter orange
Respiratory (asthma, spasm, coughs)	Lavender, bergamot

Salvia triloba – Greek or Cretan sage

This species has been used in medicine as an antispasmodic, astringent, haemostatic and diuretic, but also as a culinary herb and in perfumery. The main constituents are 1,8-cineole and limonene (around 38%) camphor at 15 per cent, terpineol and borneol at around 7 per cent and thujone at 6–7 per cent, and α- and β-pinenes at 5–6 per cent (Harvala, Menounos and Argyriadou 1987). This would indicate that it should be used with caution; however, it has been used as an antiviral for cold sores (herpes simplex Type 1, HST1) and the human papilloma virus (HPV).

Genus *Thymus*

The genus *Thymus* is botanically complex, with over 100 species and varieties or cultivars (Soulier 1995). Essential oils can be extracted from many species, including *Thymus serpyllum* (wild thyme), *T. capitatus* (Spanish oregano), *T. mastichina* (Spanish marjoram), *T. saturoides* (Moroccan thyme), *T. vulgaris* (common thyme) and *T. zygis* (Spanish thyme).

In addition, several *T. vulgaris* chemotypes are available for use in aromatic medicine and aromatherapy, including CT thymol, carvacrol, linalool and geraniol. In general, from a safety point of view, oils with a high content of the phenols thymol and carvacrol will be dermal irritants and strong mucous membrane irritants (Tisserand and Balacs 1995).

Historically, thyme is an important herb. It is a tough perennial with tiny, dark green leaves, although there are many decorative varieties too. Like many of the other members of its family, it is a bee plant – Greek honeys are characterised by its distinctive flavour. In ancient Greece thyme was burned as a fumigant to repel insects. In fact, the name comes from the Greek word meaning 'to fumigate'. As well as being a culinary and strewing herb, thyme was used medicinally, especially for the throat, chest and digestion (Gordon 1980).

Thymus vulgaris – common thyme

The essential oil is distilled from the fresh or partially dried leaves and flowering tops of the herb (Lawless 1995). The first distillate is red in colour and cloudy in appearance – this is termed 'red thyme oil'. This can be filtered and redistilled to produce 'white thyme oil'. They both have a sharp, warm herbal odour.

If the chemotype is not specified, it is likely that the essential oil will contain up to 60 per cent phenols, and also the monoterpenes *para*-cymene and γ-terpinene (Lawless 1995; Bowles 2003). Tisserand and Balacs (1995) give some detail regarding the chemistry of the thyme oils – see Table 8.19. Soulier (1995) gives more detail regarding the chemistry of the thyme oils available for use in aromatherapy. See Table 8.20 for a summary.

Table 8.19 Chemotypes of thyme (according to Tisserand and Balacs 1995)

Chemotype	Thymol	Carvacrol
Thymol	32–63%	1–5%
Carvacrol	1–13%	23–44%
Thymol/carvacrol	26%	26%

Table 8.20 Thyme oil chemistry

Thymus vulgaris – **wild CT**	**Main chemical constituent(s)**
French, wild *Thymus vulgaris*, low altitude	Thymol or carvacrol
French, wild *Thymus vulgaris*, high altitude	Linalool
French, wild *Thymus vulgaris*, high altitude on exposed slopes	Geraniol (rare)
Thymus species	
Thymus zygis (Spanish thyme)	Thymol (50–75%)
Thymus capitatus (Spanish oregano)	Carvacrol (70–85%)
Thymus mastichina (Spanish marjoram)	1,8-cineole (60–75%) and linalool (5–20%)
Thymus saturoides (Moroccan thyme)	Borneol (15–30%)
Thymus serpyllum (wild thyme)	Thymol – usually adulterated

A blend of four UK grown cultivars of *Thymus zygis*, and a single linalool chemotype of *T. zygis* in jojoba oil, was investigated with regard to activity against two strains of methicillin-sensitive and two strains of methicillin-resistant *Staphylococcus aureus*. The blend contained significant amounts of thymol and linalool, with relatively high concentrations of α-terpinene and terpinen-4-ol, which are not usually present in thyme oils – being characteristic of tea tree (Caplin, Allan and Hanlon 2009). The study showed that the blend had 'substantial' inhibitory and bactericidal activities on all of the strains of *Staphylococcus*, and was more effective than the *T. zygis* CT linalool alone. They suggested that the blend was a potential hand disinfectant for reducing staphylococci on the skin, and the decolonisation of nasal staphylococci.

Price and Price (2007) give indications and actions for seven thyme oils. All are credited with antimicrobial, warming, tonic and stimulant properties, and some are antispasmodic and mucolytic. The thyme oils have applications in many circumstances, such as muscular aches and pains, debility, fatigue, respiratory congestion and coughs and low immunity. They all blend well with other herbal oils, and should be blended with non-irritant oils, especially lavender, rosemary and marjoram; also citrus (bergamot and lemon). Thyme oils should be used with caution on hypersensitive, diseased or damaged skin, or on children under two, and thyme should not be used at more than 1 per cent concentration on mucous membranes (Tisserand and Balacs 1995). For this reason, thyme oils should not be evaporated.

Table 8.21 shows a summary of the properties of the thymes.

Table 8.21 Thyme properties and indications (according to Soulier 1995 and Price and Price 2007)

Thyme species and chemotype	Properties and indications
Thymus mastichina	Catarrhal bronchitis Viral and bacterial infections
Thymus saturoides	Arthritis Fatigue, debility
Thymus vulgaris CT linalool	Immunostimulant Counteracts fatigue Neurotonic, psychic and cerebral Stimulant Anti-tussive Anti-infectious
Thymus vulgaris CT geraniol	Cardiotonic (Price and Price 2007)
Thymus vulgaris CT thymol	Broncho-pulmonary Anti-infectious esp. chronic infections Anti-tussive Immunostimulant Mucolytic Warming

FAMILY LAURACEAE

This is a very large family of tropical and subtropical plants, which contains over 2000 trees and shrubs. Many members of this family, including the genera *Aniba*, *Cinnamomum*, *Laurus*, *Litsea* and *Ravensara*, produce essential oils of commercial and medicinal significance (Weiss 1997).

GENUS ANIBA

This genus is closely related to *Cinnamomum*, and many species produce essential oil. The most significant members of the genus *Aniba* are *A. duckei*, *A. parviflora* and *A. rosaeodora*, all of which yield rosewood, or *bois de rose*, essential oil.

The most common species, from the aromatherapy essential oil trade perspective, would appear to be *A. rosaeodora* from Brazil. The essential oil is obtained from the wood chips from the tropical evergreen. There are environmental issues associated with its production: there are major concerns over deforestation (Santana *et al.* 1997), and rosewood was included on the endangered species list, leading to the preparation of sustainable management plans; however, Burfield (2004) commented that there was no independent audit of the bio-resources and cast doubt on the actual relevance of such initiatives. The essential oil is a colourless mobile liquid with a mild, sweet, woody, floral odour (Lawless 1995).

According to Bowles, rosewood contains linalool as its major component at 85.3 per cent, followed by α-terpineol at 3.5 per cent and *cis*-linalool oxide at 1.5 per cent. According to Burfield (2004) the linalool content is usually in the region of 84–93 per cent and is a racemic mix of *d*- and *l*-linalool. Price and Price (2007) highlight rosewood's applications as an antifungal for candida and as an 'anti-infectious' agent for respiratory infections; also for its stimulating and tonic qualities, which can aid in cases of general debility, overwork, sexual debility, nervous depression and stress-related headaches. For some uses of rosewood in aromatherapy, please see Table 8.22.

Table 8.22 Rosewood essential oil in aromatherapy

System	Rosewood with
Nervous (stress, debility, etc.)	Lavender, bergamot, clary sage, geranium, lemon, palmarosa, lemongrass, jasmine
Integumentary (including infections)	Lemongrass, lavender, palmarosa, geranium
Respiratory	Sandalwood, ginger, benzoin, lemon

GENUS CINNAMOMUM

This genus contains around 200 species. Several of these are significant from an essential oil and aromatherapy perspective. These are *Cinnamomum camphora*, the botanical source of camphor essential oils, and also ravintsara (also inaccurately described as ravensara) essential oil; *C. cassia* yielding cassia or Chinese cinnamon, and *C. verum* (previously *C. zeylanicum*), which is the source of cinnamon bark and leaf oils.

CINNAMOMUM CAMPHORA – CAMPHOR AND RAVINTSARA

The Japanese *C. camphora* is known as *hon-sho* is considered to be the true camphor tree, and the botanical source of camphor essential oil. Crude camphor exudes from the wood of the tall evergreen, via the fissures in the bark; the roots also contain the volatile oil (Weiss 1997).

The essential oil is steam distilled from the crude camphor, rectified under vacuum, producing three fractions – white (lightest), brown and yellow camphor. Because of this they are not classed as true essential oils, as they are incomplete. Only the white camphor has use in aromatherapy, as the safrole content of the other fractions is high, in brown camphor at 80 per cent and 20 per cent in yellow. Safrole is a very toxic compound, associated with genotoxicity and carcinogenicity (Tisserand and Balacs 1995). White camphor is dominated by the ketone known as 'camphor' at 30–50 per cent, and the oxide 1,8-cineole at 50 per cent (Tisserand and Balacs 1995). Its camphor content confers potential convulsant and neurotoxic hazards, so white camphor essential oil is contraindicated in epilepsy, fever, pregnancy and children under two (Tisserand and Balacs 1995). White camphor is rarely used in aromatherapy, and if it is used it should be with caution.

C. camphora was introduced to Madagascar in the middle of the nineteenth century, and now grows wild in the central eastern region. This species is known to produce subspecies and four distinct chemotypes. The cineole type contains around 76 per cent 1,8-cineole, and also 20 per cent α-pinene and α-terpinene. The linalool type is dominated by linalool at around 80 per cent with 10 per cent monoterpenes – this is available as ho oil. The safrole type contains 80 per cent safrole and 10 per cent monoterpenols. Finally, the nerolidol type contains 40–60 per cent nerolidol with 20 per cent each of monoterpenoids and sesquiterpenoids (Behra, Rakotoarison and Harris 2001).

Ravintsara essential oil is obtained from the Madagascan *C. camphora* leaf; this is the cineole chemotype. It has a fresh, clean, cineolic scent, and the main components are 1,8-cineole at 53–68 per cent, sabinene at 12–15 per cent, α- and β-pinenes at up to 10 per cent, and myrcene at around 1–2 per cent. It has very low camphor content (if any), so the above contraindications do not apply to ravintsara oil. It appears to be strongly antiviral and antimicrobial and an excellent nerve tonic (Behra *et al.* 2001).

Jeannot *et al.* (2007) give a similar list of constituents; they also note an α-terpineol content of up to 8.7 per cent and terpinen-4-ol at up to 3.6 per cent. This is similar to the figures given by Price and Price (1997) for *Ravensara aromatica* essential oil. Its therapeutic properties have been described in relation to its constituents. It is indicated as an anti-inflammatory for bronchial asthma, and is also a bronchodilator – it has been suggested that 1,8-cineole inhibits cytokine and prostaglandin production by stimulating monocytes in vitro (Juergens, Stöber and Vetter 1998, cited in Jeannot *et al.* 2007).

The aromatherapy literature does give indications for ravintsara, under the guise of 'ravensara'. Price and Price (1997) highlight its anti-infectious applications – for glandular fever, bronchitis, flu, sinusitis and whooping cough. Here it is also cited as an antiviral, useful for chicken pox, dendrites, herpes zoster, viral enteritis and viral hepatitis. Schnaubelt (1995, 1999) suggests that it is a central nervous system tonic with uplifting qualities, making it a good choice in cases of flu. He also states that it is helpful for insomnia. Ravintsara can be used with the fixed oil of *Calophylum inophyllum* (also from Madagascar) to alleviate the pain of shingles. For its uses according to Schnaubelt, see Table 8.23.

Table 8.23 Ravintsara essential oil (adapted from Schnaubelt 1995, 1999)

System	Ravintsara with
Immune/Respiratory (viral infections) Asthma	*Eucalyptus radiata* (50:50 topical application over thorax, and inhalation) Inhalation, with lavender
Immune/Herpes zoster (shingles)	50:50 with tamanu fixed oil (*Calophylum inophyllum*) applied to lesions
Nervous (insomnia)	Osmanthus absolute

CINNAMOMUM CASSIA – CHINESE CASSIE (OR CASSIA)

This essential oil is not used in aromatherapy because it is a strong dermal sensitizer and mucous membrane irritant. It contains very large amounts of cinnamaldehyde, in the region of 75–90 per cent (Tisserand and Balacs 1995).

CINNAMOMUM VERUM (ZEYLANICUM) – CINNAMON BARK AND LEAF

Two cinnamon oils are available – one from the inner bark and one from the leaves. The tree is native to wet tropical regions of Sri Lanka, India and Southeast Asia (Weiss 1997). Cinnamon bark oil is not used in aromatherapy as it is a dermal irritant, a strong dermal sensitizer and a mucous membrane irritant. This is mainly due to the eugenol content of up to 18 per cent and cinnamaldehyde content of up to 75 per cent (Tisserand and Balacs 1995).

Cinnamon leaf oil can be used in aromatherapy, although the suggested maximum concentration is 3 per cent. Tisserand and Balacs cite numerous oral contraindications related to the eugenol content. Eugenol is hepatotoxic and inhibits blood clotting. The leaf oil contains 70–90 per cent eugenol and traces of safrole (<1%). Cinnamon leaf essential oil is a light yellow/brownish, mobile liquid with a somewhat harsh, warm, spicy odour. It is used in perfumery and confectionary. Because of its eugenol content, cinnamon leaf oil is rubefacient and antimicrobial. In aromatherapy, Lawless (1995) suggests that it can be used to improve circulation, aid the digestive system, support the immune system and ease conditions such as debility and stress. See Table 8.24 for some uses of cinnamon leaf oil in aromatherapy.

Table 8.24 Cinnamon leaf essential oil in aromatherapy

System	Cinnamon leaf with
Cardiovascular (poor peripheral circulation) Musculoskeletal (aches and pains, rheumatism)	Lavender, nutmeg, lemongrass, citrus oils, e.g. grapefruit, lemon
Digestive	Coriander seed, cardamom, palmarosa, sweet orange, mandarin, lime
Nervous/Immune (debility, stress-related conditions, susceptibility to infection)	Lavender, lemon, bay laurel, ravintsara, rosewood, ylang ylang, lime

GENUS LAURUS

LAURUS NOBILIS — LAUREL LEAF OR BAY LAUREL

This is a small genus. *L. nobilis* produces laurel essential oil, sometimes called bay laurel essential oil. This should not be confused with the bay essential oil from *Pimenta racemosa*. *L. nobilis* is a tree with dark green, lanceolate leaves, known as bay leaves, which are widely used in food flavouring – an important ingredient in a *bouquet garni*. It produces clusters of small flowers and black/purple berries which also yield an essential oil.

The laurel leaf is also known for its symbolism, as the victor's wreath that crowned men in ancient Greece and Rome. However, a wreath of bay leaves also was a sign of academic distinction; we still have the 'poet laureate', and European countries have the academic award of '*baccalaureate*', which means 'laurel and berries'. From the time of Hippocrates, the aromatic leaves were used to keep infection at bay, and in Elizabethan times it was used as a strewing herb in the homes of 'distinguished persons' (Gordon 1980).

The essential oil is obtained by steam distillation from the bay leaves. It is dominated by 1,8-cineole at 40–45 per cent and it also contains linalool (10%), the ester α-terpinyl acetate (9%), various monoterpenes and monoterpene alcohols. It may also contain up to 5 per cent methyleugenol. The chemical composition can vary widely, however, depending on the distillation method. It is a colourless or very pale yellow, mobile liquid, with a strong, sweet, aromatic, camphoraceous odour. It is a major ingredient in a Syrian olive oil soap (Aleppo's *sabun bi ghar*), which has been exported for over 500 years (Weiss 1997).

Laurel leaves are used topically for the relief of rheumatic pain in traditional Iranian medicine. An animal study conducted by Sayyah *et al.* (2003) indicated that the leaf oil had anti-nociceptive and anti-inflammatory actions that were comparable with conventional analgesic and non-steroidal anti-inflammatory medications. They also noted that it has mild sedative properties.

According to Tisserand and Balacs (1995), laurel leaf oil is a potential sensitizer and mucous membrane irritant. Schnaubelt (1999) suggests that it is most useful for lymphatic support during the treatment of upper respiratory tract infections – applied neat over the lymph nodes. For some uses of laurel leaf, please see Table 8.25.

Table 8.25 Laurel leaf essential oil in aromatherapy

System	Laurel leaf with
Musculoskeletal (pain, including arthritis and rheumatism)	Lavender, pine, juniperberry, rosemary, geranium, clove bud
Immune	Ravintsara, niaouli, thyme CT linalool
Respiratory	Ravintsara, sweet marjoram, spike lavender

GENUS LITSEA

LITSEA CUBEBA – MAY CHANG

This is a fairly large genus; the most significant essential oil producer is *L. cubeba*. A citral-rich essential oil known as may chang is obtained from the small fruits (resembling the cubeb pepper) of the small, fragrant tropical tree. China is the largest producer and consumer of this product. The essential oil is a pale yellow, mobile liquid with an intense, lemon, fresh-fruity odour (Weiss 1997).

The oil is characterised by its high citral content (85%). Bowles cites may chang as containing geranial (40%), neral (33.8%) and limonene (8.3%). Geranial and neral are the isomers known in combination (a racemic mixture) as 'citral'. Citral can be irritating to the skin and mucous membranes, but it is also credited with calming, sedative properties according to Franchomme and Pénoël (1990, cited in Bowles 2003, p. 83).

Lawless (1995) suggests that may chang is useful for its antiseptic and deodorant qualities, that it is a digestive and stomachic, and a sedative that can combat tension and stress-related conditions. She also mentions research that has shown that may chang can be of value in the treatment of cardiac arrhythmia; unfortunately this is not referenced. For some uses of may chang oil, especially in relation to its citral content, please see Table 8.26.

Table 8.26 May chang essential oil in aromatherapy

System	May chang with
Nervous (stress-related problems)	Lavender, rosewood, bergamot, palmarosa, geranium, rose, neroli or jasmine
Integumentary (excessive perspiration or odour)	Palmarosa, geranium, bergamot, peppermint, sandalwood
Digestive	Ginger, black pepper, mandarin

GENUS RAVENSARA

The genus *Ravensara* is native to Madagascar – a biodiversity 'hotspot'. The name is derived from the Malagasy word '*ravintsara*', which means 'good leaves'. In recent years there has been a lot of confusion around the taxonomy of the species that yield an essential oil which is often supplied to the aromatherapy profession as 'ravensara' essential oil. In an attempt to clarify this situation, Behra *et al.* (2001) suggest that *R. aromatica* leaf essential oil should be referred to as 'aromatic ravensare', *R. aromatica* bark essential oil as 'havozo' and *C. camphora* leaf essential oil as 'ravintsara'. For the aromatherapeutic applications of ravintsara, please refer to the profile of the essential oil of *Cinnamomum camphora* from Madagascar. By the late 1990s and the early 2000s the genus *Ravensara* had been over-exploited and subject to deforestation, although it was still abundant in the Madagascan rainforests. Behra *et al.* (2001) stressed the importance of only using essential oils that are produced from sustainable sources.

R. aromatica bark yields an essential oil known as 'havozo' (meaning 'aromatic tree'). This species is indigenous to Madagascar, and is easily recognised by its small green flowers; its fruits also yield an essential oil. It is also known as the Madagascar clove-nutmeg (Weiss 1997). The essential oil has an anisic odour and is dominated by phenolic ethers such as methyl chavicol (around 90%) and anethole. Generally, it is not recommended that oils with such high levels of methyl chavicol are used in aromatherapy – however, this one does have useful antimicrobial potential: it is active against *E. coli* (De Medici, Pieretti and Salvatore 1992, cited in Behra *et al.* 2001).

Aromatic ravensare is the leaf oil from *R. aromatica* and, unlike the bark oil, this does have aromatherapeutic applications. It has a sweet, fresh, lemony, cineolic odour and its main constituents are sabinene (10.2–16.4%), limonene (13.9–22.5%), myrcene (5–7.3%), linalool (3.57%) and 1–8 cineole (1.8–3.3%). It is said to be strongly antiviral, and a general tonic and anti-stress remedy (Behra *et al.* 2001).

GENUS SASSAFRAS

This very small genus contains one essential oil-producing species, *Sassafras albidum*. Sassafras essential oil is obtained from the dried root bark of this large deciduous tree. The essential oil contains 85–90 per cent safrole and thus is not used in aromatherapy due to its toxicity and carcinogenic potential.

FAMILY MYRISTACEAE

The family belongs to the order Magnoliales, and contains the large genus *Myristica*.

GENUS MYRISTICA

Generally, the *Myristica* are evergreen rainforest trees, which produce yellow, fleshy drupes. Only one is of major significance: *Myristica fragrans* – the seed is the source of nutmeg, and the aril (the membrane around the seed) is the source of mace (Weiss 1997). Nutmeg and mace essential oils are widely used in the flavour and fragrance industries; they also have aromatherapy applications. Nutmeg is more commonly used than mace.

MYRISTICA FRAGRANS – NUTMEG

Nutmeg essential oil is a pale yellow, mobile liquid with a fresh, slightly piney top note and warm, spicy middle notes (Williams 2000). It is dominated by monoterpenes – around 75 per cent (Price and Price 1997). According to Bowles (2003), nutmeg is typically composed of α-pinene (22%), sabinene (18%) and β-pinene (15.6%) with terpinen-4-ol (7.9%) and the phenolic ether myristicin at 6 per cent.

The predominance of monoterpenes may suggest that nutmeg essential oil is astringent, tonic and a mild rubefacient with analgesic potential. The presence of myristicin along with small amounts of elemicin was at one time cited as conferring stupefying and psychotropic effects to nutmeg essential oil (Lawless

1992). However, the amounts used in aromatherapy are too small to carry this risk. There are also traces of safrole and methyleugenol – both potentially carcinogenic constituents. For this reason Tisserand and Balacs (1995) suggest that it is better to use West Indian nutmeg in aromatherapy, as the East Indian oil contains more safrole (up to 3.3%).

Nutmeg essential oil is indicated as an analgesic, digestive stimulant and tonic (neurotonic, reproductive stimulant, uterine tonic) (Price and Price 1997). They also cite Reynolds (1972) with reference to nutmeg as an inhibitor of prostaglandin synthesis. In their 1994 review of nutmeg, Tisserand and Balacs confirm that this effect is due to ground nutmeg rather than the essential oil. However they do discuss the potential psychotropic effects of the essential oil at length, and suggest that the oil may certainly be of use in diarrhoea, hypertension, rheumatoid arthritis, anxiety, depression and sleep disorders. Please see Table 8.27 for some suggested uses in aromatherapy.

Table 8.27 Nutmeg essential oil in aromatherapy

System	Nutmeg with
Nervous (pain – muscles, joints, rheumatic, neuralgia, sciatica); dysmenorrhoea	Lavender, ginger, black pepper, juniperberry, sweet fennel, grapefruit
Debility, anxiety, depression	Sandalwood, cardamom, jasmine or rose
Digestive	Ginger, coriander seed, cardamom, all citrus oils

FAMILY MYRTACEAE

From the aromatherapy perspective, this family is one of the most important. It is a large family, containing 75 genera and around 3000 species. Most members of the family are tropical trees and shrubs indigenous to tropical regions of America, Asia and Australia. The genera of interest to aromatherapists are *Agonis, Eucalyptus, Leptospermum, Melaleuca, Myrtus, Pimenta* and *Syzigium* (formerly known as *Eugenia*).

GENUS AGONIS

AGONIS FRAGRANS – FRAGONIA

A. fragrans is the botanical source of a relatively new essential oil named by its discoverer, botanist Chris Robinson (Wheeler *et al.* 2001); it has since been trademarked as Fragonia™. The essential oil is steam distilled from the fresh leafy twigs/terminal branches of this small, shrubby tree that is native to Australia.

The odour is described as cineolic (eucalyptus-like) and herbaceous/balsamic, with cinnamon-like notes. It has been compared to tea tree essential oil in many ways; the general consensus is that it has a more acceptable aroma for general aromatherapy use, including massage. Fragonia is also finding its way into the phytocosmeceutical industry.

The essential oil contains roughly equal proportions of 1,8-cineole (26–33%), α-pinene (22–27%) and monoterpene alcohols such as α-terpineol (5–8%), linalool, geraniol and terpinen-4-ol. This is considered to be the ideal ratio of these compounds for the treatment of respiratory infections (Pénoël 2005, cited in Turnock 2006). Fragonia is being investigated in relation to its many potential therapeutic actions, including analgesic, anti-inflammatory, expectorant and antimicrobial properties. It would appear to be a potent antimicrobial that is active against *Escherichia coli*, *Staphylococcus aureus* and *Candida albicans* (Carson 2006, cited in Turnock 2006). Pénoël (2006) has also commented on its effects on the psyche, maintaining that it is remarkably soothing and has the ability to unblock the emotions.

Some suggested uses in aromatherapy are as an expectorant (especially if infection is present), for pain and inflammation (including arthritic pain), as a substitute for tea tree for its antimicrobial actions, and to balance the emotions.

GENUS EUCALYPTUS

This is a very large genus. Most of the Eucalypts are indigenous to Australia; however, they are adaptable and have been introduced to many countries, worldwide. Many Eucalypts yield essential oil from their leaves and twigs, most of which find applications in the pharmaceutical, flavour and fragrance industries. Many of the essential oils have aromatherapy applications.

The species that have most significance in aromatherapy and aromatic medicine, because of their expectorant and other properties, and high content of the oxide 1,8 cineole, are *Eucalyptus globulus* var. *globulus* (blue gum), *E. polybractea* (blue-leaved mallee), *E. dives* (broad leaved peppermint), *E. radiata* (narrow leaved peppermint), *E. smithii* (gully-gum) and *E. viridis* var. *viridis* (green mallee). The medicinal eucalyptus oils are often referred to as '*eucapharma* oils' (Weiss 1997). *E. citriodora*, the lemon-scented gum, produces an essential oil with a characteristically high content of citronellal. This does not possess expectorant properties, but it is strongly antimicrobial, and it too has uses in aromatherapy. *E. staigeriana*, the lemon-scented ironbark, is also being used in aromatherapy.

E. CITRIODORA — LEMON-SCENTED EUCALYPTUS OR GUM

E. citriodora is very different from all of the above, in that it is not characterised by a high 1,8-cineole content. The essential oil is a colourless to pale yellow liquid with a strong, fresh, rosy-citronella odour; the ISO specification states that it should contain a minimum of 70 per cent citronellal (Weiss 1997). Price and Price (1997) note that other significant constituents include its parent alcohol citronellol, *iso*-pulegol and 1,8-cineole – although this can range from 0.4 per cent to 17.9 per cent. Citronellal may have calming and antifungal properties (Bowles 2003). Price and Price (1997) state that its bacteriostatic properties are due to a natural synergism between citronellal and citronellol, and that the oil is active against *Staphylococcus aureus*. They also claim that it has antifungal activity. Therefore, although this is not classed as a 'medicinal' essential oil, it may have considerable use in treating some infections, perhaps even methicillin-resistant *S. aureus* (MRSA).

E. DIVES – BROAD LEAVED-PEPPERMINT

This species has several chemotypes – 1,8-cineole, piperitone and phellandrene. It is interesting that it is not cultivated in its native Australia. Price and Price (1997) give some information regarding the piperitone chemotype and its uses. They state that it contains 40–50 per cent of the ketone piperitone and 30 per cent α-phellandrene. Although it is safe for 'normal' aromatherapy use, they suggest that it is contraindicated for babies and pregnant women, citing Franchomme and Pénoël (1990). Its main uses are for infections and wound healing, but the information is scant. Price and Price also comment that Beckstrom-Sternberg and Duke (1996) state that piperitone is anti-asthmatic and an insectifuge.

EUCALYPTUS GLOBULUS VAR. GLOBULUS – EUCALYPTUS BLUE GUM

This is the most commonly available eucalyptus essential oil; it usually referred to simply as eucalyptus oil or globulus oil. The blue gum is grown for its timber as well as for essential oil production. It is grown in its native Tasmania and Southern Victoria; Spain, China and South America are also significant producers. The essential oil is rectified, as the crude globulus oil has an unpleasant odour that is caused by lower aliphatic aldehydes, which can also cause irritation and coughing when inhaled (Weiss 1997). There are standard specifications for globulus oil – published by the International Standards Organisation (ISO) and the British Standards Institution (BSI). According to these, the 1,8-cineole content should be 80–85 per cent. Globulus oil is typically water-white with a refreshing cineolic (eucalyptus-like) odour.

    E. globulus essential oil is therefore dominated by its oxide, which has been fairly well investigated with regard to safety and therapeutic actions. In large amounts, 1,8-cineole can have neurotropic effects (slurred speech, coma, convulsions), and it can cause respiratory irritation, as it is a rubefacient and mucous membrane irritant. Bowles (2003) cites Pénoël and Franchomme (1990) who suggest that *E. globulus* should be used with care in asthma.

Its therapeutic effects are considerable. 1,8-cineole is an expectorant, an anti-inflammatory in cases of bronchial asthma, and it may also be a stimulant of the trigeminal nerve – hence its ability to increase alertness (Bowles 2003). Buchbauer (1996) states that 1,8-cineole can increase cerebral blood flow, and has also suggested that it has spasmolytic properties (1993). Balacs (1997), in a comprehensive review of cineole-rich oils, explores the pharmacokinetics of 1,8-cineole, emphasising that this compound is absorbed very quickly from the air into the bloodstream.

A double-blind, placebo-controlled, randomised clinical trial conducted by Kehrl, Sonnemann and Dethlefsen (2004) investigated the potential of 1,8-cineole as a treatment for acute, non-purulent rhinosinusitis. The cineole, delivered in enteric coated capsules, was shown to thin and drain secretions and reduce inflammation, compared with the placebo.

Apart from 1,8-cineole, globulus oil contains significant amounts of α-pinene (up to 27%) and limonene (Price and Price 1997; Bowles 2003). Aromatherapy applications include a myriad of respiratory problems (thanks to its expectorant and decongestant actions), including infections, bronchitis, sinusitis, etc. It is indicated for relief of muscular aches and pains. An animal study (Silva *et al.* 2003) indicated that it has peripheral anti-nociceptive activity and dose-related central analgesic activity, in addition to having anti-inflammatory effects. *E. globulus* is also used as an antiseptic for urinary tract infections and relief of migraine (Price and Price 1997). Pénoël (1992) suggests that *E. globulus* is particularly useful for all respiratory infections, especially 'deep' ones, flu, otitis, sinusitis and rhinitis, viral infections, lymphatic node infections, bacterial and fungal dermatitis and rheumatism.

E. POLYBRACTEA – BLUE LEAVED MALLEE

In its native Australia, this is considered to be the most suitable species for large-scale production of *Eucalyptus* oil – it benefits the local economy as it does not grow well elsewhere, and it has a very high essential oil yield and a higher natural cineole content than *E. globulus* typically 70–90 per cent, and so is an excellent natural source for isolating cineole. Like globulus oil, it is usually rectified; the rectified oil has a sweet, cineolic, camphoraceous odour. Other important constituents are *p*-cymene, terpinen-4-ol, α-pinene, limonene, β-pinene and sabinene (Weiss 1997).

E. RADIATA — NARROW-LEAVED PEPPERMINT

This species is widely used in aromatherapy, often in preference to other cineole-rich oils, as it would appear to have no associated hazards or contraindications. According to Weiss (1997), the oil is colourless to pale yellow with a fresh, powerful, peppery-camphoraceous odour; and a 1,8-cineole content of up to 50 per cent and phellandrene up to 40 per cent. Price and Price (1997) emphasise its use as energizing oil for chronic fatigue and immune deficiency, but also as an expectorant/mucolytic, especially in combination with *E. smithii* (see below). They also suggest that it is important to blend it with terpene-rich oils for best results – they do not give any suggestions, but Scots pine would be appropriate. Pénoël (1992), in his article 'Winter Shield' gives a very different chemical composition from Weiss (1997) and Price and Price (1997) – giving an oxide content of 70 per cent, and no mention of phellandrene. He suggests that *E. radiata* is useful for all respiratory infections (but not as 'deep' as discussed in relation to globulus), acne, vaginitis and endometriosis, and that it can be inhaled on its own or with rosemary.

E. SMITHII — GULLY-GUM

This species yields a cineole-rich essential oil. It is not cultivated in Australia, so the oil from Australia is obtained from wild trees. It is grown commercially in South Africa and Argentina. The 1,8-cineole content is 70–80 per cent, and the rectified oil has a fresh cineolic scent (Weiss 1997). Price and Price (1997) cite properties and indications that are very similar to *E. globulus*, except that *E. smithii* also has 'balancing' qualities and that it is safe to use, undiluted, as a chest rub.

E. STAIGERIANA — LEMON-SCENTED IRONBARK

E. staigeriana is now available for aromatherapy use, although its applications are not well documented. According to Weiss (1997), the rectified essential oil is used in perfumery and toilet preparations. It has a sweet, fresh, fruity scent, and chemically it contains geraniol (9–18%), methyl geranate, geranyl acetate, limonene, β-phellandrene (12–34%) and neral. If these constituents have the properties described in Bowles (2003), it can be expected that this oil would be a useful antibacterial and antifungal, analgesic and possibly 'hormone balancing' agent in aromatherapy.

E. VIRIDIS VAR. VIRIDIS — GREEN MALLEE

This species tends to co-exist with *E. polybractea* – they are very similar and often harvested indiscriminately. Weiss (1997) indicates that its 1,8-cineole content is around 80 per cent, and that it is used in the same ways as *E. globulus*. In aromatherapy, it may be used in the same ways as other cineole-rich eucalyptus oils.

For some information on the use of the cineole-rich eucalyptus oils, please see Table 8.28.

Table 8.28 Cineole-rich *Eucalyptus* essential oils in aromatherapy

System	Eucalyptus with
Respiratory (coughs, infections, sinusitis)	Lemon, thyme, rosemary, lavender, Scots pine, sandalwood
Musculoskeletal	Black pepper, lavender, basil, rosemary
Nervous (migraine, fatigue, debility)	Lemon, lavender

Genus Leptospermum

This is a fairly large genus, containing around 80 species; however, few of these are cultivated for their essential oils.

Leptospermum petersonii — lemon-scented tea tree

This is the source of a citral- and citronellal-rich essential oil that is used in perfumery, and occasionally in aromatherapy. Citral is isolated from the essential oil and used to produce the violet-scented chemical, ionone. *L. petersonii* essential oil has a lemony, pungent, diffusive odour. Its aromatherapy uses are not well documented, but it would be reasonable to assume that it has antimicrobial, sedative and possibly anti-inflammatory properties due to its aldehydes.

L. scoparium — manuka

Manuka essential oil has been investigated with regard to its antimicrobial properties and medicinal/pharmaceutical applications. It is distilled from the leaves and twigs of a small, shrubby tree which is native to New Zealand. The indigenous Maori and early European settlers used the infusion of the leaves and twigs for a wide variety of ailments, including genito-urinary and gastro-intestinal infections, for pain relief and skin problems (Maddocks-Jennings *et al.* 2005).

Manuka oil has a distinctive odour that is reminiscent of tea tree — perhaps not a scent that has immediate appeal, so its use in aromatherapy massage is limited. However, it can be used successfully in essential oil prescriptions for topical use. The essential oil is chemically complex, and contains around 15 per cent leptospermone, a ketone, along with sesquiterpenes and their oxygenated derivatives (Price 1998). Leptospermone is a cyclic ketone, sometimes described as a ß-triketone, which apparently inactivates hyalarodinase, an enzyme that increases diffusion of toxins in the tissues (a 'spreading factor'). It is postulated that leptospermone can act as an anti-venom spreading agent, and also prevent the diffusion of toxins in the tissues due to infections (Mertz 1994). Price (1998) also states that manuka is an effective antiseptic and antifungal, with potential use against *S. aureus*, including MRSA.

The composition of manuka oil, and that of another New Zealand native – kanuka (the white or tree manuka, originally classified as *L. ericoides* and reclassified as *Kunzea ericoides*) is variable – the geographical source significantly influences this. Manuka oils from the North Island, especially from the East Coast region, typically contain higher levels (>30%) of leptospermone and flavesone (another triketone), while oils from the South Island contain higher percentages (65%) of sesquiterpenes and sesquiterpenoids. Kanuka oil from both the North and South Islands contains *para*-cymene, which is associated with analgesic properties. Both oils contain sesquiterpenes, which may confer anti-inflammatory properties. It has also been suggested that manuka oil is a useful antispasmodic (Maddocks-Jennings *et al.* 2005).

Maddocks-Jennings, Cavanagh and Shillington (2009) evaluated the effects of a mixture of manuka and kanuka (*K. ericoides*) essential oils when used as a mouthwash or gargle to prevent radiation-induced oropharyngeal mucositis. This small study had a positive outcome, in that the patients who used the mouthwash experienced delayed onset of mucositis, and their weight loss was reduced in comparison with the control and placebo groups.

Genus Melaleuca

Often, members of the genus *Melaleuca* are referred to as 'paperbark trees', as typically the bark resembles paper and can be pulled off the tree in strips. Many members are essential oil producers. The species of commercial importance and of significance in aromatherapy and aromatic medicine are *M. alternifolia* (tea tree), *M. cajuputi* (cajuput) and *M. quinquenervia* (niaouli). Essential oils from all three have been the subject of a considerable amount of research into their pharmaceutical and medicinal applications, and they are all used in aromatherapy. Other species of interest are *M. bracteata* (black tea tree) and *M. linariifolia*. A relative newcomer to aromatherapy is *M. ericifolia* (rosalina oil).

Melaleuca alternifolia – tea tree

M. alternifolia is a small, shrub-like paperbark tree, native to northern New South Wales and Queensland in Australia. It reaches 5–8 m, and the mature trees produce loose, whitish flowers with terminal spikes. *M. alternifolia* prefers a marshy soil around rivers and a subtropical climate (Faiyazuddin *et al.* 2009). The essential oil is extracted from the leaves and twigs, and is a colourless to pale yellow or green, mobile liquid (Weiss 1997) with a distinctive, warm, spicy, slightly camphoraceous odour.

The essential oil is characterised by its terpinen-4-ol content – around 45 per cent – and low 1,8-cineole content of 3–17 per cent (Weiss 1997). Price (1998) comments that in the recent past, a 1,8-cineole content of a maximum of 4 per cent was desirable; many oils in fact have a 1,8-cineole content of nearer 15 per cent. Bowles (2003) gives a figure of 3 per cent, with the other significant constituents being γ- and α-terpinene at 15.7 per cent and 7.1 per cent, respectively. *Para*-cymene is also present – usually noted for its analgesic potential, but here it may also be important in the antimicrobial/antifungal actions (Price and Price 1999).

Tea tree oil is a very useful antimicrobial agent. It has been well investigated in this respect, and as a consequence has become very popular in a wide range of skin care and antiseptic products. Tea tree oil is found in formulations for acne, gingivitis, halitosis, toenail infections, *tinea pedis*, oral candidiasis and dandruff. It has broad-spectrum action, and is active against all three groups of pathogenic microorganisms (Faiyazuddin *et al.* 2009). According to Carson and Riley (1995), cited in Bowles (2003), the constituents responsible for this are terpinen-4-ol and α-terpineol. These two compounds usually occur together, sharing the same metabolic pathway. Budhiraja *et al.* (1999), cited in Bowles (2003), suggest that terpinen-4-ol activates monocytes. It also has anti-inflammatory activity (Faiyazuddin *et al.* 2009).

However, in their review of tea tree oil Faiyazuddin *et al.* (2009) comment that in contrast to the many studies exploring the therapeutic benefits of tea tree, there have been few that look at its potential toxicity. They highlight that oral ingestion, especially in children, carries a risk, that in rats the oral LD_{50} is 2.0–2.5 ml/kg, and that doses of <1.5 g/kg can cause ataxia. In addition to this, there is an increased risk of irritation or allergic reaction if oxidised tea tree is applied to the skin. It deteriorates rapidly if not stored correctly, and the degradation products may be responsible for these adverse reactions. Finally, the review cites Bischoff and Guale (1998) who reported cases of dermal toxicity in cats, showing that undiluted tea tree oil produced symptoms of hypothermia, incoordination, dehydration, trembling and the death of one cat in three. This, coupled with unpublished reports of temporary paralysis in dogs exposed to tea tree oil in grooming products and when used as an antiseptic, would suggest that tea tree oil is perhaps best avoided in pet care.

The medicinal odour of tea tree may restrict its popularity in aromatherapy massage, but it often forms part of aromatherapy support treatments. Price and Price (1999) ascribe analgesic, antibacterial, antifungal, antiviral, anti-inflammatory and immunostimulant actions (among others) to tea tree essential oil. They suggest that it is most useful for treating many bacterial infections such as abscesses, acne, bronchitis, genito-urinary infections and MRSA (citing Carson, Hammer and Riley 1995, and Carson *et al.* 1995), and for treating candida infections. Williams *et al.* (1998) and Caelli *et al.* (2001) also give similar indications for tea tree. When using tea tree for its antimicrobial actions, it can be blended with other essential oils that complement these, such as the antiseptic and anti-inflammatory properties of lavender and geranium.

M. CAJUPUTI – CAJUPUT

Cajuput essential oil is extracted from wild trees in Malaysia, Indonesia and Australia. There has been much confusion over its naming, so literature is not always reliable – it has been frequently confused with *M. leucadendron* (Weiss 1997). The rectified product has a strong, camphoraceous, sweet odour (Williams 2000).

Chemically, the essential oil is variable. According to Bowles (2003) the botanical source of cajuput is *M. leucadendron;* and she gives the main components as 1,8-cineole at 41.1 per cent, α-terpineol at 8.7 per cent and *para*-cymene at 6 per cent. Cajuput oil is used as a panacea in its countries of origin; in aromatherapy it is considered to be a useful antimicrobial, expectorant and analgesic, with applications in the treatment of respiratory and urinary tract infections, and for pain (Price and Price 2007).

M. ERICIFOLIA – SWAMP PAPERBARK, ROSALINA

M. ericifolia is the botanical source of rosalina essential oil. This species is native to Australia, especially growing in coastal regions, and recently its essential oil has become popular in aromatherapy. This leaf oil is dominated by monoterpenoids; however, the geographical source influences the constituent profile. Oils from the North give rise to the Type 1 essential oil, which is linalool-rich and cineole-poor; Type 2 oils come from the far South and are cineole-rich and linalool poor (Brophy and Doran 2004). Rosalina has a soft, pine-like, earthy odour. It is said to have a similar therapeutic profile to that of tea tree, and many find its odour more acceptable for massage purposes.

M. QUINQUENERVIA – FIVE-VEINED PAPERBARK, NIAOULI

This species is native to Indonesia, New Caledonia and southern Papua New Guinea, and is the botanical source of essential oil. There are several chemovars, so niaouli oils vary considerably in their chemical composition. Most of the essential oil is produced on the island of New Caledonia and then exported to France, where it is preferred to eucalyptus oil (Weiss 1997). The essential oil is a colourless mobile liquid with a strong, sweet camphoraceous odour (Williams 2000), not dissimilar to eucalyptus.

Bowles (2003) gives the main constituents of niaouli from Madagascar as 1,8-cineole at 41.8 per cent, viridiflorol (a sesquiterpene alcohol) at 18.1 per cent and limonene at 5 per cent.

In aromatherapy practice, niaouli is sometimes referred to as 'MVQ oil' (*Melaleuca viridiflora quinquenervia*). Schnaubelt (1999) indicates that it is important in French aromatic medicine, where it is used for hepatitis and dysplasia of the colon, as a vaginal douche and to protect against radiation burns. He suggests that it can be used topically as an expectorant, an anti-allergenic and anti-asthmatic; he also claims that it is an endocrine tonic. Blending suggestions include tea tree, ravintsara and the fixed oil of *Calophylum inophyllum* – which is apparently successful for the alleviation of haemorrhoids and genital herpes.

A study conducted by Donoyama and Ichiman (2006) revealed that niaouli was the best oil for 'hygienic massage practice', in that it showed greater antibacterial activity than eucalyptus, lavender, sage, tea tree and thyme linalool in relation to the bacteria found on the therapists' hands and the subjects' skin.

GENUS MYRTUS

Only one member of this genus is of importance, *Myrtus communis*, which yields myrtle essential oil. This should not be confused with the toxic essential oil of the wax myrtle (*Myrica* spp.).

MYRTUS COMMUNIS – MYRTLE

M. communis is an evergreen shrub that yields myrtle essential oil from the fresh leaves. It grows in Mediterranean regions and North Africa (Weiss 1997). The essential oil is a yellow to orange or greenish, mobile liquid with a warm, fresh and woody/camphoraceous odour. Bowles (2003) states that the principle components of Spanish myrtle essential oil are myrtenyl acetate (35.9%), 1,8-cineole (29.9%) and α-pinene (8.1%) Myrtle oil is used in aromatherapy mainly for its expectorant qualities, where it can be of value in asthma, bronchitis, catarrh and chronic coughs. It also has applications for skin care, colds and flu (Lawless 1995). Schnaubelt (1999) suggests that it can be used with cypress in cases of pleurisy.

GENUS PIMENTA

This comparatively small genus of aromatic shrubs and trees is indigenous to tropical regions of America, and the Caribbean. Two species are commercially important, as their essential oils are used in the flavour and fragrance industry; they are also available for use in aromatherapy. *Pimenta racemosa*, the bay rum tree, yields a leaf essential oil, and *P. dioica*, the source of allspice, yields pimento berry essential oil (Weiss 1997).

PIMENTA DIOICA – PIMENTO BERRY

Pimento berry essential oil (sometimes known as allspice) is obtained from an evergreen tree native to the West Indies and South America. It produces fruits that are steam distilled to yield a pale yellow, mobile essential oil with a sweet, warm, spicy odour (Lawless 1995). Like bay essential oil, it has very high eugenol content – in the region of 60–95 per cent (Tisserand and Balacs 1995). The same cautions apply. Lawless (1992) gives a slightly different therapeutic profile. She highlights its uses for painful conditions affecting the muscles and joints, for poor circulation, chills, congested coughs, bronchitis and for nervous exhaustion.

PIMENTA RACEMOSA – BAY RUM, WEST INDIAN BAY

This tropical evergreen tree is the botanical source of bay essential oil – often called West Indian bay, to avoid confusion with the essential oil from *Laurus nobilis*, which is also sometimes called bay. The essential oil is obtained from the leaves; it is a yellow, mobile liquid with a fresh, spicy, sweet odour (Williams 2000).

The main chemical constituents, according to Bowles (2003) are eugenol at 56 per cent, chavicol (estragole) at 21.6 per cent and myrcene at 13 per cent – all well noted for their analgesic actions. Tisserand and Balacs (1995) suggest that the eugenol content would imply that the oil is a mucous membrane irritant, potentially hepatotoxic, and that it could inhibit blood clotting. Therefore they contraindicate the oral use of bay oil in a range of situations where there is liver impairment or anticoagulant medication. Topically, they suggest that the maximum concentration should be 3 per cent, although they do note that West Indian bay was not in fact irritating to human skin at 10 per cent.

In aromatherapy, bay oil is most often used as an analgesic for muscle and joint pains, neuralgia, and also for poor circulation. It blends very well with lime, grapefruit and lemon, ylang ylang, lavender, geranium and black pepper.

GENUS SYZYGIUM

The clove was originally classified as *Eugenia caryophyllata*, and a revision of classification placed it in the genus *Syzygium* – it is now correctly referred to as *Syzygium aromaticum*. The clove is a spice of great commercial importance (historically and currently), as is clove bud oil (Weiss 1997). The essential oil also has aromatherapy and aromatic medicine applications, notably to relieve pain and assist the digestion.

SYZYGIUM AROMATICUM – CLOVE

Weiss (1997) gives a very detailed account of the clove, a tree indigenous to the Moluccas, whose buds became an enormously important spice. Clove products include the whole and ground buds that are used as a spice, clove bud oil, clove stem oil and clove leaf oil. The essential oils are also used as a source of eugenol for the pharmaceutical industry (Weiss 1997). In aromatherapy only the clove bud oil is used, as the leaf and stem oils are considered to have too high a eugenol content to be safe (Lawless 1992).

Clove bud oil is a pale yellow, mobile liquid with a warm, fruity, spicy odour (Williams 2000). Its principle chemical constituents are eugenol at 76.6 per cent, β-caryophyllene at 9.8 per cent and eugenyl acetate at 7.6 per cent (Bowles 2003). As you would expect, all of the texts suggest that the essential oil is a powerful antibacterial and analgesic – certainly related to the eugenol content. So the same precautions given by Tisserand and Balacs (1999) for eugenol-rich oils apply to clove bud oil.

Price and Price (2007) suggest that clove bud oil is very useful as an analgesic for rheumatoid arthritis and neuralgia, as an antiseptic in many situations including abscess, acne, ulcers and wounds, as an anti-inflammatory and antispasmodic – especially for the digestive system – as an immunostimulant, and for debility and fatigue. Schnaubelt suggests that for its anti-inflammatory actions, it is most effective at a low concentration of one drop in 20 ml. *In vivo* animal studies demonstrated that the immunostimulatory activity in mice treated with clove essential oil was due to an improvement in humor-mediated and cell-mediated immune response mechanisms (Schmidt *et al.* 2009). Please refer to Table 8.29 for some suggestions for the use of clove bud oil in aromatherapy.

Table 8.29 Clove bud essential oil in aromatherapy

System	Clove bud with
Musculoskeletal/nervous (pain, inflammation)	Lavender, clary sage, geranium, bergamot, bay laurel, West Indian bay, cinnamon leaf
Digestive	Sweet orange, lime, grapefruit, palmarosa
Nervous/immune	Rose or jasmine, lavender, bay laurel, West Indian bay, rosewood, ylang ylang, lime, benzoin resinoid, vanilla absolute

Family Piperaceae

Genus Piper

This family includes 10–12 genera, and the genus *Piper* contains about 1000 species, many of which are tropical shrubs or woody climbers (Weiss 1997), but only one is of interest here.

Piper nigrum – black pepper

Black pepper is a native of the hills of Western India, and also of the wet tropical forests. Its history goes back to Ancient Greece, and in the Middle Ages it was an extremely important commodity for seasoning or preserving meats, and as a medicine. It is a perennial, woody, glabrous (devoid of surface hairs or projections) climber, according to Weiss (1997), with many greenish-purple branches, alternate, ovate, shiny leaves and spikes of small, yellowish-green to whitish flowers. The dehiscent drupe contains a single seed which is green when unripe, becoming red when ripe and black on drying. The dried, black, wrinkled skin contains a single whitish seed, a peppercorn.

Black pepper oil is steam distilled from the imported unripe fruits, which have been dried and ground. The oil is a colourless to pale green mobile liquid, and the aroma, according to Weiss (1997), is similar to the freshly ground spice – fresh and dry-woody, warm and spicy. The main components vary according to the origin and method of harvesting and drying, so as there is no such thing as typical black pepper oil, it is often said to be dominated by terpenoid hydrocarbons (about 70–80%). Limonene is present from 0–40 per cent, β-pinene 5–35 per cent, α-pinene 1–19 per cent, α-phellandrene 1–27 per cent, β-phellandrene 0–19 per cent, sabinene 0–20 per cent, δ-3-carene trace and up to 15 per cent, and myrcene trace and up to 10 per cent. Sesquiterpenes are also present, notably β-caryophyllene, from 9–33 per cent.

Price and Price (2007) highlight the analgesic, antibacterial, anticatarrhal, expectorant and febrifuge properties, and also suggest that black pepper oil is useful as a digestive stimulant. Black pepper essential oil is rubefacient and therefore useful for joint and muscle pain, and it is indicated for colds, flu and infections (Lawless 1996). Traditionally it is also used for digestive complaints as diverse as diarrhoea, flatulence, constipation, colic, loss of appetite and nausea. For the aromatherapeutic uses of black pepper, see Table 8.30.

Table 8.30 Black pepper essential oil in aromatherapy

System	Black pepper with
Muscular	Lavender, basil, marjoram, rosemary, geranium, juniperberry, lemongrass, ginger, plai
Digestive	Clary sage, sweet fennel, peppermint, citrus oils, cinnamon leaf, ginger, coriander seed, cardamom
Respiratory	Frankincense, ginger, eucalyptus, rosemary

FAMILY POACEAE

The family Poaceae was formerly known as the Gramineae. This is a fairly large family of monocots, and several genera yield essential oils of commercial importance (Weiss 1997) and of use in aromatherapy.

The genus *Cymbopogon* (previously known as *Andropogon*) consists of 50–60 species of tropical, perennial, tufted grasses, coarse-growing and with extremely aromatic foliage. The leaf oils used by aromatherapists are *C. nardus* (Ceylon citronella), *C. winterianus* (Java citronella), *C. citratus* (West Indian lemongrass), *C. flexuosus* (East Indian lemongrass) and *C. martinii* (palmarosa). In the genus *Vetiveria* the only oil used by therapists comes from the rhizome and roots of *V. zizanioides*. These oils all come from the Far East – India, Sri Lanka, Indonesia and Malaysia – and the oils are usually steam or hydro-distilled (Weiss 1997).

GENUS CYMBOPOGON

CYMBOPOGON CITRATUS – WEST INDIAN LEMONGRASS

This is only produced under cultivation. It is grown mainly in Argentina, Brazil, Guatemala, Honduras, Haiti and other Caribbean islands, Java, Vietnam, Malaysia, Sri Lanka, Madagascar and the Comoro islands, and also in the Philippines, China, India, Bangladesh, Burma, Thailand and Africa.

C. FLEXUOSUS – EAST INDIAN LEMONGRASS

This species is grown in Southern India, mainly in Kerala. There are two varieties, the white-stemmed and the red-stemmed – and it is usually the latter that produces the 'typical' oil. Both varieties have long, narrow leaves and they rarely flower. The young leaves contain the most oil.

Prior to distillation the leaves are harvested and then allowed to wilt for two days, in order to give a higher yield and increased citral content. They are also finely chopped prior to extraction (Lawless 1996). The oil has a strong lemony odour due to the high citral content and it remains stable for a long time if correctly stored. The essential oil is usually a yellow to dark yellow or amber, slightly viscous liquid.

The major constituents are shown in Table 8.31; however, there is variability.

Table 8.31 Major constituents of lemongrass essential oils (adapted from Weiss 1997)

Component	*C. flexuosus*	*C. citratus*
Citral	85%	80%
Geraniol	5%	3%
Methyl heptenone	6%	0.3%
Myrcene	0.8%	20%
Dipentene	0	4%
Nerol	0	2%

Lemongrass oil is fungicidal and potentially anticarcinogenic (Weiss 1997). Lawless (1996) lists an impressive number of properties, and suggests uses in skin care (acne, athlete's foot, excessive perspiration, scabies and as an insect repellent), for poor circulation, joint and muscle pain, for the digestive system (colitis, indigestion and gastro-enteritis), fevers and infectious diseases, headaches, nervous exhaustion and stress.

The high citral content would also suggest that the essential oil has anti-inflammatory, sedative and antifungal properties (Franchomme and Pénoël 1990; Lis-Balchin 1995). Lawless (1996) suggests that it may cause dermal irritation or sensitisation in susceptible individuals, and so should be used with care. This might be due to the high citral content, but other components, such as monoterpenes, might reduce the potential for irritation.

Some possible therapeutic uses of lemongrass essential oil have been investigated. An early animal study conducted by Seth *et al.* (1976) suggested that injected lemongrass oil had a central nervous system depressant (tranquillising) effect and an analgesic effect. Faiyazuddin *et al.* (2009) reviewed the antimicrobial activity of lemongrass, and recommended it for the treatment and control of acne. They conducted a study that suggested that a 5 per cent dilution of lemongrass essential oil delivered in a nanoemulsion 'carrier' could be an effective treatment.

For some suggestions of how lemongrass may be used in aromatherapy, please see Table 8.32.

Table 8.32 Lemongrass essential oil in aromatherapy

System	Lemongrass with
Integumentary (acne, athlete's foot and fungal infections)	Lavender, sandalwood, palmarosa, patchouli, geranium, ocimum, tulsi
Nervous (stress, anxiety)	Sandalwood, patchouli, vetivert, geranium, lavender, rose
Musculoskeletal (muscles/circulation, joint pain)	Sandalwood, juniperberry, black pepper, ginger, basil

CYMBOPOGON MARTINI – PALMAROSA

Palmarosa essential oil is obtained from one of the two varieties of *Cymbopogon martinii*, or *C. martinii* var. *martinii* (motia), which grows in India. The closely related *C. martini* var. *sofia* is gingergrass; however, this oil is rarely used in aromatherapy.

Palmarosa essential oil is produced mainly from wild plants, and has been known at least since the arrival of the Portuguese in India in the late sixteenth century. It is often the basis for inexpensive scents and soaps. It is produced by steam or hydro-distillation of the fresh or dried grass (Weiss 1997).

The grass has many stiff stems of a yellow or greenish-yellow colour and the smooth leaves are long and narrow, of a lighter green than the stems. Older leaves generally have a higher oil content than young ones. The oil is pale yellow to olive with a sweet, floral, rosy geranium-like aroma, but can vary greatly depending on origin, age or method of distillation. The major components are monoterpene alcohols (geraniol (<95%), citronellol (<2%), linalool (<4%) and nerol) with some monoterpenes (limonene, myrcene and γ-terpinene), esters (geranyl acetate) and the sesquiterpene alcohol, elemol (Weiss 1997).

Lawless (1996) recommends palmarosa for skin care (acne, dermatitis, infections, sores and wrinkles), and for nervous exhaustion and stress. She also cites Maury (1989 [1961]) as testifying to its effect on the intestinal flora, and therefore its usefulness in combating intestinal infections. For some aromatherapeutic uses, please see Table 8.33.

Table 8.33 Palmarosa essential oil in aromatherapy

System	Palmarosa with
Integumentary	Lavender, geranium, lemongrass, ocimum, sandalwood, patchouli, vetivert
Nervous system (stress)	Lavender, geranium, lemongrass, sandalwood
Immune	Lavender, rosewood, thyme geraniol or linalool

C. NARDUS – CITRONELLA

Citronella essential oil is characterised by citronellal, its dominant aldehyde. *C. nardus* is grown mainly in Sri Lanka, and another species that produces an essential oil, *C. winterianus*, is grown throughout the Far East, and now also in Central and South America. The two types are generally known as Ceylon and Java types. The difference lies mainly in their geraniol content; see Table 8.34. Like the other members of the Poaceae family, the oil comes from a tufted perennial grass with a fibrous root system, and in this case it is the leaves that are used. Prior to steam distillation they are usually wilted and chopped (Weiss 1997).

Table 8.34 Comparisons of *C. nardus* and *C. winterianus* (adapted from Weiss 1997)

Characteristic	*C. nardus*	*C. winterianus*
Colour	Yellow to brown/ greenish-yellow	Colourless to pale yellow
Aroma	Floral, woody, grassy, leafy – due to camphene-borneol-methyleugenol mix	Sweet, fresh and lemony
Main constituents	Geraniol (60%) Citronellal (15%) Citronellol (10%)	Geraniol (45%) Citronellal (50%) Citronellol (20%)
Uses	Insecticides, cheap perfumes and household cleaners, and as raw material for geraniol, citronellol, citronellal and menthol production	Perfumes, toiletries and household cleaners and for raw materials (as for *C. nardus*)

Lawless (1996) recommends citronella for skin care, and for supporting the immune system and the nervous system. Schnaubelt (1995) says that it is sedative, anti-inflammatory and antispasmodic, while Bowles (2003) suggests that the geraniol content will contribute to an anti-infectious (antifungal), analgesic and sedative effect. The antifungal effect of geraniol might well be augmented by the presence of antifungal aldehydes.

Genus Vetiveria

Vetiveria zizanioides – vetivert (vetiver)

Vetivert (or vetiver) is native to India. It is used there, and in other countries, for soil conservation because of its extensive root mass. It is also used to make fans, mats, screens and thatch. In Sri Lanka vetivert is known as the 'oil of tranquillity'. It is also produced commercially in China and some oil comes from Central America, the Caribbean and Brazil. Oil from wild plants is known as '*khus*' in India. The best quality essential oil frequently comes from Réunion.

Its stems and leaves are erect and develop from a branched and spongy rhizome. The leaves do not contain volatile oil, and they are usually burned before the roots are harvested.

Vetivert volatile oil is produced in mature roots, in secretory cells in the first cortical layer, outside of the endodermis. Alifano *et al.* (2010) suspected that root bacteria may have a role in the biogenesis of the oil. Their research revealed that there is an ecological significance between vetivert and its root-associated bacteria, which can influence gene expression and the composition of the volatile oil.

The essential oil is produced by steam distillation from the roots and rhizome. The roots may be dried prior to distillation, as this promotes an increased oil yield, and then they are chopped and soaked in water. Distillation is often by direct-fired stills.

Vetivert oil is dark brown to dark amber, and viscous. Its odour is strong, sweet, woody and earthy. The odour is influenced by α- and β-vetivone and khusimone. It contains mainly sesquiterpenoids, the major component being vetiverol (50–75%), although Price and Price (2007) suggest that this component is less dominant.

Lawless (1996) lists a wide variety of applications for vetivert – in skincare for acne, cuts, wounds and oily skin; for arthritis, muscular pain, rheumatism, sprains and stiffness; and for the nervous system, encompassing debility, depression, insomnia and nervous tension. Price and Price (2007) suggest that it is an anti-infectious agent, a circulatory and glandular tonic and an immunostimulant. They also state that it is emmenagogic, but cite no research to support this. Schnaubelt (1995) echoes this view of vetivert as a stimulant for the endocrine, immune and circulatory systems. Mojay (1996) suggests that vetivert can be used to treat eczema, and this might be related to its ketone and sesquiterpene content.

Table 8.35 Vetivert essential oil in aromatherapy

System	Vetivert with
Integumentary	Lavender, bergamot, helichrysum, geranium, patchouli, sandalwood
Nervous system (stress)	Lavender, rose, sandalwood, violet leaf, ylang ylang
Musculoskeletal	Lavender, ginger, black pepper, lemongrass
Immune	Lavender, palmarosa

FAMILY ROSACEAE

The family Rosaceae is very large indeed, comprising around 115 genera. However, one genus is of particular significance: the genus *Rosa*, which comprises a group of herbaceous shrubs.

GENUS ROSA

Fossilised rose tissues, estimated to be around 35 million years old, have been found in Montana, Colorado and Oregon. The rose is native to the northern hemisphere, although its exact origins are disputed. All species in the southern hemisphere have been introduced and cultivated. Initially it was the use of rose as a medicine that established its importance to man; Pliny listed 32 rose-based remedies. Early on, the rose also became important in cosmetics and perfumes (Gordon 1980). By the time of the Romans (a period well noted for its excesses), roses were symbols of pleasure and were used in many circumstances – as decorations at banquets, for strewing floors, for floating in wine, to crown bridal couples and garnish statues of Cupid, Venus and Bacchus, at festivals of Flora and Hymen, and for scattering in the paths of chariots (Grieve 1992 [1931]). It was embraced by many other cultures too – for example, the Greek poetess Sappho called the rose the 'queen of flowers', and the white rose was adopted as a Jacobean emblem. Today it is used in herbal medicine, and it is one of the most important raw materials of perfumery, as well as an ornamental shrub of significance and value.

There are around 150 species of rose, and a myriad of named cultivars. Essential oils, concretes and absolutes may be produced from the flowers – all finding applications in perfumery. The products vary in specification and odour, depending on the botanical source, geography and ecology and method of extraction. Three species are recognised as being important for the fragrance industry – *Rosa damascena* (the damask rose, common to Bulgaria and Turkey),

R. centifolia (the cabbage or Provence rose) and *R. gallica* (known as the apothecary rose). These, and their hybrids, are extracted to produce essential oils, concretes and absolutes. Essential oils available for the aromatherapy profession include the most desirable Bulgarian and Turkish rose otto (here the essential oil is distilled from *R. damascena*), rose oil from Morocco (where the essential oil is distilled from *R. damascena*), rose oil from Morocco and France (where the essential oil is distilled from *R. centifolia*), rose oil from Egypt (distilled from *R. gallica* var. *aegyptiaca*), and rose oil from China (from *R. rugosa* and others). Absolutes are also available for aromatherapy use – for example, rose absolute 'centifolia', and *rose de mai* absolute, which is produced in France and Morocco.

Chemically the essential oil and absolutes are quite distinct. Rose essential oil is characterised by the presence of monoterpenes and their alcohols – geraniol at 15.8–22.2 per cent and citronellol at 22.5–60 per cent, and small amounts of the aromatic alcohol, phenyl ethanol, at around 0.9–3 per cent (Price and Price 1999). The essential oil is colourless to pale yellow, with a deep, sweet, warm, rich, tenacious odour; the Moroccan (*R. centifolia*) oil has a less spicy note than the oils from Bulgaria or Turkey (Weiss 1997). For information on rose absolute, see Chapter 10 (page 251).

In aromatherapy the most commonly cited properties attributed to rose essential oil are antibacterial, astringent, anti-inflammatory and cicatrisant actions, so it is often used to help the skin. Rose is also reputed to be of great assistance in problems pertaining to the female reproductive system, including premenstrual stress and menopause. The aroma is also thought to be antidepressant and an aphrodisiac. Hongratanaworakit (2009) demonstrated that transdermal absorption of rose can produce a state of relaxation, and supported its use in aromatherapy for the alleviation of stress. For some uses of rose essential oil in aromatherapy, please see Table 8.36.

Table 8.36 Rose essential oil in aromatherapy

System	Rose essential oil with
Integumentary (indicated for mature skin, dry, oily or sensitive skin, eczema, thread veins)	Lavender, geranium, neroli, helichrysum, sandalwood, patchouli, vetivert, bergamot
Female reproductive system	Clary sage, sweet fennel, cypress, juniperberry
Respiratory (hay fever, asthma, coughs)	Sandalwood, ginger, benzoin or peppermint, eucalyptus (1,8-cineole types)
Nervous (anxiety, depression, stress)	Geranium, jasmine, patchouli, bergamot, lavender, benzoin

Family Rutaceae

Genus Citrus

The large Rutaceae family is divided into seven subfamilies. The subfamily Aurantioideae contains the Citreae, within which the most important genus, from the fruit and volatile oil perspective, is the genus *Citrus*. Oils obtained from this genus are widely used in the flavour and fragrance industries. Citrus has two subgenera, containing 16 subspecies. The genus probably originated in Southeast Asia and the Pacific Islands, although the exact origins are not known, due to extensive hybridisation and cultivation. It is thought that all species are derived from *Citrus medica*, *C. maxima* and *C. reticulata* (Svoboda and Greenaway 2003).

The genus is very variable in appearance, containing some large and some small trees, some bearing large fruits and others small fruits. They are widely grown in the Mediterranean region; the only one to come from the Americas is grapefruit. *Citrus* is now cultivated on a large scale (Weiss 1997). All *Citrus* species are small, spiny, evergreen trees with fragrant white flowers and leaves and edible fruits. The leaves are dotted with volatile oil glands and 'petitgrain' leaf oil is produced in some species. The fruit oils are found in numerous volatile oil sacs in the flavedo (peel). With the notable exception of bitter orange, the peel oils are generally a by-product of the juice and canned fruit industry.

Citrus oils fall into two categories – cold pressed and distilled. Most lemon and sweet orange oil is cold pressed, a process in which pressure is applied to the fruit, and oils and juice are drawn off simultaneously, but into separate channels. If the essential oil is extracted prior to the juice, then both abrasion (scarification) and pressure are used. Lime is usually distilled, but distilled lemon and orange oils are not common. Most citrus oils are used in foods, condiments, drinks, perfumery, cosmetics and pharmaceuticals. Seed oils are also produced, and these may have pharmaceutical applications due to their potential antimicrobial activity (Weiss 1997).

The aroma of citrus oils comes mainly from aldehydes, but the oils also contain large amounts of terpenes, especially *d*-limonene. Some oils are de-terpenated for the flavour and fragrance industry, as the removal of terpenes can solve solubility problems without adversely affecting the aroma. However, these are not recommended for aromatherapy use, which is based on using 'complete' oils, produced according to Viaud's criteria. Cold pressed oils often contain furanocoumarins – constituents that are implicated in phototoxicity (Tisserand and Balacs 1995). The distilled oils do not contain furanocoumarins, as these are not volatile and therefore do not distil over into the essential oil. Because of the high percentage of monoterpenes in citrus oils they are prone to deterioration (Weiss 1997) and therefore require careful storage and protection from air, heat and light.

In the genus there are 16 species and many more cultivars. Cold pressed or distilled citrus fruit oils include sweet orange (*C. sinensis*), bitter orange (*C. aurantium*), lemon (*C. limon*), grapefruit (*C. paradisi*), mandarin (*C. reticulata*), bergamot (*C. aurantium* subsp. *bergamia*) and lime (*C. aurantifolia*). The most significant essential oil obtained from citrus leaves is petitgrain oil, from *C. aurantium* ssp. *amara*, although leaf oils are obtained from the other citrus species. The highly scented flowers of the bitter orange yield an essential oil known as neroli bigarade, obtained by distillation or by enfleurage. This oil is widely used in perfumery. Neroli oil can also be obtained from the flowers of the sweet orange (neroli Portugal) and from lemon flowers (neroli citronier). Orange flower water is a distillation by-product that is of value in skin care. The flowers can also be extracted with solvent, the product being an absolute – this is more correctly known as orange blossom absolute, not neroli. Please refer to Chapter 10 (page 252) for information on this absolute.

All of the citrus fruit oils, petitgrain and neroli oils have aromatherapy applications. Generally, they are noted as being 'uplifting' oils, with antibacterial activity and astringent action. They are often cited as being helpful to the digestion. The peel oils may have anti-inflammatory activity (Baylac and Racine 2003). Neroli oil is considered to be one of the most calming oils, and also is widely used to help in cases of fragile, sensitive skin. There has been some research into the impact of citrus scents on mood. For example, Hongratanaworakit and Buchbauer (2007) demonstrated that transdermal absorption of sweet orange oil decreased autonomic arousal, while promoting feelings of cheerfulness and vigour, leading them to support the use of sweet orange oil for the relief of depression and stress.

Citrus aurantifolia/C. medica var. acida – lime

Lime possibly originated in northern India, where it is still widely grown. It is a small tree with drooping branches and many short, stiff spines. Its sharply scented flowers grow singly, and its fruit is nearly spherical, small and greenish to light yellow in colour. Distillation is the usual method of extraction, although small amounts of expressed oil are available. Distilled oil is produced from both ripe and unripe fruits, while expressed oil comes mainly from green unripe fruits. Extraction can be by steam distillation of the slurry from crushed whole limes and finely chopped peel, or by distilling the juice from fruit pressing. Cold pressed oil is more expensive. The expressed oil is obtained by pressing whole fruits and passing the extract through centrifuges to separate the oil quickly. The manual method was to use an *écuelle à piquer* to scarify the fruit (Weiss 1997).

The chemical composition of lime oil is variable. Distilled oils have less citral, β- pinene and γ-terpinene, and more *p*-cymene, terpinen-4-ol and α-terpineol than the expressed oil (Weiss 1997). Franchomme and Pénoël (1990) suggest that the expressed oil is composed of approximately 73 per cent monoterpenes, with alcohols, esters, aldehydes around 12 per cent, and coumarins. Bowles (2003) states that distilled Persian lime essential oil contains 58 per cent limonene, 16 per cent γ-terpinene and 6 per cent β-pinene.

It has been reported that inhalation of limonene, a major chiral component of many citrus oils, stimulates the sympathetic nervous system and evokes alertness (Heuberger *et al.* 2001, cited in Saiyudthong *et al.* 2009). However, a study examining the effects of massage with lime essential oil (Saiyudthong *et al.* 2009) demonstrated that systolic blood pressure was decreased after a single massage with lime, suggesting the reduction of sympathetic activity and potentiation of the parasympathetic response. While it was acknowledged that massage alone could produce these effects, it was also suggested that the lime essential oil potentiated the parasympathetic response; it was noted that the mode of administration of an essential oil can affect the therapeutic outcome: the fragrance alone can increase alertness, but if applied topically with massage the same oil could have a relaxing, stress-relieving effect.

Much citrus research has focused on the effects of these oils on the autonomic nervous system and mood. Citrus oils are also important in the food industry, and they are thought to have health-promoting effects, for example as dietary anti-oxidants. In 2009 Patil *et al.* conducted an *in vitro* study of lime essential oil to investigate its possible use in the prevention of colon cancer. The lime oil that they used contained *d*-limonene at 30.13 per cent and d-dihydrocarvone at 30.47 per cent along with 'verbena', β-linalool, α-terpineol and *trans*-α-bergamotene. It was demonstrated that the lime oil was able to inhibit the proliferation of colon cancer cells, and that the likely mechanism was the induction of apoptosis. So although this may not have immediate applications in aromatherapy practice, it highlights the wider potential health benefits of lime essential oil.

Lawless (1996) suggests that lime has uses in skin care, for circulatory problems such as high blood pressure, varicose veins and poor circulation, and for arthritis, cellulite, obesity and rheumatism. She also recommends it for asthma, throat infections, bronchitis and catarrh, for dyspepsia, colds, flu, fever and infections. Franchomme and Pénoël (1990) state that it is sedative, anti-inflammatory, anticoagulant and antispasmodic and suggest that is indicated for anxiety and stress, and inflammatory and spasmodic problems of the digestive system. Please see Table 8.37.

Table 8.37 Lime essential oil in aromatherapy

System	Lime with
Integumentary	Lavender, bergamot, geranium, patchouli, sandalwood, vetivert
Nervous system (stress, depression)	Basil, laurel leaf, frankincense, sandalwood, patchouli, ylang ylang, vetivert
Musculoskeletal	Lavender, laurel leaf, bay, pimento, black pepper, ylang ylang, lemongrass
Digestive	Coriander seed, cardamom, clary sage, sweet fennel, black pepper, ginger

C. AURANTIUM SSP. AMARA – BITTER ORANGE
PEEL, PETITGRAIN AND NEROLI

Bitter orange, also known as the sour or Seville orange, is native to Southeast Asia, but has now become established in the Mediterranean, especially Spain – hence its name of Seville orange. The bitter orange tree, *Citrus aurantium* var. *amara*, has been cultivated for its fragrance products for many years. Its highly fragrant flowers produce neroli oil (*C. aurantium* ssp. *amara* flos.). The leaves and twigs produce a true petitgrain bigarade (*C. aurantium* ssp. *amara* fol.); petitgrain Paraguay is obtained from similar leaves in Paraguay. Neroli and petitgrain are important ingredients in classic colognes.

The bitter orange fruit is spherical, medium to dark green, becoming more yellow as it ripens, and yields bitter orange oil. The fruits have a long history of culinary and medicinal uses. The main use for the whole fruit is for marmalade. The liqueur curaçao, is flavoured with the unripe fruits. The tree is native to Asia; therefore its flowers and fruits form part of Oriental medicine – mainly as remedies for the myriad of disorders of the digestive system, as a cardiac tonic, and for anxiety.

The peel oil is a yellow, mobile liquid; waxy, crystalline sediment may appear with age (Weiss 1997). The aroma is fresh and delicate, with sweet floral undertones, and a green note can be detected. The major components include terpenes at around 90 per cent (particularly *d*-limonene), linalool, esters (linalyl acetate) and decanol. Due to the presence of furanocoumarins this oil is considered phototoxic (Lawless 1996). Bitter orange oil has indeed a citrus odour, but in contrast with its close relation sweet orange, it is subtle and fresh with a fairly tenacious floral undertone (Aftel 2008).

Lawless (1996) gives its uses as for sweet orange in the areas of skin care, especially for oily skin, and also for mouth ulcers, obesity and fluid retention, bronchitis, chills, cold and flu, constipation, spasm of the digestive system, indigestion and palpitations, nervous tension and stress. Price and Price (2007) suggest that it is anti-inflammatory, anticoagulant, sedative and tonic, and recommended for poor circulation, gastric pain, palpitations, constipation, anxiety and care of the gums.

Oils from citrus fruits such as bitter orange have a distinct uplifting effect, and are also indicated for moving forward/moving on from redundant behaviour and making a fresh start (Rhind 2009). Bitter orange oil also has a 'green' note, and so can also be used to counteract feelings of anger and frustration by promoting regulating, cooling, relaxing, clarifying sensations (Holmes 1997; Rhind 2009).

The production of the leaf oil of *C. aurantium* var. *amara*, 'petitgrain bigarade', is carried out mainly in Europe and North Africa. It has a floral sweet, orange-like odour that is widely used in perfumery. The Paraguay product is stronger in odour, sweet and woody-floral (Weiss 1997).

The main constituent of the leaf oil is the ester, linalyl acetate, but it also contains monoterpenes and 30–40 per cent monoterpene alcohols (Franchomme and Pénoël 1990). Schnaubelt (1995) recommends this oil to balance the autonomic nervous system; Franchomme and Pénoël (1990) support this, in addition to citing its antispasmodic, anti-inflammatory, anti-infectious and antibacterial properties. They suggest uses for rheumatism (of nervous origin), respiratory infections and infected acne, and consider this oil to be without hazard.

The highly scented flowers of the bitter orange yield an essential oil known as neroli bigarade, obtained by distillation or by enfleurage. Neroli first become popular as a fragrance in the sixteenth century. The scent was named after a town called Neroli, near Rome, whose princess used the scent and so made it popular. Over the years its use became widespread in Europe, from princesses to prostitutes (Lawless 1994). It is one of the most expensive natural materials in perfumery. Aftel (2008) describes its fragrance as 'cool, elegant and intense…with suave strength and understated sexuality'. Many of the floral oils, including neroli, do contain trace amounts of indole, a compound found in animal faeces. This is thought to have a sexual attraction for the animals involved in pollination (Calkin and Jellinek 1994). (Many of the plant aromatics categorised as aphrodisiacs do contain animal pheromones such as indole.)

The flowers are hand-picked early in the morning, when they have just opened; this produces the best quality oil. 'Neroli' oil can also be obtained from the flowers of the sweet orange (neroli Portugal) and from lemon flowers (neroli citronier). Orange flower water is a distillation by-product that is of value, and it may be used in aromatherapy skin care.

Neroli essential oil is regarded as one of the most calming oils, and is also widely used to help in cases of fragile, sensitive skin. It is a pale yellow liquid that darkens when it deteriorates, with a sweet, spicy, orange blossom odour (Jouhar 1991). It must be kept cool and protected from light.

Chemically, neroli bigarade essential oil is dominated by *l*-linalool at 37.5 per cent, with *d*-limonene at 16.6 per cent and β-pinene at 11.8 per cent (Bowles 2003). Linalool is antibacterial, analgesic, sedative and antispasmodic – all associated with the use of neroli in aromatherapy. Price and Price (1999) suggest that neroli bigarade is of most use as an antidepressant: a lightly tranquillising and 'neurotonic' essential oil useful for fatigue, to aid sleep and to redress sympathetic nervous system imbalance. Jäger *et al.* (1992) reported that inhalation of neroli has sedative effects. Weiss (1997) states that neroli bigarade is a weak antiseptic, but has strong bactericidal action on *Staphylococcus aureus*, and that in traditional medicine it was believed to induce a semi-trance state when inhaled warm. Please see Table 8.38 for some aromatherapeutic uses of neroli.

Table 8.38 Neroli bigarade essential oil in aromatherapy

System	Neroli essential oil with
Integumentary (indicated for fragile or sensitive skin, acne, varicose veins)	Lavender, geranium, helichrysum, sandalwood, patchouli, bergamot, petitgrain, lemon
Nervous system (nervous depression, anxiety, insomnia)	Lavender, geranium, petitgrain, vetivert, sandalwood, all citrus oils
Musculoskeletal (muscular tension and spasm)	Lavender, rosemary, basil, marjoram, ginger, black pepper, lemongrass

C. AURANTIUM SSP. BERGAMIA – BERGAMOT

Bergamot essential oil production became established in Italy in the sixteenth century, and even today the most significant producer is Italy, with oils from Calabria still regarded as the best available. The tree is similar to other citrus trees, the fruit being spherical and yellow when ripe. It is less widely distributed than its close relative, the bitter orange. There is some doubt as to its botanical origins and whether this valuable sub-species is a mutation or a hybrid. The fruit is not edible, but the oil is widely used in perfumery and to flavour Earl Grey tea, tobacco and many foods (Weiss 1997).

Bergamot essential oil has a light olive green hue that fades with time, becoming yellow/pale brown in colour. It does not have the typical citrus, zesty aroma of the other citrus peel oils. The artisan perfumer and therapist Aftel (2008) describes the aroma as having 'an extremely rich, sweet lemon-orange scent that evolves into a more floral, freesia-like scent, ending in an herbaceous-balsamic dryout'. The fragrance of bergamot is almost universally liked, and it also has several properties that combine to make it one of the most useful aromatherapeutic essential oils.

There is a great deal of variation in its composition, usually related to its geographical origins (Weiss 1997). According to Price and Price (2007) the major components are alcohols (45–60%) including linalool, esters (30–60%) including linalyl acetate, and monoterpenes including limonene, α- and β-pinene and γ-terpinene. Bergamot oil also contains phototoxic furanocoumarins, in this case one known as bergapten (5-methoxypsoralen or 5-MOP), therefore care should be taken when using it on the skin, and exposure to sunlight must be avoided following use. It is of interest that 5-MOP sometimes forms part of the ultraviolet light treatment for psoriasis, and that it was included in sun protection/tanning preparations in the 1960s and 1970s before its use was restricted. A furanocoumarin-free essential oil is available, which effectively removes this risk.

Price and Price (2007) assign an impressive array of properties to this oil, suggesting that it is antibacterial, antiviral, antiseptic, antispasmodic and sedative. They recommend the oil for wounds, herpes simplex (cold sores), insomnia, burns, loss of appetite and psoriasis. It is also indicated, along with German chamomile, lavender and sandalwood, as a local wash for cystitis.

Lawless (1996) suggests uses in skincare (for acne, boils, cold sores, eczema, as an insect repellent and for insect bites, oily skin, psoriasis, scabies, varicose ulcers and wounds), for the respiratory system (halitosis, mouth infections, sore throat and tonsillitis), flatulence and loss of appetite, cystitis, leucorrhoea, pruritus and thrush, for colds, fever, flu and infectious diseases, and for anxiety, depression and stress.

Table 8.39 Bergamot essential oil in aromatherapy

System	Bergamot with
Integumentary	Lavender, geranium, helichrysum, patchouli, sandalwood, vetivert
Nervous system (stress)	Frankincense, sandalwood, ylang ylang, rose, jasmine, vetivert
Musculoskeletal	Lavender, pimento, black pepper, lemongrass
Digestive	Coriander seed, cardamom, black pepper, ginger
Genito-urinary	Sandalwood, juniperberry, lavender, German chamomile, geranium
Respiratory (asthma, infections)	Clary sage, pine, fir, cypress, Atlas cedarwood

C. HYSTRIX — KAFFIR LIME LEAF AND PEEL

This species yields both leaf and peel oils. Hongratanaworakit and Buchbauer (2007) investigated the effects of massage with the peel oil on human autonomic and behavioural parameters. It caused an increase in blood pressure and decrease in skin temperature, compared with the placebo group; and the kaffir lime group rated themselves as more alert, cheerful and vigorous than the control. Based on this study, it would seem that kaffir lime peel oil has activating effects and could be used in the context of aromatherapy massage to alleviate depression and stress.

C. LIMETTA — SWEET LIME

This species is grown in southern Italy. It is very similar to lemon oil in aroma, and only very small volumes of the essential oil are produced.

C. LIMON — LEMON

Although the lemon tree is from Asia, the main producer of essential oil is now Sicily. The fruit is ovoid, and yellow when ripe, with a smooth or rough peel, depending on the variety. The cold pressed oil is clear, a pale to greenish yellow which turns brown with age, and the odour is fresh, sweet and lemony (Weiss 1997).

The major components of the oil are monoterpenes, at 90–95 per cent (Price and Price 2007) and citral. The principle monoterpene is *d*-limonene at approximately 70 per cent; however, citral has a major impact on the odour. The oil is also phototoxic due to the presence of non-volatile furanocoumarins, and it may cause dermal irritation in some people (Lawless 1996).

Citrus oils are usually associated with uplifting effects. Following previous studies on the antidepressant effects of the inhalation of citrus fragrances, Komori (2009) conducted a study on the effects of the inhalation of lemon and valerian essential oils on the autonomic nervous system in healthy and depressed male subjects. Depression is associated with an increase in sympathetic nervous activity and decreased parasympathetic nervous activity, and dysregulation of the psychoneuroimmunological balance. This study showed that in the healthy subjects, lemon stimulated both sympathetic nerve activity and the parasympathetic nervous system. However, the depressed subjects, who already had enhanced sympathetic activity, showed a decrease relative to the enhanced parasympathetic activity, after inhalation of lemon. Valerian has a long tradition of use as a sedative. In this study, inhalation of the essential oil did not stimulate sympathetic activity in any of the test subjects. The findings support the use of lemon as an antidepressant essential oil.

Price and Price (2007) comment that lemon essential oil is anti-infectious, antibacterial, antifungal, antiviral and anti-inflammatory. It is also thought to

be astringent, diuretic and immunostimulant. Brudnak (2000) suggested that
d-limonene is anti-carcinogenic. Please see Table 8.40 for some suggestions for
the use of lemon in aromatherapy.

Table 8.40 Lemon essential oil in aromatherapy

System	Lemon with
Integumentary	Lavender, bergamot, lime, geranium, helichrysum, ylang ylang, neroli, rose, jasmine, cypress, patchouli, sandalwood, vetivert
Nervous system (stress, depression)	Frankincense, bergamot, sandalwood, ylang ylang, geranium, patchouli, rose
Musculoskeletal	Lavender, eucalyptus (cineole types) black pepper, juniperberry
Digestive	Coriander seed, cardamom, black pepper, ginger, sweet fennel, lime, grapefruit
Respiratory	Eucalyptus (cineole types), fir, pine, cypress, bergamot, sweet fennel, rosemary, marjoram, basil, thyme linalool, sandalwood, ginger

C. PARADISI – GRAPEFRUIT

Grapefruit is the only citrus species that is native to the New World and it may
be descended from hybrid plants which were introduced to Barbados in the
seventeenth century. The tree is large and vigorous, with sturdy branches and
angular twigs. It has large leaves and white, highly fragrant flowers. An essential
oil may be produced from the leaves. The fruit is large, light yellow to orange in
colour, and is the source of the peel oil (Weiss 1997).

Grapefruit essential oil is a relative newcomer to perfumery, only becoming
available at the beginning of the nineteenth century (Aftel 2008). It can be
produced by steam distillation or cold expression of the peel. The cold pressed
oil is yellow to pale orange, and the aroma is sweet and fresh, similar to the fruit
itself. It will deteriorate rapidly on exposure to the air (Weiss 1997).

The major constituent of the peel oil is limonene (approximately 84%);
nootkatone (a sesquiterpene ketone) and traces of a sulphur-containing compound
give the oil its distinctive aroma (Williams 1996). Monoterpenes make up about
95 per cent of the oil (Weiss 1997). It does not appear to be strongly phototoxic.

Tisserand and Balacs (1995) suggest that the maximum concentration of grapefruit should be 4 per cent, due to the potential for phototoxicity.

Grapefruit in the diet has acquired popular associations with weight loss. Harris (2005) cites Shen *et al.* (2005), who demonstrated that the scent of grapefruit could affect autonomic nerve activity, increasing lipolysis and metabolism, thus reducing weight in rats. (Lavender, which was investigated in a similar manner, had the opposite effects.) In general terms, this can be interpreted as the fragrance of grapefruit having activating effects.

Table 8.41 Grapefruit essential oil in aromatherapy

System	Grapefruit with
Integumentary	Lavender, bergamot, geranium, ylang ylang, neroli, rose, jasmine, sandalwood, cypress
Nervous system (stress)	Rosemary, ylang ylang, geranium, jasmine, neroli, palmarosa
Musculoskeletal	Lavender, eucalyptus (cineole types), sweet fennel, black pepper, juniperberry, ginger, lemon
Digestive	Coriander seed, cardamom, black pepper, ginger, sweet fennel, lime
Circulatory–lymphatic	Sweet fennel, juniperberry, black pepper, rosemary, lemon

According to Lawless (1996) grapefruit is useful in skin care (for acne, oily skin, and for toning the skin) and for cellulitis, obesity, stiffness and fluid retention, cold and flu, depression, headaches, nervous exhaustion and performance stress. Franchomme and Pénoël (1990) suggest that the oil is a good air antiseptic. For some aromatherapeutic uses, please see Table 8.41.

C. RETICULATA – MANDARIN, TANGERINE

Mandarin and tangerine are usually considered as one species. 'Tangerine' is the name used in English-speaking countries, and 'mandarin' elsewhere (Weiss 1997). The tree is normally small, with a spreading habit and thin drooping branches, with or without spines. The leaves are narrow and lanceolate. Mandarin petitgrain is produced by steam distillation of the leaves; its main constituents are citral and linalool. The tree produces single white flowers and the fruit is a flattened sphere, with a peel that may vary from yellow to deep orange-red.

The peel oil is pale to mid-yellow or orange, depending on the cultivar, and the aroma is intense, sweet and, very occasionally, not very pleasant – a fishy note can be present. Aftel (2008) asserts that the oil sold as tangerine is much preferable to mandarin for perfumery, and indeed the same applies in aromatherapy. According to Price and Price (2007), the major constituents are usually monoterpenes, dominated by limonene at 65 per cent or more, alcohols including linalool, short chain fatty aldehydes at around 1 per cent, trace amounts of thymol and sometimes anthranilates. Anthranilates are nitrogen-containing esters, which can give rise to the fishy note. Thymol and dimethyl anthranilate contribute to the aroma, even although they are only present in traces (Weiss 1997).

Lawless (1996) recommends mandarin essential oil for skin care, notably acne, oily skin, scars and stretch marks, and as a 'toner', and for fluid retention and obesity, digestive problems and the nervous system (insomnia, nervous tension and restlessness). She considers it useful for children and pregnant women, as it carries little hazard, and states that it blends well with other citrus oils (especially neroli), and spice oils.

Price and Price (2007) consider it to be antifungal, antispasmodic, anti-epileptic and hepatic. They highlight its calming qualities and its applications in cases of insomnia and nervous tension. Tisserand and Balacs (1995) consider it to be without hazard, but Franchomme and Pénoël (1990) suggest that it does contain furanocoumarins and therefore is phototoxic. For some aromatherapeutic uses of mandarin/tangerine in aromatherapy, please refer to Table 8.42.

Table 8.42 Mandarin/tangerine essential oil in aromatherapy

System	Mandarin/tangerine with
Integumentary	Lavender, geranium, neroli, rose, frankincense
Nervous system (stress)	Lavender, geranium, neroli, Roman chamomile
Digestive	Coriander seed, cardamom, black pepper, ginger, sweet fennel, marjoram, lime
Circulatory–lymphatic	Sweet fennel, juniperberry, black pepper, rosemary, grapefruit

C. SINENSIS – SWEET ORANGE

This species is probably a native of the southwest China–Burma borders, but is now grown throughout the world. It is a medium-sized tree with ovate, glossy green leaves. The branches may be spiny. Sweet orange petitgrain oil is produced by distilling the leaves; monoterpenes are the main constituents of this type of petitgrain. The flowers are white and fragrant, occurring singly or in clusters. The yellow-orange fruit is oval or ellipsoidal with a smooth peel.

Sweet orange essential oil is produced by cold pressing the peel or whole fruit, or by steam distilling the residues from the segmenting or juicing processes (Weiss 1997). Cold pressed orange oil is pale yellow-orange to dark orange, but the colour does vary according to the cultivar used and the country in which it is grown. The aroma is fresh, fruity and similar to the peel when scarified.

The main constituents are monoterpenes (around 90%), mainly limonene, and the aldehydes octanal and decanal. Alcohols are present, mostly linalool, as are esters, mainly octyl and neryl acetates (Weiss 1997). Franchomme and Pénoël (1990) also include furanocoumarins and ketones (β-carvone and α-ionone), and suggest that the oil may be phototoxic. They recommend it for dyspepsia, insomnia, anxiety and as an air disinfectant.

Like most citrus oils, sweet orange is considered to be a useful antiseptic, a digestive stimulant and a circulatory and lymphatic system stimulant. It certainly is well regarded as an uplifting essential oil. Hongratanaworakit and Buchbauer (2007) demonstrated that the transdermal absorption of sweet orange oil decreased autonomic arousal, while promoting feelings of cheerfulness and vigour, leading them to support the aromatherapeutic use of sweet orange oil for the relief of depression and stress.

For some aromatherapeutic uses of sweet orange (and bitter orange), see Table 8.43.

Table 8.43 Sweet and bitter orange essential oils in aromatherapy

System	Orange with
Digestive	Sweet fennel, marjoram, clary sage, coriander seed, cardamom, black pepper, ginger
Nervous system (stress)	Jasmine, geranium, neroli, Roman chamomile, sandalwood
Circulatory–lymphatic	Sweet fennel, juniperberry, black pepper, rosemary, grapefruit

C. TACHIBANA

This is a species that is cultivated at Japanese shrines. Its flower oil has a floral, jasmine-like and orange flower-like scent; its main constituents are linalool at

28 per cent and γ-terpinene at 25 per cent. The peel oil has a sweet, green, juicy odour; it is dominated by limonene at 71 per cent and linalool at 9 per cent (Ubukata *et al.* 2002, cited in Svoboda and Greenaway 2003).

So far, there have been no reports of this essential oil being used in aromatherapy, however its scent and constituents indicate that it would be safe to use, and that it may well have applications in perfumery.

FAMILY SANTALACEAE

This family belongs to the order Santalales. The Santalaceae is the sandalwood family; it contains around 25–30 genera – however, classification is difficult. The genus of interest, genus *Santalum*, contains 16–20 tropical, evergreen, semi-parasitic trees and shrubs (Weiss 1997).

GENUS SANTALUM

The most important species is *Santalum album* ('East Indian sandalwood', or white sandalwood), which is highly valued for its aromatic wood and oil. The use of both can be traced back over 2500 years in India, and before then it undoubtedly had ritual and ceremonial uses (Weiss 1997). Traditionally the wood was used for carving ornaments and furniture, and as incense, and the fragrant oil was used in perfumery (Erligmann 2001). Sandalwood essential oil still has a very important place in perfumery. It has virtually no top note, and is remarkably persistent – acting as a fixative but also supporting and enhancing other notes, and contributing incomparable soft, woody, powdery notes to the dryout (Aftel 2008).

There are more than 15 species that produce an essential oil, but only three of these are of significance in aromatherapy. These are the white sandalwood *Santalum album* and two sandalwoods from Australia, *S. spicatum* and *S. austrocaledonicum*.

S. album is an evergreen tree that can reach 12 m in height at maturity, at around 60 years of age. The heartwood and roots do not rot or decay, due to the presence of the volatile oil. The tree is variously described as an obligate root parasite that becomes more independent as it matures, or as having a semi-parasitic habit. In its early stages of growth, the seedling's roots contact the roots of other plants ('host' plants); a structure known as a haustorium develops from these roots and acts as a sucker, absorbing nutrients for the sandalwood from the host. Once the tree is established, the parasitic habit continues, but becomes less important for survival once the true roots are established (Weiss 1997; Erligmann 2001).

The volatile oil is contained in the heartwood and the larger roots, and the essential oil is obtained by hydro- or steam distilling the pulverised heartwood and major roots. Due to over-harvesting, exploitation and fraud, white sandalwood is now very scarce. The main production areas are Mysore and also Madras.

Sandalwood harvesting is now officially controlled in India, but as trees should be over 30 years old before they contain significant quantities of volatile oil, the situation is not likely to change for a considerable time. However, sandalwood oil is also produced in Australia, from *S. spicatum* and *S. austrocaledonicum*, and these oils are now used in aromatherapy, despite differences in odour and chemistry. West Indian sandalwood is not sandalwood – this oil is obtained from *Amyris balsamifera* (Weiss 1997), and it is not a substitute in aromatherapy.

S. album essential oil is a pale yellow, viscous liquid, with a soft, sweet, woody, animal-balsamic odour (Weiss 1997). According to Bowles (2003), the main chemical constituents are sesquiterpene alcohols – α-santalols (50%) and β-santalols (25%). The woody notes are contributed mainly by the (Z)-β-santalols and traces of 2-α-*trans*-bergamotol, a sesquiterpenoid. The constituent responsible for the tenacity is β-santalene, and trace constituents such as phenols (eugenol and *para*-cresol), monoterpene alcohols (such as linalool) and ketones (nor-α-*trans*-bergamotone) also have a subtle impact (Erligmann 2001).

S. spicatum is extracted initially with solvents, followed by vacuum distillation of the residue. It could therefore be argued that this is not a true essential oil. The cost in 2001 was around half the price of Indian sandalwood (Erligmann 2001). *S. spicatum* has an extremely tenacious soft, woody, balsamic, sweet odour with a dry, spicy, resinous top note (Valder *et al.* 2003). It contains over 70 constituents and, like *S. album*, is dominated by sesquiterpenes. Like *S. album*, it contains similar levels of (Z)-β-santalol, but much less Z- α-santalol. However, it contains a sesquiterpenol that is not found in *S. album*: ll-farnesol, at over 5 per cent. This same compound is found in rose and ylang ylang. It also contains an isomer of bisabolol; this is not the same one that is found in German chamomile. A sesquiterpenoid known as dendrolasine may be present at up to 2 per cent, and this is only found in trace amounts in *S. album*. So given the differences in some major, minor and trace components, the oil does smell different to that of *S. album* – it has a top note, floral notes and green notes. Erligmann (2001) classifies *S. album* as amber-like, and *S. spicatum* as resinous.

S. album has a very important role in Ayurvedic medicine. However, recent research has indicated that some components of the oil (alcohols, diols, and triols) have antitumour properties (Kim *et al.* 2006, cited in Baldovini *et al.* 2011). Other potential medical uses include the topical treatment of human papillomavirus and pre-cancerous skin lesions, and as a skin cancer preventative (Baldovini *et al.* 2011).

Hongratanaworakit, Heuberger and Bachbauer (2004) studied the effects of transdermal absorption of α-santalol and *S. album* oil. The subjects were prevented from olfactory stimulation. It was shown that α-santalol brought about significant physiological changes suggestive of relaxation or sedation. The essential oil elicited similar physiological deactivation, but at the same time behavioural activation. They suggested that this indicated that sandalwood oil had uncoupled physiological and behavioural processes. In 2006 the same team, this time led by Heuberger, investigated the effects of inhalation of α-santalol and *S. album* oil, compared with an odourless placebo. In this study *S. album* oil had an activating effect – increasing pulse rate, skin conductance and systolic blood pressure – compared with the α-santalol and the placebo. However the α-santalol produced higher ratings of attentiveness and mood than the essential oil or the placebo. It appears that such effects on arousal and mood are related to perceived odour quality. Both studies support the use of *S. album* as a relaxing, antidepressant oil in aromatherapy.

From the therapeutic perspective, there has been little research concerning *S. spicatum*, and it does not share the same tradition of aromatherapeutic use as *S. album*, which is used as a general tonic and as a sedative; its antimicrobial properties are indicated for genito-urinary tract infections, and its bronchodilatory actions indicate its use in respiratory infections. It is used in skin care and phytocosmeceuticals for maintaining skin health and alleviating acne, dermatitis and eczema. It is also said to be a diuretic, and a lymphatic and venous decongestant (Price and Price 2007).

Based on the similarities (in the santalols) between the oils, Erligmann (2001) suggested that *S. spicatum* would share *S. album*'s sedative and antiviral (herpes simplex I) properties. She postulates that its main uses are as a urinary antiseptic and for the relief of dry, irritating coughs. For some suggestions concerning the use of sandalwood essential oils in aromatherapy, please see Table 8.44.

Table 8.44 Sandalwood essential oils in aromatherapy

System	Sandalwood with
Musculoskeletal (pain, spasm)	Juniperberry, lemongrass, black pepper, clove bud, ginger, geranium, lavender
Circulatory (venous, lymphatic)	Patchouli, cypress, lemon, grapefruit
Nervous system (debility, anxiety, depression)	Rose, jasmine, geranium, benzoin, patchouli, rosewood, bergamot, sweet orange
Respiratory (asthma, spasm, coughs, congestion)	Bergamot, ginger, benzoin, Atlas cedarwood, cypress, ravintsara, niaouli
Urinary (cystitis, urinary tract infections or UTI)	Juniperberry, cypress, bergamot, thyme linalool

Family Umbelliferae

This family, also known as the Apiaceae, has many essential oil-producing species that are of significance for aromatherapy practice. The members of this family, colloquially known as the 'carrot family', are mainly found in temperate regions, or in mountainous areas of the tropics. They may be herbs, shrubs or trees, and they all produce flowers where all of the petioles arise from the top of the stem – this form is known as an 'umbel'. Many of the essential oils obtained from this family have characteristically sweet, often anisic odours, partly due to the presence of constituents known as phenolic ethers.

It is impossible to assign general therapeutic actions to such a diverse group, but it is worth noting that many essential oils from the Umbelliferae are derived from spices, flavourings, etc. that are reputed to be digestive aids – such as dill, caraway, parsley and aniseed. Many of these aromatics, including sweet fennel and lovage, are also said to have diuretic and depurative properties. As the essential oils are from a wide range of genera, the individual species of importance are presented below.

Genus Anethum

Anethum graveolens – dill

Dill essential oil is obtained from the fruit or seeds of the herb. The feathery leaves are used as a culinary herb, and its main use in herbalism is as a digestive aid, and also to aid sleep. The essential oil has a light, fresh, spicy, caraway-like odour. Dill seed oil contains 30–60 per cent *d*-carvone. According to Lawless (1992, 1995) its main uses in aromatherapy are to support the digestive system (colic, dyspepsia, flatulence and indigestion).

Genus Angelica

Angelica archangelica – angelica

Angelica essential oil is obtained from the roots or occasionally the seeds of this large, hairy, aromatic plant. According to folk tradition, it was named after the archangel Michael, who revealed its medicinal uses to a monk. It was claimed that the herb flowered on Michael's holy day, 8 May. It grows well in northern Europe, and has been cultivated in Britain since the sixteenth century; its main uses were as a food (like celery), as a general tonic, to reduce flatulence and as an antidote to the plague. Angelica fruits are an important flavour in some liqueurs, such as Chartreuse, and it is used as a flavour in some gins (Gordon 1980).

Angelica root essential oil has a rich, herbaceous, earthy odour (Lawless 1992, 1995). The main chemical constituents are α-pinene at 25 per cent, 1,8-cineole at 14.5 per cent and α-phellandrene at 13.5 per cent (Bowles 2003). However, angelica root oil is strongly phototoxic, due to the presence of bergapten. It is indicated for the respiratory system, circulation, and the muscles and joints, for especially toxic accumulations, for the digestive system and also for anorexia, fatigue and stress/tension (Lawless 1992). The presence of α-pinene and 1,8-cineole would certainly support its reputed expectorant and antispasmodic properties and indications for the respiratory system.

GENUS ANTHRISCUS
ANTHRISCUS CEREFOLIUM – CHERVIL

Chervil essential oil is distilled from the seeds, fruit or leaves of this annual herb. The essential oil has a sweet, anisic odour and is dominated by estragole (methyl chavicol). For this reason, both Lawless (1992) and Tisserand and Balacs (1995) suggest that chervil essential oil does not have a place in aromatherapy. It is not commercially available.

GENUS CARUM
CARUM CARVI – CARAWAY

Caraway essential oil is obtained from the seed of the large biennial herb. The seeds are often added to bread and baked goods; traditionally it was used to cure flatulence, hiccups and headaches, and it was also used in early perfumery.

Caraway essential oil is often rectified to improve the odour. The rectified oil has a strong, warm, sweet, spicy odour that is closely related to the smell of the dried seed. The dominant constituent is *d*-carvone – present at 50 per cent. It also contains 46 per cent limonene and small amounts of *cis*-dihydrocarvone, myrcene and others (Bowles 2003). According to Lawless (1996), its main uses in aromatherapy are for the respiratory system – the dominant ketone might confer mucolytic properties (Bowles 2003) – and the digestive system – the indications being very similar to those for dill and angelica essential oils.

GENUS CORIANDRUM
CORIANDRUM SATIVUM – CORIANDER SEED

Coriander essential oil is distilled from the seeds of the tall annual herb. The herb was and is widely used all over Europe and the Middle East, and now it is cultivated worldwide. It has a long tradition of use, and was possibly one of the very first culinary herbs, with both leaves and ripe seeds now figuring in many cuisines, especially Asian and Middle Eastern.

Coriander seed oil is a colourless to pale yellow, mobile liquid with a sweet, spicy, woody odour. Most coriander oil is produced in Europe, notably in Croatia

(Lawless 1995). The chemical composition varies according to source and ripeness of seeds. Price and Price (1999) report that the linalool content varies from 60–87 per cent, making this the dominant constituent, followed by monoterpenes at 10–20 per cent. In this case, it is *d*-linalool rather than *l*-linalool; and this form is sometimes referred to as 'coriandrol'.

Emamghoreishi *et al.* (2005) had identified that 100 mg/kg coriander seed oil has an anxiolytic effect in mice, and following this, Mahendra and Bisht (2011) explored the potential for coriander seed essential oil and hydroalcoholic extracts as natural anxiolytics to replace benzodiazepines. They confirmed the earlier study, and proposed that the essential oil components and the flavonoids act via the GABA sub A receptor complex, in a similar way to diazepam. They have suggested that because of these anxiolytic effects and also memory-improving effects and anti-cholinesterase activity, coriander seed oil and extracts may have applications in the management of CNS disorders and neurodegenerative diseases.

Price and Price (2009) highlight several therapeutic uses for coriander seed oil. Antibacterial and anti-infectious actions indicate that it is useful for respiratory and urinary tract infections, while its antispasmodic, stomachic and carminative properties are useful for the digestive system. Like angelica, it is indicated for anorexia. It is also indicated as an analgesic for osteoarthritis and rheumatic pain. Coriander seed may also be able to impart a sense of euphoria (Schnaubelt 1995), and together with its other properties, it is considered to be a useful aromatherapeutic oil. For some uses, please see Table 8.45.

Table 8.45 Coriander seed essential oil in aromatherapy

System	Coriander seed with
Digestive	Dill, caraway, angelica root, sweet fennel, cardamom, nutmeg, lavender, black pepper, citrus oils
Musculoskeletal (arthritis, rheumatism)	Nutmeg, sweet fennel, grapefruit, black pepper, juniperberry, lavender
Nervous (tension, stress, anxiety, depression, fatigue, lethargy, debility, convalescence)	Lavender, citrus oils, palmarosa, geranium, rosewood, rose, jasmine

GENUS CUMINUM
CUMINUM CYMINUM – CUMIN

Cumin essential oil is obtained from the ripe seeds of this annual herb. It is closely related to coriander and, like coriander, its seeds are widely used in Asian cuisine.

However, its essential oil is very different, being dominated by cuminaldehyde at 20–40 per cent (Tisserand and Balacs 1995). It can be used to support the digestive system and nervous system and aid with 'toxic accumulations' (Lawless 1992). Cumin essential oil is not widely used in aromatherapy – mainly as it is strongly phototoxic, and possibly because of its distinctive aroma, reminiscent of curry.

Genus Ferula

Ferula galbaniflua – galbanum

Galbanum essential oil is obtained by distillation of the oleoresin that exudes from this large perennial herb. Like all of the other resins and gums, it has an ancient tradition of use as a medicine and incense. The oleoresin is from the Middle East; most of the essential oil is distilled in Europe. The essential oil is a colourless to pale yellow, mobile liquid with a very powerful, fresh green odour, reminiscent of green bell peppers. This distinctive green note is due to the presence of trace amounts of a nitrogen-containing pyrazine, 2-methoxy-3-1-butylpyrazine (Gimelli 2001). Galbanum essential oil is dominated by monoterpenes, including the pinenes and limonene.

Its main uses in aromatherapy, according to Lawless (1992) are for the skin (cicatrisant, anti-inflammatory and antiseptic qualities), the musculoskeletal system (analgesic, circulatory stimulant) and the respiratory system (expectorant and antispasmodic) and as a general tonic. Galbanum essential oil is not included in most aromatherapy texts; therefore it is underused in current aromatherapy practice. For some suggested aromatherapeutic uses, please refer to Table 8.46.

Table 8.46 Galbanum essential oil in aromatherapy

System	Galbanum with
Integumentary (indicated for mature skin)	Lavender, geranium, sandalwood, patchouli, jasmine, violet leaf
Musculoskeletal (aches and pains)	Lavender, black pepper, Roman/German chamomile, clary sage
Nervous (tension, stress, fatigue, lethargy)	Lavender, geranium, rosewood, hyacinth, violet leaf
Respiratory	Scots pine, fir, rosemary, Atlas cedarwood, lemon

Genus Foeniculum

Foeniculum vulgare var. dulce — sweet fennel

The essential oil is obtained from the seeds of this tall biennial herb. Fennel is an ancient and important medicinal herb for the digestion and the respiratory system, as well as having a reputation for aiding weight loss. The whole plant is aromatic, and all parts are used in cooking.

Sweet fennel essential oil is produced in France, Italy, Spain, Turkey and Bulgaria. It is a pale yellow, mobile liquid with a characteristic fresh, sweet, anise and earthy aroma. The proportions of its main chemical constituents can be variable and dependent on the source material (Lawless 1992). According to Bowles (2003) they are typically *trans*-anethole at 80 per cent, limonene at 6 per cent and estragole at 4.5 per cent. A ketone, fenchone, may also be present as a minor constituent; this is dominant in the essential oil obtained from the bitter fennel, *F. vulgare* var. *amara*. It has been suggested that sweet fennel oil may also have mild oestrogenic qualities, possibly conferred by the *trans*-anethole (Price and Price 1999). This compound is a phenolic ether that, in large doses, can produce psychotropic effects; however, this is highly unlikely when used at low levels in aromatherapy practice. *Trans*-anethole has also been shown to exert analgesic and antispasmodic effects (Tisserand and Balacs 1995).

Sweet fennel oil has been ascribed a wide range of therapeutic actions, and is cited in most texts as being of value in several areas of aromatherapy practice. These are for the respiratory system, the digestive system, and the female reproductive system.

Sweet fennel seeds were traditionally used to treat dysmenorrhoea; it was thought that this was due to the antispasmodic effect of the volatile oil. Animal studies have demonstrated that sweet fennel oil has a direct, relaxing effect on the uterine muscle; therefore the oil could be used in the treatment of dysmenorrhoea, but may also increase bleeding due to the relaxation effect (Ostad *et al.* 2001, cited in Harris 2001).

According to Price and Price (1999), sweet fennel oil is particularly useful for its therapeutic actions on the digestive system (antispasmodic, carminative). It is also indicated for PMS and menopause symptoms, because of not only its possible oestrogenic qualities, but also its other properties that may alleviate associated symptoms, such as oedema (diuretic), breast engorgement (decongestant) and bloating (carminative); cellulite, a common female complaint, is also mentioned, because the oil is also said to be diuretic. It is cited as a respiratory tonic, but its bronchodilatory action is not emphasised. The analgesic quality is not highlighted. Sweet fennel oil also has antifungal activity, and could be used in the treatment of fungal nail infections (Patra *et al.* 2002). The inhalation of sweet fennel essential oil can produce a decrease in mental stress, fatigue and depression (Nagai *et al.* 1991).

Therefore, this is a very versatile and useful oil in aromatherapy. Most authors suggest caution in pregnancy (apart from the last two months), avoidance in oestrogen-dependent cancer and if liver function is compromised, and that it should be used in low doses. For some uses, please see Table 8.47.

Table 8.47 Sweet fennel essential oil in aromatherapy

System	Sweet fennel with
Female reproductive	Geranium, juniperberry, clary sage (use sage with caution)
Digestive	Sweet marjoram, black pepper, sweet orange, mandarin, lime, clary sage, peppermint
Respiratory	*Eucalyptus* spp. (1,8-cineole types), lemon

GENUS LEVISTICUM
LEVISTICUM OFFICINALE – LOVAGE

An essential oil can be distilled from both the roots and the aerial parts of this large, aromatic perennial herb. The oil from the roots is reminiscent of celery. Little information is available, as it is not used much in aromatherapy practice. The essential oil is composed mainly of phthalides, 70 per cent (Lawless 1992) – these include butylidene and its derivatives and ligostilides; coumarins and furocoumarins are also present (Lawless 1995). Lawless suggests that it may have uses for the accumulation of toxins, the digestive system and the genito-urinary system.

GENUS PETROSELINUM
PETROSELINUM SATIVUM – PARSLEY

Parsley seed oil is not often used in aromatherapy, mainly due to the presence of apiol, a phenolic ether that can, if abused, cause many serious problems including coma, respiratory depression, cyanosis, hypotension and other consequences, such as kidney damage. There are three chemotypes – however, a 'typical' parsley seed essential oil will contain myristicin (a phenolic ether) at around 28 per cent, 2,3,4,5-tetramethoxyallylbenzene (TMAB) at 23 per cent and parsley apiol at 21 per cent (Tisserand and Balacs 1995). Parsley seed oil should only be used with caution externally, it is contraindicated in pregnancy and it should not be taken orally.

Genus Pimpinella

Pimpinella anisum – aniseed, anise

This is misnamed as it is actually the whole fruit, not just the seed that is used. Anise has a long history, reaching back to ancient Egypt, Greece and Asia Minor. It was used in baked goods and confections, and as a carminative and expectorant, and also an aphrodisiac. Today it is used to flavour many alcoholic drinks of the pastis and ouzo types. Aniseed essential oil has a warm, spicy, sweet odour, very characteristic of the herb. It has a very high proportion of *trans*-anethole – up to 90 per cent. Although this has therapeutic actions (see sweet fennel) the very high level here means that aniseed should be used with caution, avoiding it in alcoholism, breastfeeding, oestrogen-dependent cancers, liver disease, pregnancy, endometriosis and paracetamol use (Tisserand and Balacs 1995).

Family Valerianaceae

This is a family of herbs that includes the genus Valerian. *Valeriana officinalis* is the common valerian, whose root has been used since earliest times to heal a myriad of problems. It is perhaps best known as a gentle tranquilliser, and for aiding sleep.

Genus Nardostachys

Nardostachys jatamansi – spikenard

Spikenard is an aromatic herb, native to India, China and Japan. It has pungent, aromatic rhizomes which can be steam distilled to yield an essential oil. The tuberous root of 'nard' has been used over the centuries as incense, medicine and perfume. The herbalist Dioscorides considered it to be a warming and drying herb; it is mentioned in the Old and New Testament as an anointing oil, and the Romans used it in perfumery.

Spikenard has a pungent, earthy, valerian-like odour. According to Lawless (1992) its principal constituents are bornyl acetate, *iso*-bornyl valerianate, borneol, patchouli alcohol, terpinyl valerianate, α-terpineol, eugenol and pinenes. These constituents suggest uses for the respiratory system, as well as for skin care (allergies and inflammation) and insomnia, stress and tension (Lawless 1992).

Spikenard oil is a useful sedative, but its well-documented historical uses suggest that it is suited to calm the individual who is experiencing times of change and transition. In contemporary aromatherapy practice spikenard is rarely used, perhaps due to its cost and availability, as well as its intense scent. However, if an individual needs an aroma that can help with emotional and spiritual release or freedom issues, or needs help adjusting to major transitions in life, it is perhaps one of the most appropriate oils to use.

Family Zingiberaceae

This family includes around 47 genera of about 1500 species of perennial tropical and subtropical herbs (Weiss 1997). There are two subfamilies, the Costoideae and the Zingiberoideae. Cardamom (*Elettaria cardamomum*), plai (*Z. cassumunar*) and ginger (*Zingiber officinalis*) belong to the latter.

Genus Elettaria

Elettaria cardamomum – cardamom

Cardamom is a strong perennial herb growing from a rhizome as ginger does, but producing dark green, lanceolate leaves, and pale green flowers in panicles. The fruit is a spherical, pale green to yellow, trilocular capsule containing an essential oil, mainly in the dark brown seeds. The fruits are first sun-dried, or dried in a flue to avoid mould forming. The oil may also be distilled from fresh fruits and CO_2 extraction is possible. The major producer of the essential oil is India (Weiss 1997).

Cardamom has an ancient history – reference to it has been found on a clay tablet from ancient Sumaria (Weiss 1997). Cardamom has been used for thousands of years; it is very important in Arabic cultures (Classen, Howes and Synnott 1994) and Eastern traditional medicine (Lawless 1994). Like neroli and several other plant aromatics, it is often considered to be an aphrodisiac – but not to the same extent, and usually in combination with other aromatics. Lawless (1994) comments that cardamom, 'the Fire of Venus', was used as a mediaeval love potion, and that according to Vedic texts it had a reputation as a powerful aphrodisiac. Cardamom features in incenses too – for example, in Tibetan practice it is used medicinally for anxiety, and in Hindu ceremonies it forms part of a powdered incense formula called '*Abir*'. It has been distilled to yield the essential oil since the sixteenth century, and is used in perfumery to give spicy, warm notes in floral fragrances (Aftel 2008).

The essential oil is colourless to pale yellow with a warm and spicy aroma, with an added camphoraceous or cineolic note (Weiss 1997). The major constituents of the distilled oil are 1,8 cineole at around 50 per cent, α-terpinyl acetate at 24 per cent and limonene at 6 per cent (Bowles 2003).

Lawless (1996) states that its main uses are for the digestive system (anorexia, colic, cramp, dyspepsia, flatulence, halitosis, heartburn, indigestion and vomiting) and the nervous system (mental fatigue and nervous strain). Franchomme and Pénoël (1990) state that it is tonic and stimulating, antispasmodic, anticatarrhal and expectorant – probably because of the high 1,8-cineole content. For some uses of cardamom in aromatherapy, see Table 8.48.

Table 8.48 Cardamom essential oil in aromatherapy

System	Cardamom with
Digestive	Coriander seed, black pepper, ginger, cinnamon leaf, clove bud, all citrus oils (especially sweet orange and mandarin)
Nervous system (fatigue, debility)	Jasmine, ylang ylang, rose, sandalwood, bergamot, frankincense, rosewood
Respiratory	Lavender, Atlas cedarwood, bergamot, sandalwood

GENUS ZINGIBER

ZINGIBER CASSUMUNAR – PLAI

Plai essential oil is a fairly recent introduction to the West, but has been used for some time by Thai massage therapists, primarily for joint and muscle complaints. The plant is native to Thailand, Indonesia and India and the oil is steam distilled from the fresh rhizome. It has a cool, green, peppery, tea tree-like aroma. The main active components are terpinen-4-ol (25–45%) sabinene (25–45%), γ-terpinene, α-terpinene and trans-1-(3,4-dimethoxyphenyl) butadiene (1–10%) (Price and Price 2007; Leelarungrayub and Suttagit 2009), and also α-pinene, cassumunin A and B and curcumin (Leelarungrayub and Suttagit 2009). Each of these compounds has anti-inflammatory activity.

In 2009 Leelarungrayub and Suttagit conducted a study that revealed that plai essential oil has a high antioxidant activity, and an anti-inflammatory action which was optimal at high dilutions of 1:100 and 1:1000v/v. They concluded that plai could be useful in medical treatments, in conjunction with phonophoresis or iontophoresis for the relief of pain and inflammation.

Wells (2003) attributes numerous properties to this oil and cites research into its anti-inflammatory action (Pongprayoon 1997) and its ability to reduce oedema and pain for up to 18 hours using a dilution of 10 per cent. A 10 per cent blend has also been used for post-operative swelling after knee surgery. Wells suggests that it has a cooling action on inflammation and might, in conjunction with tarragon or rosemary and cypress, reduce the intensity of an asthmatic attack induced by exercise or allergy. Wells also recommends it for irritable bowel syndrome (IBS) and menstrual cramps, and suggests that there have been no adverse reactions to its use.

Price and Price (2007) note that it has been suggested for use in ME and for pain relief; however, it is perhaps its anti-inflammatory potential that is most significant; they cite research by the Thailand Institute which demonstrated that trans-1-(3,4-dimethoxyphenyl) butadiene was twice as potent as Diclofenac

(Voltarol). For some suggestions on the aromatherapeutic use of plai, please see Table 8.49.

Table 8.49 Plai essential oil in aromatherapy

System	Plai with
Digestive (IBS)	Black pepper, orange, lime, tarragon, mandarin, cardamom, peppermint
Articular system	Black pepper, juniperberry, lemon, neroli, Atlas and Himalayan cedarwood, orange, nutmeg, lemon
Respiratory (asthma)	Tarragon, rosemary and cypress
Reproductive system (menstrual cramps)	Clary sage, sweet marjoram, sweet fennel, orange
Immune system (ME)	May chang, rosewood, palmarosa, Spanish lavender

ZINGIBER OFFICINALIS – GINGER

Ginger is native to tropical India and Southeast Asia, Australia and Japan. It has an ancient use as a spice, being mentioned in the earliest Sanskrit literature and in writings in China. It was used by the ancient Middle Eastern cultures too, and was introduced to the New World by the Portuguese.

Ginger is an erect, leafy perennial with purple flowers, growing from a horizontal rhizome near the surface of the soil. The rhizome is firm with a corky and scaly skin, and varies in colour from buff to dark brown through to black. The oil-containing cells are scattered throughout the cortex and the pith of the rhizome. The oil is obtained by distilling the preferably unpeeled, dried and powdered rhizomes (Weiss 1997).

The oil is a pale yellow to orange, mobile liquid, becoming more viscous with age or exposure to the air. The aroma is rich, warm and spicy, with a citrus-like top note and a woody undertone (Aftel 2008). The odour is powerful too, and it should be used very sparingly in a prescription. In perfumery, ginger is used as a 'toner', and its odour is very difficult to imitate (Jouhar 1991). Its main constituents are sesquiterpenes (zingiberene at <40%, α-curcumene at <20%, farnesene at <9%) and sesquiterpene alcohols (<18%). Monoterpenes (1–20%) and aldehydes influence the distinctive aroma.

Ginger essential oil is an analgesic, general tonic, digestive tonic and expectorant (Price and Price 2007). Franchomme and Pénoël (1990) suggest that it is anti-inflammatory, a bronchodilator and antipyretic. It is indicated for digestive pain, chronic bronchitis and flatulence, and as a general tonic.

It is also useful for mitigating nausea and vomiting. Geiger (2005) demonstrated that a 5 per cent solution of ginger in grapeseed oil, applied naso-cutaneously, benefited patients who have a high risk of post-operative nausea and vomiting. A study conducted by de Pradier (2006) looked at the efficacy of a mixture of equal parts of essential oils of ginger, cardamom and tarragon on 86 post-operative patients. One or two drops of the oil mixture was applied, with light friction to the sternocleidomastoid area of the neck and the carotid-jugular axis, immediately following surgery, and at the first sign of nausea. Overall, 75 per cent had a favourable response – especially those who has also received one single dose of a pro-emetic drug. If more than one drug had been administered, there was still a positive response in 50 per cent of the patients, i.e. a complete blocking of nausea and vomiting within 30 minutes. A negative response was recorded in 19 patients. It was not established whether the results were due to percutaneous effects or inhalation.

Ginger essential oil has also been investigated with regard to its effects on immune responses. Schmidt *et al.* (2009) demonstrated that it could restore the humoral immune response in immunosuppressed mice, so it is possible that the essential oil could be of support to those with compromised immune systems.

For some aromatherapeutic uses of this well-researched oil, please see Table 8.50.

Table 8.50 Ginger essential oil in aromatherapy

System	Ginger with
Digestive	Sweet fennel, marjoram, clary sage, coriander seed, cardamom, black pepper, ginger, all citrus oils (especially sweet orange and mandarin)
Nausea	Coriander seed and tarragon (caution)
Nervous system (fatigue, debility)	Jasmine, geranium, neroli, sandalwood, frankincense, rosewood, lime
Musculoskeletal (tension, pain)	Lavender, lemongrass, clove bud or cinnamon leaf, black pepper, grapefruit, Atlas cedarwood

CHAPTER 9

Essential Oils of the Gymnospermae

Introduction

It is thought that 300 million years ago, the first aromatic plants appeared on the planet. These were the coniferous trees. Some of these species continue to thrive today; many are notable sources of essential oils, such as species of *Pinus* (pine), *Picea* (spruce), *Abies* (fir) and *Cupressus* (cypress).

The Coniferales is the largest order of gymnosperms and the most widely distributed. Most of its 49 genera are evergreen trees and contain around 570 species. There are six families: the Araucariaceae, Cephalotaxaceae, Cupressaceae, Pinaceae, Podocarpaceae and Taxodiaceae. These trees generally grow at high altitude in northern latitudes, most showing a pyramidal growth pattern, with simple leaves, needles or scales; they all produce cones. Most are monoecious (having the female and male reproductive organs separated in different structures on the same plant) and produce pollen grains.

The Coniferales includes several families containing aromatic genera. The families Cupressaceae and Pinaceae include genera that are notable for the production of essential oils used in aromatherapy.

FAMILY CUPRESSACEAE

This family contains many species that produce essential oils, several of which have aromatherapy applications, and a few of which are toxic. The genera of interest to aromatherapists are *Thuja*, *Chamaecyparis*, *Cupressus* (true cypress), *Juniperus* (juniper) and *Pseudotsuga* (Douglas fir).

Thuja has a long herbal tradition; however, most aromatherapy books state that the essential oil is considered too toxic to have applications in aromatherapy. At the other end of the scale, Mediterranean cypress is the most commonly used cypress in aromatherapy practice. There are several areas of application, such as aiding the respiratory system, the urinary system and the skin. There are several essential oils obtained from the genus *Juniperus*. Applications common to this group of essential oils are for pain, the respiratory and urinary systems, and as depuratives and diuretics.

Genus Chamaecyparis

Chamaecyparis obtusa – Hinoki leaf or wood

This tree is known as the Hinoki false cypress; there are no documented accounts of the therapeutic use of its essential oil. However, the oil is used in perfumery (it is well tolerated on the skin) and the tree has been protected since 1982 by the Japanese government (Burfield 2002).

Genus Cupressus

Cupressus sempervirens – cypress

C. sempervirens is the Mediterranean cypress. This is a tall, evergreen tree with graceful, slender branches and a conical shape, which bears small flowers and round, brownish-grey cones. There are many species of cypress, but it is mainly *C. sempervirens* that is of interest to aromatherapists.

In aromatherapy this is the most commonly used true cypress essential oil. The essential oil is produced in France, Spain, Croatia and Morocco, from the needles and twigs. It is a pale yellow to green/olive, mobile liquid with a lingering, smoky, balsamic odour. Chemically it is dominated by α-pinene, δ-3-carene and cedrol (Bowles 2003), therefore it has both monoterpenes and a sesquiterpenol as major constituents.

Price and Price (2007) give a full profile of this chemically complex oil, suggesting many uses in aromatherapy. They highlight its usefulness as a neurotonic for debility and also as a phlebotonic with astringent action, making it useful for broken capillaries. Other areas of application include the respiratory system for coughs and spasm; the urinary system because of its diuretic action; and for its toning astringent and phlebotonic actions on the skin. Schnaubelt (1999) suggests that cypress has antispasmodic properties, and is therefore useful for all bronchial complaints. He also concurs with Price and Price (2007) regarding its efficacy as a venous and lymphatic decongestant, aiding oedema and varicose veins. For some aromatherapeutic uses of cypress, please see Table 9.1.

Table 9.1 Mediterranean cypress essential oil in aromatherapy

System	Cypress with
Respiratory – bronchitis, pleurisy* (Schnaubelt 1999)	Sandalwood, *Eucalyptus* spp. (1,8-cineole types), myrtle,* frankincense, bergamot
Circulatory–lymphatic (varicose veins, oedema)	Patchouli, geranium, juniperberry, rosemary, lemon, grapefruit
Integumentary (broken capillaries, oily skin, acne)	Ylang ylang, geranium, rose, helichrysum, bergamot, sandalwood, patchouli

*Asterisks indicate a particular relationship between the condition and the oil thus identified.

GENUS JUNIPERUS

JUNIPERUS ASHEI – MEXICAN CEDAR, TEXAS CEDAR

Despite its name, this is not a true cedar. The essential oil obtained from *J. ashei* is also called Texas cedarwood oil, as it is here that the essential oil is distilled. It is dominated by α-cedrene and cedrol (Lawless 1996). Bowles (2003) states that Texan cedar oil is obtained from *J. mexicana*, and contains thujopsene, a sesquiterpene, at 32 per cent. The essential oil can be irritating to the skin; the main aromatherapy applications reported are for articular pain, respiratory congestion and urinary tract infections (Lawless 1996).

JUNIPERUS COMMUNIS – JUNIPERBERRY

Juniper essential oil is widely used in aromatherapy practice. The essential oil for aromatherapy use is obtained from the berries (although 'inferior' oil is extracted from the needles and twigs) and it is produced in Italy, France and Croatia. Juniperberry is a well-known flavouring in gin, and it is currently enjoying resurgence in popularity as a culinary ingredient. The essential oil is a colourless or pale green, mobile liquid with a fresh, resinous, woody aroma. The needle/twig product has a turpentine note.

Chemically, the dominant constituent is α-pinene at 33 per cent. Myrcene, a monoterpene, said to have analgesic properties, is present at around 11 per cent; β-farnesene is present too, at 10.5 per cent. This is a sesquiterpene with potential pheromonal effects (Bowles 2003). Terpinen-4-ol and α-terpineol are also found, and these are said to have diuretic action.

Price and Price (2007) cite several uses for juniperberry essential oil – most of which are echoed in popular aromatherapy books. These include its applications for muscle and joint pain (including gout) because of its analgesic, rubefacient and depurative qualities. For the urinary system it is an antiseptic, depurative and diuretic, and so can aid problems such as cystitis, oedema and cellulite. Juniperberry can also be used for skin problems such as acne and weeping eczema. For some uses, refer to Table 9.2.

Table 9.2 Juniperberry essential oil in aromatherapy

System	Juniperberry with
Urinary	Sandalwood, bergamot, cypress
Circulatory–lymphatic (cellulite, oedema)	Sweet fennel, geranium, cypress, rosemary, lemon, grapefruit, sage, black pepper
Musculoskeletal (muscular and articular aches and pains, gout)	Rosemary, sweet marjoram, eucalyptus, basil, black pepper, grapefruit

JUNIPERUS OCYCEDRUS – CADE

Juniperus oxycedrus is commonly known as medlar (not to be confused with *Mespilus germanica*, the well-known deciduous fruiting tree also known as medlar). A rectified essential oil, known as cade oil, is obtained from *J. oxycedrus*. Cade oil is an ingredient of some pharmaceutical preparations for skin disorders such as psoriasis, and it is also used in the fragrance industry. It is used in aromatherapy, but not widely, due to a reputation for causing sensitisation reactions (Lawless 1996).

JUNIPERUS SABINA – SAVIN

This is often called simply 'juniper' or shrubby red cedar. It yields an essential oil known as savin oil, which is not used in aromatherapy, as it is embryotoxic (Tisserand and Balacs 1995) due to its high content of sabinyl acetate, and it is also irritating to the skin. In addition, it has an unpleasant odour (Lawless 1996).

JUNIPERUS VIRGINIANA – VIRGINIAN CEDARWOOD

This tree and its wood, and the incense derived from the wood, hold an important place in Northwest/Pacific Indian tradition. Virginian cedarwood oil is distilled from the waste, powdered wood from sawmills, as the wood itself is an important commodity. The main use is in the manufacture of pencils, but it is used in furniture manufacture, including the traditional 'cedar chest'.

Virginian cedarwood essential oil is used widely in the fragrance industry. It is also commonly used in aromatherapy. However, it is often named 'cedarwood' and therefore confused with Atlas cedarwood essential oil. Virginian cedarwood has a smell reminiscent of pencil shavings, clean, woody/oily. Its dominant constituents are α-cedrol at up to 15 per cent, α- and β-cedrene, thujopsene, β-caryophyllene and γ-eudesmol (Burfield 2002).

The commonly cited uses are very similar to those of Atlas cedarwood, except that it is not recommended in pregnancy (Lawless 1996). There does not seem to be a basis for this (Burfield 2002).

GENUS PSEUDOTSUGA
PSEUDOTSUGA TAXIFOLIA – DOUGLAS FIR

This is known as the Oregon Douglas fir, or the Oregon balsam. The tree is widely distributed in North America. An essential oil is distilled from its leaves, and sometimes the resin. This has a very fragrant odour which is reminiscent of pineapples. It is dominated by geraniol at 31–32 per cent – unusual for a coniferous oil – and also bornyl acetate and traces of citral (Jouhar 1991).

Holmes (2001) describes Douglas fir as having an appetite-stimulating lemony note, which can counteract mental and emotional confusion. This was one of the fragrances explored by Warren and Warrenburg (1993), where it was reported as being distinctly relaxing, its effects being similar to those of meditation. The words are different, but essentially they describe the same quality – that of a still mind and calm vitality.

GENUS THUJA
THUJA OCCIDENTALIS – THUJA

Thuja is also known as 'cedar', or *arbor vitae*, the 'tree of life'. This is one of the tallest conifers. Its name '*thuja*' is derived from the Greek word meaning 'to fumigate': or *thuo*, also meaning 'to sacrifice' (as ancient cultures were thought to burn the wood with sacrifices). The wood is used for construction and furniture making, and in earlier times it was used as an astringent, a diuretic and an abortifacient.

The essential oil is considered too toxic to have applications in aromatherapy. It is dominated by the ketone thujone at around 60 per cent (Lawless 1996) – in this case α-thujone, and around 10 per cent β-thujone. Thujone is one of the ketones that may cause convulsions and produce liver and CNS damage; even small doses can result in nausea, hallucinations and coordination difficulty (Bowles 2003). Schnaubelt (1999) suggests that it can be used externally in small amounts, citing its use on warts, but commenting on the lack of evidence for this practice.

FAMILY PINACEAE

In this family the four most important genera, from the essential oil perspective, are *Abies* (fir), *Cedrus* (cedar), *Picea* (spruce) and *Pinus* (pine).

The volatile oils are produced in resin canals, and can be extracted from the wood, needles and cones. Essential oils from the family Pinaceae are widely used in the flavour and fragrance industry, and in pharmaceutical preparations. The essential oils are also used in household antiseptic products and disinfectants.

In aromatherapy the main applications of the pine essential oils are to aid the respiratory system (especially if infection is present), to aid convalescence and to help in cases of general debility. The pine oils are used as analgesics for articular and muscular pain, and are also indicated in cases of urinary system infections. Spruce and fir oils are less frequently used, despite their very pleasant, typical conifer fragrance; their principal application is to aid the respiratory system. Essential oils from the true cedars are also applied to aid the respiratory system and to alleviate muscular and articular pain. In addition, they may be used to help with skin problems, and are considered to be very effective for reducing stress.

GENUS ABIES (THE TRUE FIRS)

The fir oils are not widely used in aromatherapy practice, although they are used extensively in the fragrance industry for their fresh, conifer scents; they lack the resinous base notes of the pines and junipers. They are all dominated by monoterpenes.

ABIES ALBA – SILVER FIR

The essential oil is a pale/colourless, mobile liquid with a pleasant, sweet, lemony-balsamic odour. It contains santene, the pinenes, limonene and bornyl acetate (an ester). Its aromatherapy applications are for the respiratory, musculoskeletal and immune systems (Lawless 1996), and its scent can also impart mental clarity (Holmes 2001).

ABIES BALSAMIFERA – CANADIAN BALSAM FIR

According to Bowles (2003) this essential oil typically contains α-pinene at 33 per cent, δ-3-carene at 21.5 per cent and bornyl acetate at 11.9 per cent. These constituents would suggest that Canadian fir has similar applications to the other coniferous oils; Lawless (1996) suggests that it may be used in skin care, respiratory conditions, cystitis and depression.

ABIES SACHALINENSIS

This species of fir is widely distributed in Hokkaido, Japan. Although it is not a well-known essential oil in the west, it has been the subject of several studies in Japan. Satou et al. (2011) state that its main constituents had previously been identified as α-pinene, camphene, β-pinene, β-phellandrene and bornyl acetate.

Their 2011 animal study (using mice) attempted to clarify the mechanisms whereby essential oils such as that of *A. sachalinensis* produce their anxiolytic effects. It was found that inhalation of *A. sachalinensis* was a better route of administration than intraperitoneal injection for eliciting an anxiolytic-like response, and that the response was probably mediated by brain concentrations of its constituents and possibly the olfactory sense. This species of fir, amongst others, is prevalent in areas where *Shinrin-yoku* ('taking in the forest atmosphere') is a traditional practice for maintaining health and well-being. In this context, the results of this study would certainly support the use of *A. sachalinensis* for reducing anxiety.

ABIES SIBIRICA – SIBERIAN FIR

Matsubara *et al.* (2011) cite studies that indicate that Siberian fir essential oil has antibacterial and antiviral activity, and they comment that the tree is part of traditional Siberian medicine, helping to maintain health during the severe winters. Their 2011 study revealed that inhalation of air containing the essential oil reduced arousal levels after a prolonged visual display terminal (VDT) task. The participants were aware of the presence of the odour, and commented that it induced feelings of pleasure, so there is an element of hedonic valence to consider. However, the results obtained via physiological measurements and EEG readings were nonetheless significant. Prolonged VDT work can lead to mental fatigue, sleep disorders and anxiety, therefore it was suggested that Siberian fir essential oil has the potential to prevent such problems without influencing task performance.

GENUS CEDRUS
CEDRUS ATLANTICA – ATLAS CEDAR

This is the most commonly used true cedarwood essential oil. *C. atlantica* is a tall, evergreen tree with a highly aromatic, hard wood, which is native to the Atlas Mountains of Algeria. It has close relations with *C. libani* (Lebanese cedarwood) and *Cedrus deodara* (Himalayan cedarwood). Atlas cedarwood essential oil is from Morocco, extracted from the woodchips and sawdust left over from wood used for construction and furniture. It is a pale amber, slightly viscous liquid with a woody, warm, camphoraceous odour. Burfield (2002), in a review of cedar oils, suspects that many of the 'cedar' oils sold to aromatherapists are not genuine, and are probably adulterated with the cheaper and readily available Chinese cedar, *Cupressus funebris*.

It is dominated by sesquiterpenes. Price and Price (2007) note that cedrene is present at 50 per cent, sesquiterpene alcohols atlantol and cedrol at 30 per cent, and ketones α-atlantone and γ-atlantone at 20 per cent. However, Burfield (2002) gives a different analysis. He states that the sesquiterpenes α-, β- and γ-himalchenes constitute almost 70 per cent of the oil, while other components include α- and γ-atlantone isomers at 10–15 per cent. These have sweet woody odours (especially the *d*-α-atlantone) that make a significant contribution to the odour profile.

Price and Price (2007) highlight its applications as an antiseptic for skin problems (especially scalp problems and eczema), for the urinary tract, and as an antipruritic when combined with bergamot. They also recommend it as a lymphatic stimulant and as a mucolytic with applications for the respiratory system. Schnaubelt (1999) suggests that it is a gentle but powerful circulatory stimulant, useful for fluid retention and helpful for cellulite. The scent, which is sweeter and woodier than the other conifers, can help ground and calm the mind (Holmes 2001).

In aromatic medicine and for internal use, Atlas cedar is contraindicated in pregnancy and for children (Price and Price 2007); however, its external use in aromatherapy does not appear to carry a risk (Tisserand and Balacs 1995). For some suggestions on the use of Atlas cedarwood essential oil in aromatherapy, please see Table 9.3.

Table 9.3 Atlas cedarwood essential oil in aromatherapy

System	Atlas cedarwood with
Respiratory (bronchitis)	Sandalwood, *Eucalyptus* spp. (1,8-cineole types), benzoin resinoid, ginger, frankincense
Integumentary – scalp (seborrhoea, stimulant) Integumentary (eczema, itching, pruritus)	Juniperberry, rosemary, lavender, ylang ylang Sandalwood, vetivert, bergamot, lavender
Circulatory–lymphatic	Sweet fennel, juniperberry, rosemary, grapefruit, lavender, patchouli, cypress, black pepper

CEDRUS DEODARA – HIMALAYAN CEDAR

C. deodara produces a very similar essential oil to *C. atlantica* (Lawless 1996). This tree grows on the Himalayan slopes of Northern India, Afghanistan and Pakistan. In India it is used for external structures such as railway sleepers, and it has now been over-exploited. Himalayan cedar oil is used in Ayurvedic medicine as an anti-helmintic, and in the treatment of ulcers and skin diseases. The oil is yellow to reddish-brown and slightly viscous, with a 'dirty', slightly crude note, woody and also with sweet, resinous and urinous notes; rectified oils are used in aromatherapy.

The notable chemical constituents are *para*-methyl-δ-3-tetrahydroacetophenone, *para*-methyl acetopheneone, *cis*- and *trans*-atlantone, α- and β-himalchenes, ar-dihydroturmerone, *d*-himachalol and *d*-allohimachalol (Burfield 2002).

Burfield (2002) considers that the aromatherapeutic uses of Atlas and Himalayan cedarwood oils, based on their sesquiterpene and sesquiterpene derivatives, are broadly confirmed by a few studies. For example, himachalol and other sesquiterpenes from *C. deodara* were shown to have spasmolytic activity (Kar *et al.* 1975; Patnaik *et al.* 1977, cited in Burfield 2002), and *C. deodara* was shown to have analgesic and anti-inflammatory activity in animal studies (Schinde *et al.* 1999a, b, cited in Burfield 2002). Baylac and Racine (2003) confirmed that it might have anti-inflammatory activity, as it was an inhibitor of 5-lipoxyoxygenase.

In the last two chapters we have looked at most of the aromatherapeutic essential oils, and a few that are perhaps more hazardous than therapeutic. In the next chapter we will explore some aromatic extracts with considerable therapeutic potential which have been avoided or underused in aromatherapy, and which deserve consideration and recognition.

GENUS PICEA

PICEA ALBA – WHITE SPRUCE

This is not used in aromatherapy practice.

PICEA EXCELSA – NORWAY SPRUCE

This is not used in aromatherapy practice.

PICEA MARIANA – BLACK SPRUCE

Information on its use is scarce, but Schnaubelt (1999) suggests that it is a bronchial decongestant and an even more powerful adrenal stimulant than *P. sylvestris*. It can be combined successfully with Scots pine and blackcurrant bud absolute in cases of adrenal exhaustion (Schnaubelt 1999). Holmes (2001) suggests that its fragrance confers a sense of endurance and stamina, especially if combined with grand fir or Scots pine.

GENUS PINUS

PINUS MUGO VAR. PUMILIO – DWARF PINE

The essential oil is extracted from the needles and twigs. It can be irritating due to the presence of δ-3-carene at 35 per cent (Bowles 2003), and is therefore largely avoided in aromatherapy (Lawless 1996).

PINUS PALUSTRIS – LONGLEAF PINE

This species of pine produces an oleoresin (turpentine) that is steam distilled and rectified to yield a product also known as turpentine. The wood, needles and twigs of the tree can be steam distilled to yield an essential oil, which is used in aromatherapy (Lawless 1996).

PINUS SYLVESTRIS – SCOTS PINE

The essential oil is steam distilled from the needles. In aromatherapy this is probably the most commonly used of the pine oils, possibly due to its odour being less like disinfectant than that of *P. palustris*. The essential oil is produced in Hungary, Siberia and the Balkans. It is a colourless/pale yellow, mobile liquid with a strong, coniferous, fresh odour.

The essential oil is dominated by monoterpenes, notably α- (42%) and β-pinene and δ-3-carene at 20.5 per cent (Bowles 2003). These constituents are said to be mucolytic (Franchomme and Pénoël 1990); but also may be irritating to the respiratory tract (Bowles 2003). Perhaps this is why they have the effect of making mucus thinner, as they may stimulate the goblet cells of the respiratory tract. However, Bowles (2003) suggests that such monoterpene-rich essential oils should be used with caution on those who suffer from asthma. The same constituents are said to be rubefacient and therefore analgesic, hence their use for muscle and joint pain.

Schnaubelt (1999) suggests that Scots pine is an endocrine stimulant containing 'hormone-mimicking, polycyclic terpenoids', and is a 'forceful tonic and adrenal stimulant' that can be used at 10 per cent over the kidney/adrenal area for adrenal support.

For some aromatherapeutic uses, please see Table 9.4.

Table 9.4 Scots pine essential oil in aromatherapy

System	Scots pine with
Respiratory (especially colds, flu, rhinitis, sinusitis)	Cypress, Atlas cedarwood, rosemary, marjoram, eucalyptus, lemon, galbanum
Musculoskeletal (muscle and/or joint pain	Juniperberry, rosemary, black pepper, marjoram, lavender
Nervous/Immune/Endocrine (adrenal support, stress, debility, convalescence)	Basil, rosemary, ravintsara, lemon, grapefruit, lavender, black pepper

CHAPTER 10

Absolutes and Resinoids in Aromatherapy

Introduction

Absolutes and resinoids are the most highly concentrated and unaltered aromatic materials produced for use in the perfumery industry, and most do not have documented therapeutic uses, certainly not in the way that essential oils have. With the possible exceptions of jasmine, rose and neroli absolutes and benzoin resinoid (rose and neroli are also available as essential oils), few absolutes and resinoids have even acquired an aromatherapy tradition of use. With one or two exceptions, they are not usually used at all in aromatic medicine.

Concretes, absolutes and resinoids are products of solvent extraction, as essential oils are products of distillation, enfleurage or expression. Solvent extraction can be used to remove the odorous component from any aromatic plant material. However, it is generally used for the flowers of plants whose volatile oils would be extensively degraded by the heat, pressure and steam of distillation – for example, jasmine and tuberose. The final residue of the process is often a viscous, reddish-brown coloured liquid or paste. The colour depends on the pigments in the plant material – for example, lavender absolute is bright green in colour. Some absolutes are decolourised with activated charcoal, which absorbs some of the pigments.

Solvent extracted plants are considered to be closer in scent to the natural plant than their steam distilled counterparts. However, it is imperative that only high quality absolutes are used, as poor quality products might contain traces of solvent.

Resistance to the use of absolutes in therapeutic practice, and defence of their use and potential, is summarised by Baylac and Racine (2003). The first reason that aromatherapists give is the concern that benzene and chlorinated solvents may remain in the product. However, modern solvent extraction does not use these solvents, and the process also involves ethanol extraction, which will remove any residual primary extraction solvent remaining in the concrete. In reality the final absolute will only contain a few parts per million of the primary solvent, and much less than 3 per cent ethanol. The second line of resistance is that the composition of absolutes and resinoids is less accessible, and that they contain small proportions of non-volatiles with as yet unknown properties. However, molecular distillation of absolutes yields products known as incolores, which do not contain these non-volatiles; so perhaps these would be acceptable to aromatherapists.

Following on from a 2003 study on the 5-lipoxyoxygenase (5-LOX) inhibitory capacity, which is a possible mode of action for some anti-inflammatory essential oils and absolutes, Baylac and Racine (2004) investigated the potential for aromatic extracts to inhibit human leukocyte elastase (HLE) *in vitro*. This enzyme is also important in the pathophysiology of inflammation, and is involved in the degradation of the matrix proteins collagen and elastin. UV exposure will stimulate HLE activity, hence the ultimate visible effect of sun damage to the skin, including wrinkles and loss of elasticity. In this study, the absolutes outperformed the essential oils in their ability to inhibit HLE. Only two of the essential oils tested, myrrh and ylang ylang, showed even weak activity. Turmeric oleoresin (*Curcuma longa*) showed the strongest activity (even greater than the reference), and poplar bud absolute, rosemary extract and benzoin resinoid showed very strong inhibitory activity. Also active were the absolutes and resinoids of gentian, linden, violet leaf, myrrh, cocoa, artichoke, fucus (a genus of seaweed), jasmine, blackcurrant bud, rice and tea. It was noted that curcumin oleoresin contains curcuminoids – three complex diones with antioxidant and anti-inflammatory activity – which are not found in the essential oil. It was concluded that absolutes, resinoids and oleoresins do have a place in aromatherapy practice.

If some absolutes and resinoids have physiological actions, most appear to exert effects on the psyche. Their highly concentrated odours mean that they can be used in very low concentration, so their psychotherapeutic effects will probably be due to inhalation and the limbic system rather than via direct pharmacological activity – but this is only a hypothesis.

Of interest is that one of the early criticisms of aromatherapy was in relation to the direct translation of the herbal uses of aromatic plants into the aromatherapy materia medica, so that the essential oils were ascribed the same properties as the whole plant or herb. As absolutes often contain constituents that are absent in the essential oil, and so are closer to the plant, it will be interesting to see how the therapeutic use of absolutes develops in the future. However, as the aromatherapy mode of delivery is via inhalation and transdermal absorption, this may best be developed in prescriptions and products for the skin. It is also doubtful that practitioners who advocate the energetic approach will use absolutes, because of the involvement of solvents including alcohol.

We will now explore just a few of the absolutes and resinoids that have potential aromatherapeutic use; as before, these are organised according to their botanical families and genera.

Family Amaryllidaceae

Genus Narcissus — narcissus

This genus contains *N. jonquilla* (jonquil) and *N. poeticus* (narcissus), from which an essential oil (ex-enfleurage) and an absolute can be obtained. The plant is cultivated in the Mediterranean, Morocco and Egypt for its aromatic extracts.

Narcissus absolute is used in aromatherapy, and it has many applications in perfumes. It is a dark orange/olive green, viscous liquid with a heavy, sweet, herbaceous, hay-like, earthy, floral odour. It only smells like narcissus on extreme dilution. Like all absolutes, it is chemically very complex, containing aromatic alcohols (phenyl ethanol, α-terpineol, *l*-linalool), methyl ionone, anisic aldehyde and benzyl acetate (Jouhar 1991). There are trace amounts of indole. Indole (a cyclic imine) itself smells of mothballs, but it is faecal at 10 per cent and jasmine-like in trace amounts (Williams 2000). According to Lawless (1992, 1995) it has antispasmodic, aphrodisiac and narcotic actions, and can be used in aromatherapy for its fragrance alone.

Sub-family Agavaceae

Genus Polyanthes — tuberose

The most significant species in this family is the night-blooming *Polyanthes tuberosa*, which yields tuberose extract by enfleurage (the flowers continue to emit their scent after picking), or an absolute from its flowers. Tuberose is a tall perennial with lily-like flowers – the double flower variety is used as a cut flower. It is native to Central America, and cultivated in France, India (where it acquired an importance in ritual), Morocco and Egypt. Tuberose absolute is an expensive product that is widely used in perfumery.

The absolute is a soft, dark brown paste with a heavy, honey-like, sweet-caramel, floral aroma. When absolutes such as tuberose have a paste-like consistency, it is not possible to dispense them in drops into fixed plant oil or other carrier medium, and there may be additional solubility problems which can result in the formation of an undissolved residue. To facilitate their use in aromatherapy, it is best to prepare a 5 per cent w/w solution in a stable carrier such as jojoba; the diluted absolute should then be left to stand until any precipitate has formed and settled, then the clear portion can be decanted carefully into a clean container. This stock solution can then be used with ease in oil-based formulae.

Chemically, tuberose is very complex, containing alcohols (nerol, farnesol, geraniol, and benzyl alcohol), aromatic esters (methyl benzoate, methyl anthranilate, benzyl benzoate and methyl salicylate), eugenol and tuberone, a ketone (Jouhar 1991). Like many intense florals, it contains traces of indole. The scent of tuberose is said to have narcotic properties. This word is widely used in perfumery to denote a heavy, sleep-inducing scent, and overuse of such aromatics may have a stupefying effect. In aromatherapy tuberose is used mainly for its fragrance, and to promote relaxation and sleep (Lind 1998).

FAMILY APOCYNACEAE

GENUS PLUMERIA

PLUMERIA ALBA — FRANGIPANI

Plumeria alba is a small tree with scented flowers; their fragrance is more intense at night, in order to attract their pollinators, the sphinx moths. It is believed that *P. alba* is native to South and Central America or the Caribbean, and then introduced to Australia. In the South of India it is often planted near shrines; it is sometimes called the 'temple tree'. The flowers are beautiful, and have acquired a variety of meanings in various cultures – such as new life, creation, dedication and devotion. The Hawaiian culture regards the frangipani flower as a symbol of everything good. In Ayurvedic medicine it is used to calm fear and anxiety, and also to treat tremors and insomnia (McMahon 2011a).

Frangipani absolute has a rich, exotic, heady, floral aroma, with sweet, honey-like notes and fruity notes. It is said to bring comfort, impart inner peace and release tension; it has been used in terminal care.

FAMILY CARYOPHYLLACEAE

GENUS DIANTHUS

DIANTHUS CARYOPHYLIUS — CARNATION

There is only one genus relevant to perfumery or aromatherapy – the genus *Dianthus*. *Dianthus caryophylius* is the carnation, and *D. plumarius* is known as the pink. Carnation absolute has been used in aromatherapy, and is of importance in perfumery, although as a dominant note it has been less popular in recent years. It has a very powerful fragrance and is extremely costly to produce. The absolute is a green or brown, highly viscous liquid or paste, with sweet, herbaceous, honey-like, minty floral and spicy notes. Most carnation oil on the market is synthetic; synthetic carnation is usually derived from clove oil (Jouhar 1991). Its psychotherapeutic effects have not been explored in the literature, however several individuals who have had the opportunity to experience its scent, in an aromatherapy context, have expressed feelings of 'comfort' and 'joy' or of 'being carefree', and a few have commented that it evoked positive childhood memories of playing in a garden.

Family Fabaceae
Genus Spartium
Spartium junceum – genet

Spartium junceum is commonly known as Spanish or weaver's broom, because the twigs were used for sweeping; it is the botanical source of genet absolute. It should not be confused with broom absolute, which is sweet and honey-like, and is obtained from the shrub *Cytisus scoparius* (common broom), in the south of France and Morocco. Genet absolute is obtained from the yellow-golden flowers and is a dark brown, very viscous liquid with a tenacious, sweet, rosy, floral odour with green, herbaceous and hay-like notes (Jouhar 1991). It blends well with orange blossom and linden blossom.

Family Liliaceae

This family contains, amongst others, onions, chives, leeks, garlic (all genus *Allium*), bluebells, lilies and hyacinths. Essential oil of garlic, onion, etc. is obtainable, and these oils do have many uses in the flavour industry. They also have clinical and pharmaceutical significance, notably as antiseptics. These oils are not normally used in aromatherapy because of their pungent odours.

Genus Hyacinthus
Hyacinthus orientalis – hyacinth

This is sometimes called *jacinthe* oil. Hyacinth oil has been used in aromatherapy as well as in the fragrance industry, for which it is produced. It is cultivated commercially in both Holland and France. The absolute is a dark greenish liquid that has a very powerful, sharp, green, leaf-like odour, only pleasant on dilution, and only resembling hyacinth on extreme dilution (Jouhar 1991). At the time of writing, hyacinth absolute is very scarce; however, synthetic hyacinth is easily obtained. There is a marked difference in the fragrance: the synthetic version lacks the deep green/earthy note, and sweet green-floral notes dominate; it is obviously not 'natural'.

Chemically, hyacinth absolute is complex, containing phenylethanol, eugenol, methyl eugenol, benzoic acid, benzyl acetate, benzyl alcohol, cinnamic alcohol, cinnamyl acetate, benzaldehyde, cinnamic aldehyde, methyl- and ethyl- *ortho-*

methoxybenzoate, methyl methyl anthranilate, dimethyl hydroquinone and
N-heptanol. There is very little to support any claims of pharmacological effects
such as those suggested by Lawless (1995) and Rose (1999), who write that
hyacinth is antiseptic, styptic and sedative – unless they are basing this on the
possibilities afforded by the dominant phenyl ethanol.

Its odour is said to be narcotic, uplifting, refreshing and invigorating, and
it may enhance creativity. The scent was used in ancient Greece to refresh the
mind, and the Romantic poets such as Byron and Shelley reputedly enjoyed the
narcotic effect of its fragrance. In a study by Warren and Warrenburg (1993),
hyacinth fragrance evoked happiness, sensuality, relaxation and stimulation, while
decreasing feelings of apathy, irritation, stress and depression. This certainly gives
a sense of its therapeutic potential.

FAMILY MAGNOLIACEAE

GENUS MICHELIA

MICHELIA CHAMPACA – CHAMPACA

Champaca is native to the Philippines and Indonesia. In traditional customs,
women wear the flowers in the hair, or behind the ears, where they open and
release their scent. Champaca flowers are also used in garlands and for floating in
water to scent rooms. The absolute is a light yellow-reddish oil with an intense,
floral scent that is used to enhance jasmine accords. The absolute is scarce, and it
is not widely used as the dominant floral in perfumery.

Its constituents are identified as 1,8-cineole, *para*-cresyl methyl ether,
benzaldehyde, benzyl alcohol, benzoic acid and phenyl ethanol (Jouhar 1991).
Its fragrance is penetrating, warm, smooth and rich; it has a neroli-like floral note
accompanied by spicy, tea-like undertones. It is suggested that champaca will have
a relaxing, euphoric effect, perhaps similar to that of jasmine or neroli.

FAMILY MIMOSACEAE

GENUS ACACIA

ACACIA DEALBATA – MIMOSA

Acacia dealbata is a small tree that belongs to the order Leguminosae; it is native
to Australia, but also grown in France, Italy and India. Its flowers and twig ends
yield an absolute that has a powerful, green-floral odour; this is mainly produced
in the south of France (Jouhar 1991). Mimosa is recommended for anxiety, stress,
tension and over-sensitivity (Lawless 1992).

ACACIA FARNESIANA — CASSIE

Acacia farnesiana is a thorny bush or small tree that is cultivated in southern France and Egypt. The yellow flowers have a fluffy appearance, and are solvent extracted to yield cassie absolute.

The odour is described as 'exquisite' by Jouhar (1991), with spicy and floral notes; it finds applications in violet or jasmine and rose accords in perfumery and it is available as attar in India. Like all absolutes, it is chemically very complex, however Jouhar (1991) mentions just two of its constituents: farnesol and methyl salicylate — which might indicate the potential for anti-inflammatory actions.

FAMILY NELUMBONACEAE

GENUS NELUMBRO

NELUMBO NUCIFERA — LOTUS

N. nucifera is known as the Indian or sacred lotus and the 'Bean of India'. It is an aquatic perennial, whose seeds can remain viable for over 1000 years. The lotus was also noted as growing in the River Nile; and it was known to the Greek historian Herodotus. The lotus has acquired a symbolic quality representing patience and calmness. It grows in muddy waters, reaching the surface and producing beautiful large, flat leaves and exquisite pink, blue or white flowers whose petals unfurl to release a beautiful fragrance. The flowers symbolise immortality, resurrection and transcendence too, as they emerge from dried up pools following the monsoon. The symbol of the lotus is prominent in Buddhism.

Lotus absolute needs to mature in order to develop its fragrance. McMahon (2011b) describes pink lotus absolute as a deep pink, viscous liquid with a rich, sweet floral heart, fruity/leathery notes and a powdery, spicy dryout. White lotus is a dark brown, viscous liquid with a similar odour but an animalic, herbaceous dryout.

FAMILY OLEACEAE

The Oleaceae belong to the order Schrophulariales. The most important genera to study, from the essential oil and aromatherapy perspectives are the genus *Jasminum* and the genus *Osmanthus*.

GENUS JASMINUM — JASMINE

There are over 40 species of jasmine, and three are cultivated specifically for essential oil, concrete and absolute production — *Jasminum auriculatum* (mainly cultivated in India), *J. grandiflorum* (known as Spanish jasmine, cultivated in India, France and the Mediterranean region) and *J. sambac* (the most commonly cultivated jasmine in India, known as 'Moonlight of the Grove' and also used in jasmine tea). There are also many cultivars. In some plantations *J. grandiflorum* is grafted onto the sturdier, wild *J. officinale.*

Jasmine is an evergreen climbing shrub that produces white, star-shaped, highly fragrant flowers, whose scent becomes more intense at night. This is a fascinating genus to study for many reasons, ranging from botanical, geographical and ecological through to the essential oil and absolute production, its aesthetic and clinical uses and its distinctive and celebrated fragrance. Jasmine absolute is a dark, orange/brown liquid. Jasmine absolute has over 100 constituents, but is dominated by aromatic esters such as benzyl acetate, methyl jasmonate and methyl anthranilate, and benzyl benzoate. Monoterpenoid alcohols such as linalool are present, as are the aromatic alcohols, such as benzyl alcohol and the sesquiterpenol farnesol. The ketone *cis*-jasmone is found and there are trace amounts of indole. The aroma varies according to its source, but is typically floral, fruity, heavy and animalic with a waxy, spicy dryout (Williams 2000).

Jasmine has a long tradition as an aphrodisiac fragrance. In aromatherapy its main uses are for counteracting depression, stress and lack of confidence (Lawless 1995; Holmes 1998). In 2007 Hirsch *et al.* demonstrated that the aroma of jasmine could dramatically improve bowling scores. They suggested that it might do this by regulating mood, enhancing alertness, and reducing anxiety, and improving self-confidence and hand–eye coordination. They concluded that a similar effect could be expected in other activities that involve hand–eye coordination and precision.

Lawless (1995) and Holmes (1998) also suggest the use of jasmine for skin care, muscular aches and pains, spasm, coughs, as a uterine tonic and for dysmenorrhoea. An unpublished *in vitro* study indicated that, due to its free radical scavenging ability, jasmine absolute could protect against UV-B damage on human keratinocytes (Baylac and Racine 2003); this would certainly support its use in anti-ageing phytocosmeceuticals. For some aromatherapeutic uses of jasmine absolute, please see Table 10.1.

Table 10.1 Jasmine absolute in aromatherapy

System	Jasmine with
Integumentary (indicated for mature skin, dry, oily or sensitive skin)	Lavender, geranium, helichrysum, sandalwood, patchouli, violet leaf
Musculoskeletal (muscular stress, tension)	Lavender, lemongrass, black pepper, Roman or German chamomile, clary sage, ginger
Nervous (depression, tension, stress, fatigue, lethargy)	Sandalwood, ginger, cardamom

Genus Osmanthus

Osmanthus fragrans — osmanthus

This genus of evergreen shrubs and small trees has one species, *Osmanthus fragrans*, whose flowers are extracted to produce an absolute that has become increasingly popular in perfumery. This evergreen shrub is native to the Himalayas, Japan and China, where the powerfully scented flowers are used to scent tea. Osmanthus absolute is an amber or green viscous liquid which has a distinctive, complex odour; it is rich, sweet, honey-like and ethereal-floral, reminiscent of plums and raisins (Leffingwell 2000) and apricot (Warren and Warrenburg 1993).

The absolute contains linalool, linalool oxide and other constituents, including phenolic alcohols, acids and ionones. Osmanthus fragrance has been investigated in relation to its effects on mood. Warren and Warrenburg (1993) found that osmanthus fragrance's 'stimulating and happy qualities are further supported by prominent reductions in the negative moods of apathy and depression'. It has been suggested that osmanthus may also enhance collagen formation, soothe skin sensitivity and help restore and refine the skin (Leffingwell 2000) – hence its recent inclusion in commercial skin care products.

Family Orchidaceae

Genus Vanilla — vanilla

There are three species that yield vanilla as a product – Bourbon or Réunion vanilla is obtained by extraction from *Vanilla planifolia* Andrews, Tahiti vanilla is obtained from *V. tahitensis* J.W. Moore, and West Indian vanilla from *V. pompona*. Vanilla is a perennial herbaceous vine, with an epiphytic habit (an 'air plant'). It has dark green, tough leaves, and produces pale green/yellow or white flowers that occur in large racemes of 20 or more blossoms. Its long, green, slender, capsule-like fruits are known as pods, and are harvested while immature. They are filled with an oily mass, containing numerous small, black, shiny seeds. The pods are cured over a period of six months, and treated by solvent extraction to yield a resinoid and absolute.

Vanilla absolute is a brown viscous liquid with the characteristic sweet, rich, balsamic odour of vanilla. It is chemically very complex. Vanillin, a phenolic aldehyde, is present at around 2 per cent (Jouhar 1991), and other constituents include hydroxybenzaldehyde, acetic acid, *iso*-butyric acid, caproic acid, eugenol and furfural (Klimes and Lamparsky 1976; Lawless 1992).

Although vanilla is widely used as food flavouring and in perfumery, its applications in aromatherapy are not well documented. It is used mainly as a balsamic agent and for its soothing odour. It blends well with floral essential oils and absolutes (ylang ylang, geranium, rose and jasmine), sandalwood and the spice oils (ginger, clove and cinnamon).

FAMILY PANDANACEAE

GENUS PANDANUS

PANDANUS ODORATISSIMUS – KEWDA OIL

P. odoratissimus grows wild in India and Malaysia. It produces creamy-white or yellow, very large, highly scented blossoms which can weigh up to 100 g. Kewda oil is light yellow in colour, with a powerful, sweet, lilac, green, honey-like fragrance. Some of the constituents include the aromatic benzyl alcohol and its esters, benzyl acetate, benzyl benzoate and benzyl salicylate, also monoterpene alcohols such as linalool and geraniol, linalyl acetate, and some sesquiterpenoids – phenyl ethanol, santalol, guaicol and an unusual constituent, ω-bromstyrene, which has a harsh, hyacinth-like odour (Jouhar 1991).

FAMILY ROSACEAE

GENUS ROSA

Please refer to the rose essential oil profile (see page 204). The main species used for absolute production are *R. centifolia* and *R. damascena*. Rose absolutes are orange-yellow to orange-brown viscous liquids. The absolutes from Morocco and France are known as 'rose de mai' absolute; in Bulgaria it is usually *R. damascena* that is grown. The absolutes have much greater amounts of phenyl ethanol than the essential oils – usually around 60 per cent (Tisserand and Balacs 1995), along with geraniol, citronellol, nerol and farnesol (Jouhar 1991). Rose absolute is usually used to counteract depression and anxiety, irritability and mood swings. For some suggestions about some uses of rose absolute, please refer to Table 10.2.

Table 10.2 Rose absolute in aromatherapy

System	Rose absolute with
Nervous (depression, anxiety, debility)	Lavender, geranium, sandalwood, patchouli, benzoin, bergamot and citrus essential oils
Female reproductive system (PMS, irritability, mood swings)	Clary sage, bergamot, geranium, Roman chamomile

FAMILY RUTACEAE

Please refer to the Rutaceae family in Chapter 8 (pages 206–218) and the essential oils of the genus *Citrus*.

GENUS CITRUS

CITRUS AURANTIUM VAR. AMARA – ORANGE BLOSSOM ABSOLUTE

The flowers of the bitter orange are distilled to yield neroli essential oil, but they are also solvent extracted to give orange blossom absolute. This is a dark, orange-brown, viscous liquid with a warm, rich, tenacious odour – similar to the flower itself – and is of great value in perfumery. Chemically, it is also dominated by linalool (32%) and linalyl acetate (16.8%) and nerolidol and farnesol at around 7 per cent – these are sesquiterpene alcohols that have been associated with anticancer effects (Bowles 2003). It also contains phenyl ethanol at 4.5 per cent and methyl anthranilate, a nitrogen-containing ester at 3.0 per cent (Weiss 1997). In aromatherapy it is used in the same way as neroli.

FAMILY SALICACEAE

GENUS POPULUS

POPULUS BALSAMIFERA – POPLAR BUD

The poplar tree has sticky, resinous, aromatic buds and its bark contains salicylin, a glycoside that is the precursor of salicylic acid (aspirin). As you might expect, the bark is used in folk medicine as an analgesic, anti-inflammatory and febrifuge. The balsam poplar has a long tradition of use, notably by the North American Indians, who used it for skin and lung ailments. The resin from the sticky buds was used as a salve, hence the name 'Balm of Gilead'. It is also used in contemporary herbal medicine as an expectorant.

Poplar bud absolute is an opaque, golden, viscous substance, with a tenacious, sweet, cinnamon-like, balsamic odour, with resinous and coumarinic undertones (McMahon 2011c). It was one of the absolutes investigated by Baylac and Racine (2004), and had a very high capacity to inhibit 5-LOX; it therefore has good anti-inflammatory potential.

FAMILY STYRACEAE

GENUS STYRAX – BENZOIN

There are several members of this genus that exude aromatic balsamic resins if the trunk is cut or damaged. Resinoids may be produced from the resin by solvent extraction. *Styrax benzoin*, *S. paralleloneuris* and *S. tonkinensis* are tall, rapidly maturing, birch-like trees native to tropical Asia. Two types of product are obtained, depending on the geographical and botanical origins. Siam benzoin is produced from *S. benzoin* and *S. tonkinensis* trees that grow in Laos, Vietnam, Cambodia, China and Thailand; Sumatra benzoin is produced from *S. benzoin* and *S. paralleloneuris* trees growing in Sumatra, Java and Malaysia (Jouhar 1991; Lawless 1992).

Siam benzoin occurs in brittle, yellow-brown to white 'tears', while Sumatra benzoin is a milky, resinous sap which hardens before it is scraped off the bark. This is formed into rectangular blocks, which break into almond-shaped pieces (Jouhar 1991). Siam benzoin resin has a sweet, balsamic, chocolate-like scent, and Sumatra benzoin resin is warm, sweet and powdery (Jouhar 1991).

The term 'benzoin' relates to the balsamic resin, while benzoin extract is a further extraction of the resin. Benzoin resinoids are brown in colour, viscous, with odours reflecting the resins. The main chemical constituents are coniferyl cinnamate in Sumatra benzoin, and coniferyl benzoate in Siam benzoin (Lawless 1995). Both contain traces of the aromatic aldehyde, vanillin, which contributes to the sweet, vanilla-like odour.

As it is not an essential oil (the odorous molecules are not sufficiently volatile to distil over), it is disregarded by many authors. However, benzoin resinoid has many well established areas of use – for example, in pharmaceutical preparations for the gums and skin, as a component of tinctures to aid the respiratory system, and in perfumery. In aromatherapy it is primarily used for its calming, comforting scent, for stress-related problems, for skin problems and respiratory problems (Lawless 1996).

Benzoin does have a reputation as a sensitiser, and it is sticky to touch. It is advisable to prepare a 'carrier' oil containing benzoin, to which other essential oils can then be added. The carrier should be of known concentration, and decanted after the resinous material has precipitated. If the resinoid is added directly to a blend for massage, the preparation will be sticky, and leave the skin feeling sticky too.

For some suggested uses of benzoin in aromatherapy, please see Table 10.3.

Table 10.3 Benzoin resinoid in aromatherapy

System	Benzoin with
Nervous system (stress, debility, anxiety, depression)	Rose, jasmine, sandalwood
Respiratory (asthma, spasm, coughs, congestion)	Bergamot, ginger, sandalwood, frankincense
Integumentary (inflammation and irritation, wounds)	Myrrh, poplar bud, patchouli, lavender, helichrysum

FAMILY TILIACEAE

GENUS TILEA

TILEA VULGARIS – LINDEN BLOSSOM

The linden or lime tree is native to Europe. It is a tall deciduous tree with bright green, heart-shaped leaves. It bears clusters of strongly scented, yellow-white flowers, sometimes called lime flowers. These flowers have a long herbal tradition. Linden tea, made from the dried flowers (*tilleul*), is widely used as a calming tea, and its other uses in herbalism are for indigestion, palpitations and nausea, migraine, hypertension and fevers. Grieve (1992 [1931]) notes that if the lime blossoms are old, a tea made from them has a narcotic effect.

Linden blossom concrete and absolute may be obtained from the blossoms – this is used in perfumery. The absolute is a yellowish, semi-solid paste with a green-herbaceous aroma. It is dominated by farnesol, and in aromatherapy is indicated for cramps, indigestion and headaches (Lawless 1992).

FAMILY VIOLACEAE

GENUS VIOLA – VIOLET

Viola alba is the Parma violet, *V. odorata* is the sweet violet and *V. suavis* is the Russian violet. The violet is a small, tender, perennial plant, with heart-shaped, slightly downy leaves that arise on stalks from a creeping rhizome. It propagates by producing runners; these species rarely set seed. The flowers are single and usually deep purple, although there are lilac and pale pink varieties too. Violet has a long tradition of use as a fragrance and a medicine, and in confectionery. The Greeks used the scent to 'moderate anger, to procure sleep and to comfort and strengthen the heart' (Homer and Virgil, paraphrased by Grieve 1992). The ancient Britons and Celts harnessed its cosmetic powers, and the violet even acquired symbolic significance – it was, like the primrose, associated with the death of the young (Grieve 1992 [1931]).

Violet is cultivated in southern France for production of a concrete and absolute from the fresh leaves and flowers. These are used in perfumery and for flavouring confectionery. The *V. odorata* leaf absolute has 'an intense, rather unattractive, green and peppery odour' (Jouhar 1991).

It is chemically complex; 2-trans-6-cis-nonadien-1-al is the component largely responsible for the odour. It also contains n-hexanal, n-octen-2-ol-1, benzyl alcohol and others, and traces of eugenol (International School of Aromatherapy 1993).

Absolutes of both *V. alba* and *V. odorata* are available for aromatherapy use. The main indications for the use of violet leaf absolute are in skin care, stress, insomnia and headache (Lawless 1995). Violet leaf absolute showed the ability to inhibit the enzyme HLE (Baylac and Racine 2004), so may have applications for sun-damaged skin and as an anti-ageing absolute. It is interesting that this research is in some way verifying the uses developed by the early Britons and the Celts. For some suggestions, please refer to Table 10.4.

Table 10.4 Violet leaf absolute in aromatherapy

System	Violet leaf with
Integumentary (indicated for fragile, sensitive, wrinkle-prone or ageing skin, eczema, acne, thread veins, sun-damage)	Linden blossom, jasmine, lavender, geranium, sandalwood, patchouli, galbanum, bergamot, vetivert
Nervous system (dizziness, headache, insomnia)	Lavender, clary sage, basil, hyacinth

FAMILY ZINGIBERACEAE

GENUS HEDYCHIUM

HEDYCHIUM CORONARIUM – WHITE GINGER LILY

The genus *Hedychium* consists of around 50 species. Hedychiums grow in Southeast Asia, southern China and the Himalayas, and they are also cultivated in the USA (Jouhar 1991; McMahon 2011d). The genus name is derived from the Greek word *hedys*, meaning 'sweet', and *chion*, meaning 'snow'. All flowers produced by members of this family produce just one stamen. *H. coronarium* produces fragrant white flowers. It is also called the butterfly or garland lily.

The flowers themselves possess a fragrance reminiscent of tuberose and gardenia (Jouhar 1991), and they can be extracted to yield an absolute – an amber liquid with warm, sweet, honey-like, exotic floral notes and a spicy, fruity, balsamic undertone. It is thought that the constituents responsible for the scent are linalool, methyl jasmonate, eugenols, *cis*-jasmone, β-ionone and lactones (McMahon 2011d). Aromatherapy uses could be for relaxation and stress relief, possibly pain relief, and to aid sleep.

Appendix E contains a summary of the indications and actions of many of the essential oils, absolutes and resinoids explored in Part III. It also contains some subjective comments, and so should be consulted in like spirit.

Glossary

Abortifacient: Induces abortion.

Absolute: A highly concentrated aromatic extract obtained by alcoholic extraction of the concrete, by means of the process of solvent extraction (or enfleurage) of aromatic plant material.

Accord: In perfumery, a combination of aromatics that combine to give a particular fragrance effect.

Agrestic: An odour that is reminiscent of the countryside.

Amber: A perfume note that is powdery and reminiscent of vanilla.

Analgesic: Pain-relieving.

Annual: A plant whose life cycle is completed within one growing season.

Anthelmintic: A remedy that destroys intestinal worms.

Antibacterial: Destroys and/or inhibits bacterial growth.

Anticoagulant: Inhibits the coagulation of blood.

Antidepressant: Counteracts depression.

Antiphlogistic: Counteracts inflammation.

Antipruritic: Relieves itching.

Antisclerotic: Prevents the hardening of tissue.

Antiseborrhoeic: Restrains sebum production.

Antispasmodic: Relieves spasm in smooth muscle tissue. (This is now taken to include skeletal muscle.)

Antitussive: Relieves coughing.

Antiviral: Destroys viruses.

Anxiolytic: Reducing anxiety.

Apoptosis: Programmed cell death; a normal physiological process in maintaining homeostasis and tissue development in multicellular organisms.

Aril: The membrane covering a seed.

Aroma-chology: The study of the psychological effects of odours.

Aromatherapy: The therapeutic application of essential oils and aromatic plant extracts in a holistic context, to maintain or improve physical, emotional and mental well-being.

Aromatic medicine: The application of essential oils in the medical field, as developed and practised in France, by medically qualified persons.

Aromatology: The intensive, clinical use of essential oils to treat disorders.

Astringent: Causes contraction of tissues; can reduce secretions, e.g. sebum.

Balsamic: Soothing.

Biennial: A plant whose life cycle is completed over two growing seasons, with seed formation at the end of the second year.

Biosynthesis: The building up of more complex chemical compounds from simpler ones within a cell.

Boiling point: The maximum, constant temperature at which a liquid evaporates, at a given pressure.

Bract: Modified leaves at the base of a flower. The flowers of clary sage, for example, have large bracts.

Carminative: Relieves flatulence.

Catalyst: A substance that can alter the rate of a chemical reaction, which remains unaltered in mass and composition at the end of the reaction.

Cephalic: Benefits the head and mind; stimulating to the thought processes.

Cholagogue: Promotes bile flow by stimulating the gallbladder.

Choleretic: Promotes the secretion of bile by the liver.

Cicatrisant: Promotes healing by formation of scar tissue.

Cineolic: A eucalyptus-like odour.

***Cis-* and *trans*-isomerism:** A type of geometrical isomerism: *cis*-isomers have groups of similar atoms on one side of a double bond, *trans*-isomers have the same groups of atoms on opposite sides of a double bond. An example is geraniol (*cis-*) and nerol (*trans-*).

Cohobation: The process of re-distilling the distillation water to recover the water-soluble components of the essential oil.

Colation: A coarse filtration process, where a liquid is strained through a coarse filter to remove extraneous, insoluble particulate matter.

Colloidal solution: A dispersion of ultra-fine particles in a liquid medium.

Concrete: An aromatic, solid or semi-solid extract containing essential oil, waxes and pigments, obtained by solvent extraction of aromatic plant material.

Condensation: The change in state from gas or vapour to liquid or solid.

Corps: Purified fat, e.g. suet or lard, used in enfleurage.

Cytophylactic: Promotes healing and repair of tissue, encourages growth of skin cells.

Decongestant: Relieves congestion, e.g. of sinuses, of the respiratory system.

Depurative: Removes impurities from the blood (detoxifying).

Diaphoretic: Increases perspiration, assists excretory function of the skin.

Digestive: Aids the process of digestion.

Distillate: The product of distillation, collected in the receiver of the still.

Diuretic: Increases urination.

Drupe: A fleshy fruit in which the seed is surrounded by a hard endocarp, e.g. a plum or a cherry.

***E-* prefix:** Abbreviation of the German *entgegen*, meaning 'opposed to', in relation to the *trans*-isomer.

Emmenagogue: Promotes menstruation.

Emollient: Soothes and softens the skin.

Enantiometer: An optical isomer.

Enfleurage: The process of absorbing the fragrance from fresh flowers of a single species into a purified fatty medium over a period of time.

Enzyme: A biochemical catalyst.

Epiphyte: A plant which does not have roots in the soil, but lives above the ground, supported by another plant or object. It obtains its nutrients from the air, rainwater and organic debris. Many orchids are epiphytes and the typical habitat is the canopies of tropical rain forests.

Essential oil: A volatile product, obtained by a physical process, from a natural source of a single botanical species, which corresponds to that species in name and odour.

Evaporation: The change in physical state from liquid to gas or vapour.

Expectorant: Aids the expulsion of mucus from the respiratory tract.

Expression: A mechanical process of scarification and compression for obtaining the volatile oil from the flavedo (coloured rind) of citrus fruits.

Extract: The soluble matter obtained from an aromatic plant by washing with a solvent that is then recovered by vacuum distillation. Extracts include concretes, absolutes and resinoids.

Exudate: A resinous substance produced by the cambium of some woody plants. Aromatic exudates include benzoin, frankincense and myrrh.

Febrifuge: Reduces fever.

Fraction: A group of essential oil constituents which have similar volatility and boiling points; these can be separately collected portions of a distillate.

Functional group: A group of bonded atoms within a molecule, the most reactive part of the molecule, used in classification of molecules.

Genus (*plural* genera): The taxonomic category between family and species.

Glabrous: A plant surface devoid of hairs or other projections.

Glands (essential oil-producing): Glandular cells, glandular hairs: a group of one or more cells whose main function is to secrete a plant's volatile oil, e.g. glandular trichomes common in the Lamiaceae; vittae or resin canals in the Umbelliferae; secretory cells in flower petals, secretory cavities in the peel of citrus fruits, etc.

Glaucous: A plant surface with a blue/grey, waxy bloom.

Haemostatic: An agent that helps to stop bleeding.

Headspace: The space above the surface of a liquid, bounded by the surrounding container. 'Headspace analysis' is the analysis of the vapour present in the headspace.

Hepatic: Aiding liver function, assisting in the detoxification process.

Hepatotoxic: Toxic to the liver.

Hydrophilic: Attracts or mixes easily with water.

Hypertensive: An agent that raises the blood pressure.

Hypnotic: Inducing sleep.

Hypotensive: An agent that reduces blood pressure.

Isolate: A single chemical constituent separated from an essential oil.

Isomer: One of two or more compounds where the molecular formula is identical, but the atoms are arranged differently, e.g. α- and β-pinenes are identical, apart from the position of a double bond.

Latent heat of vaporisation: The amount of heat required to vaporise a given mass of liquid at the boiling point. The same quantity of heat is given out by the same weight of vapour when it condenses, at the boiling point.

Laxative: Promoting bowel movement.

Lipophilic: Denotes that a substance is fat-soluble.

Lymphatic stimulant: Assisting the tissue-cleansing function of the lymphatic system.

Maceration: The process of soaking a known weight of matter in a known volume of solvent such as a vegetable oil, in a closed vessel, over a given period of time, after which the suspension is filtered, the soluble portion of the matter having dissolved in the solvent. This solution may be standardised to a given strength. If the solvent is alcohol, the resultant liquid is known as a tincture.

Molecular weight: The ratio of the weight of one molecule of a substance to the weight of one atom of hydrogen, taken as one atomic weight unit.

Mucolytic: Reduces the thickness of mucus in the respiratory tract.

Necrotic: Causes tissue damage and tissue death.

Nephrotoxic: Toxic to the kidneys.

Nervine: Nerve tonic, neurotonic, strengthens the nervous system.

Neurotoxic: Toxic to the nervous system.

Oleo-gum resin: A plant exudate, which is composed of water-soluble gum, resin and volatile oil.

Oleoresin: A plant exudate consisting of resin and volatile oil.

Optical isomerism: Where the molecule of one form is the mirror image of the other form, e.g. *d*- and *l*-limonenes and *d*- and *l*-carvones. Also known as 'stereoisomerism'.

Para- prefix: Refers to two positions on a benzene ring which are opposite to one another e.g. the 1,4-positions; e.g. *para*-cymene.

Parturient: Aids childbirth.

Phagocytosis: The process where a cell such as a white blood cell engulfs and breaks down a foreign particle or microorganism.

Phlebotonic: Tonic (strengthening, astringent) to the veins.

Phototoxicity: A photosensitising substance applied to the skin, followed by exposure to UV light, will result in skin damage, burning (and a condition known as berloque dermatitis if bergaptene (in bergamot oil) is the agent).

Polar molecule: A molecule where there is an uneven distribution of the electrical charge, e.g. water, alcohol, aldehyde, that is usually water-soluble and fat-insoluble. Non-polar molecules tend to be fat-soluble and water-insoluble.

Pomade: A product of the enfleurage process – a fragrance-saturated fat.

Prophylactic: Prevents disease or infection.

Psychotropic: Mood altering.

Racemic mix: A naturally occurring mix of two enantiomers (optical isomers) of a compound, e.g. *d-* and *l-*linalool.

Receiver: In distillation, the vessel that collects the distillate from the condenser outlet.

Rectification: A process of re-distillation of an essential oil to eliminate unwanted constituents, or to standardise the product.

Resinoid: The product of solvent extraction of an oleo-gum resin or an oleoresin, which contains the odorous constituents.

Rubefacient: Increases local blood circulation, causing redness of the affected area.

Scarification: The process of scraping the surface of citrus fruits to allow mechanical expression of the volatile oil.

Sedative: Relaxing in effect, reducing activity, promoting sleep.

Sessile: Without a stalk.

Sialogogue: Promotes salivation.

Solute: The dissolved substance in a solution.

Solvent extraction: The separation of soluble matter from a natural source of plant material, oleo-gum resin or oleoresin, using a pure, volatile solvent. At the end of the process, the solvent is recovered by vacuum distillation, leaving behind the product containing the odorous portion of the material. The product is a concrete, which can be further treated to produce an absolute, or a resinoid, which in some cases may be distilled to produce a volatile oil.

Soporific: Induces sleep.

Spasmogenic: Inducing spasm in muscle tissue.

Spasmolytic: Reduces spasm in muscle tissue.

Steam distillation: A process of distillation in which steam, under pressure, is used to heat a charge in a still, to release and vaporise the volatile molecules. The volatile portion is then condensed back into liquid form and collected in a receiver vessel.

Still note: A vegetable (cabbage-like) note that may be present in freshly distilled essential oil, which can be eliminated by brief aeration.

Stimulant: An agent that temporarily increases the function of a system, e.g. circulatory stimulant, immunostimulant.

Sublimation: The physical change in state from solid to vapour or gas phase, without going through the liquid phase.

Sudorific: Promotes perspiration.

Surface tension: The stretching force observed at the surface of a liquid.

Tincture: A preparation of plant material in alcohol or an alcohol/water solution; the ratio of plant to fluid is generally higher than that of infusions or macerations.

Tonic: Generally supporting and restorative.

Transpiration: The evaporation of water from the leaves of a plant.

Uterine: Tonic to the uterus.

Vacuum distillation: Fractional distillation under a vacuum, which reduces the temperature required for the charge to reach boiling point; this eliminates thermal stress.

Vacuum stripping: Evaporation of the product of solvent extraction in a vacuum, to remove traces of solvent that remain in the product.

Vapour: A gas, under specific conditions where a slight increase of pressure, or decrease in temperature, will result in condensation into the liquid phase.

Vasoconstrictor: Causes narrowing of the blood vessels.

Vasodilator: Causes dilation of the blood vessels.

Vesicant: Irritating to the skin; causes burning and blistering.

Viscosity: The thickness of a liquid; the internal friction within a liquid substance that opposes its tendency to flow freely.

Volatile: Descriptive of a substance which evaporates when exposed to air. The term also applies to the low boiling point constituents of natural aromatic materials, e.g. plant volatile oils.

Volatility: The rate at which a substance evaporates. The concept of volatility has led to the classification of essential oils and aromatic extracts as top, middle and base notes, which correspond to high, medium and low volatility respectively.

Vulnerary: Promotes healing of damaged tissue.

Water distillation: A distillation process suitable for a limited range of aromatic materials, where boiling water is in direct contact with the charge in the still.

Z- prefix: Abbreviation of the German term *zusammen*, meaning 'together', and referring to the *cis*-form of a pair of isomers.

Significant Chemical Constituents in Essential Oils

Table A1 Monoterpenes

Key points	Examples	Characteristic essential oils
• 10 carbon atoms • Cyclic, acyclic, chains, bicyclic, bridged carbon frameworks • Molecular weight 136 • Low polarity • Common essential oil constituents • Comparatively high volatility	Camphene δ-3-carene *Para*-cymene *d*- and *l*-limonene ß-myrcene, ocimene α- and ß-pinene ß-phellandrene Sabinene α- and ɤ-terpinene Terpinene Terpinolene *Note*: 'Dipentene' is the name given to a mixture of *d*- and *l*-limonene	*Boswellia carteri* *Citrus* spp. (limonene) *Juniperus communis* *Origanum majorana* *Pinus* spp. (α- and ß-pinene) *Piper nigrum*

Table A2 Monoterpenoid alcohols

Key points	Examples	Characteristic essential oils

• 10 carbon atoms
• Cyclic, acyclic, chains, and bicyclic carbon frameworks
• Hydroxyl functional group
• Moderate to high volatility
• High polarity
• Very common essential oil constituents, derived from the hydrolysis of various monoterpenes, e.g.
  ○ camphene → borneol
  ○ ocimene → linalool
  ○ sabinene → thujan-4-ol
  ○ ɤ-terpinene → terpinen-4-ol
  ○ limonene → menthol
	Borneol
	d- and *l*-citronellol
	Geraniol
	Lavandulol
	d- and *l*-linalool
	Menthol
	Nerol
	α-, ß- and ɤ-terpineol
	Terpinen-4-ol
	Thujan-4-ol
		Aniba rosaeodora (*d*- and *l*-linalool)
		Lavandula angustifolia (*l*-linalool)
		Coriandrum sativum (*d*-linalool)
		Cymbopogon martinii (geraniol)
		Pelargonium graveolens (citronellol)
		Mentha piperita (menthol)
		Melaleuca alternifolia (terpinen-4-ol)
		Melaleuca viridiflora (α-terpineol)

Table A3 Monoterpenoid aldehydes

Key points	Examples	Characteristic essential oils
• 10 carbon atoms • Cyclic, acyclic, chains, bicyclic and bridged carbon frameworks • Aldehyde (-CHO) functional group • Moderate to high volatility • High polarity • Common essential oil constituents – there are not as many aldehydes as alcohols, they occur as major constituents of a few oils and minor constituents in many oils • They are derived from primary alcohols such as nerol, geraniol and *iso*-geraniol, citronellol, and lavandulol	Citral – a mixture of the isomers geranial (citral a) and neral (citral b) Citronellal Cuminaldehyde Geranial Neral Perillaldehyde	*Cymbopogon citratus, C. flexuosus* and *C. nardus* (citral) *Litsea cubeba* (citral) *Eucalyptus citriodora* (citronellal) *Cuminum cyminum* (cuminaldehyde) *Melissa officinalis* (citral and citronellal)

Table A4 Monoterpenoid ketones

Key points	Examples	Characteristic essential oils
• 10 carbon atoms • Cyclic, acyclic, bicyclic and chain carbon frameworks • Ketone (-C=O) functional group • Moderate to high volatility • High polarity • These are common essential oil constituents – which occur as major constituents of a few oils and minor constituents in many oils • Formed from monoterpenes, e.g. α-pinene → verbenone ↔ verbenol; and also from certain monoterpenoid alcohols (secondary alcohols), e.g. borneol → borneone (camphor) • The ketones cannot be further oxygenated, and do not give rise to other metabolites	α- and ß-asarone Camphor d- and l-carvone Cryptone Fenchone α-ionone α-, ß- and ɣ-irone cis-jasmone Menthone and iso-menthone Methyl amyl ketone Methyl heptenone Methyl nonyl ketone α- and ß-thujone Perilla ketone Pinocamphone and iso-Pinocamphone Pinocarvone Piperitone d-pulegone Santolinenone Verbenone	*Anethum graveolens* (carvone) *Artemisia vulgaris* (thujone) *Cinnamomum camphora* (camphor) *Foeniculum vulgare* var. *amara* (fenchone) *Hyssopus officinalis* (pinocamphone) *Iris pallida* (irones) *Mentha piperita* (menthone) *Mentha pulegium* (pulegone) *Salvia officinalis* (thujone) *Thuja occidentalis* (thujone) *Viola odorata* (α-ionone)

Table A5 Terpenoid esters

Key points	Examples	Characteristic essential oils
• Reaction products of primary or tertiary alcohols and carboxylic acids. For example, tertiary alcohol linalool reacts with acetic acid to from the ester linalyl acetate and water • Cyclic, acyclic and chain carbon frameworks • Ester (-C=O) functional group • Moderate to high volatility • High polarity, also lipophilic • Common essential oil constituents, which occur as major constituents of a few oils and minor constituents in many oils	*iso*-amyl angelate *iso*-butyl angelate Citronellyl acetate Citronellyl formate Geranyl acetate Lavandulyl acetate Linalyl acetate Linalyl propionate Menthyl acetate Neryl acetate Sabinyl acetate Terpinyl acetate *iso*-amyl tiglate	*Anthemis nobilis* (angelates and tiglates) *Citrus bergamia* (linalyl acetate) *Helichrysum angustifolium* (neryl acetate) *Juniperus sabina* (sabinyl acetate) *Lavandula angustifolia* (linalyl acetate) *Salvia lavandulaefolia* (sabinyl acetate) *Salvia sclarea* (linalyl acetate)

Table A6 Monoterpenoid oxides

Key points	Examples	Characteristic essential oils
• Oxide functional group integrated within a cyclic carbon framework. Carbon atoms are numbered to indicate oxygen bonds, e.g. 1,8- and 1,4- • Few oxides exist, only one significant monoterpenoid oxide – 1,8-cineole • 1,8-cineole is widespread, occurring in many essential oils. It is sometimes called eucalyptol • 1,8-cineole is a dominant constituent in a few essential oils • Moderate to high volatility	1,8-cineole 1,4-cineole Linalool oxide Rose oxide *Note:* Ascaridole is an unsaturated terpene peroxide. A peroxide is identified by two oxygen atoms in the link between two carbons	Many *Eucalyptus* spp., e.g. *E. globulus* (1,8-cineole) *Melaleuca* spp., e.g. *M. viridiflora* (1,8-cineole) *Hyssopus officinalis* var. *decumbens* (linalool oxide)

Table A7 Monoterpenoid phenols

Key points	Examples	Characteristic essential oils
• Hydroxyl functional group and a short chain attached to an aromatic ring • Polar • Only three monoterpenoid phenols occur in essential oils, mainly in plants from temperate regions • Powerful antibacterial activity and irritant to skin and mucous membranes	Australol Carvacrol Thymol	*Satureja hortensis* and *S. montana* (carvacrol and thymol) *Thymus capitatus* (carvacrol) *Thymus vulgaris* (thymol and carvacrol chemotypes) *Origanum vulgare* (carvacrol)

Table A8 Sesquiterpenes

Key points	Examples	Characteristic essential oils
• 15 carbon atoms • Chain, monocyclic and bicyclic structures • Molecular weight 204 • Less volatile than monoterpenes • Low polarity • Common, but less so than monoterpenes • Derived from the intermediate farnesyl pyrophosphate	α-bisabolene α-cadinene α-caryophyllene ß-caryophyllene (humulene) α-cedrene chamazulene α- and ß-copaene Farnesene Patchoulene α- and ß-santalene α- and ß-zingiberene	*Commiphora myrrha* (α-bisabolene) *Matricaria recutita* (chamazulene) *Piper nigrum* (caryophyllene) *Syzigium aromaticum* (α-caryophyllene) *Juniperus virginiana* (α-cedrene) *Pogostemon cablin* (patchoulene) *Santalum album* (α- and ß-santalene) *Zingiber officinalis* (α- and ß-zingiberene)

Table A9 Sesquiterpenoids

Key points	Examples	Characteristic essential oils
<ul><li>15 carbon atoms</li><li>Chain, monocyclic and bicyclic structures</li><li>Derived from sesquiterpenes</li><li>Polar</li><li>Less volatile than monoterpenes</li><li>Fairly widespread, some oils contain significant levels</li><li>As sesquiterpenoids are larger molecules than monoterpenoids, and the carbon framework is more complex, the functional group influence is less dominant</li><li>Oxygenated derivatives of sesquiterpenes largely occur as alcohols, oxides and lactones (cyclic esters)</li></ul>	*Alcohols* α-bisabolol Carotol Cedrol Farnesol Paradisiol Patchoulol α- and ß-santalol Viridiflorol Vetiverol Zingiberol *Oxides* Bisabolol oxide Bisabolone oxide Caryophyllene oxide *Lactones* Alantolactone Costuslactone	*Citrus paradisi* (paradisiol) *Daucus carota* (carotol) *Juniperus virginiana* (cedrol) *Matricaria recutita* (α-bisabolol) *Melaleuca quinquenervia/ viridiflora* 'MVQ' (viridiflorol) *Pogostemon cablin* (patchoulol) *Santalum album* (α- and ß-santalol) *Vetiveria zizanoides* (vetiverol) *Zingiber officinalis* (α- and ß-zingiberol) *Matricaria recutita* *Inula helenium* *Saussurea costus*

Table A10 Diterpenoids

Key points	Examples	Characteristic essential oils
<ul><li>20 carbon atoms</li><li>Not common constituents, as they are generally too large to distil over</li></ul>	Salviol Sclareol	*Salvia officinalis* *Salvia sclarea*

Table A11 Phenylpropanoids

Key points	Examples	Characteristic essential oils
• Formed via the phenylpropane pathway • Molecules have one (or more) aromatic rings • Polar • Phenylpropanoids are found as phenols, alcohols, esters, aldehydes and ethers • Bifunctional and polyfunctional molecules exist, which can make classification difficult. For example, vanillin has an aldehyde group, an hydroxyl group and an ether group	*Phenylpropanoid phenols* Eugenol *iso*-eugenol Methyleugenol *para*-cresol	*Syzigium aromaticum* (eugenol) *Cinnamomum zeylanicum* (leaf) (eugenol) *Juniperus oxycedrus* (*para*-cresol) *Melaleuca bracteata* (methyl eugenol) *Pimenta dioica* and *P. racemosa* (eugenol)
	Phenylpropanoid alcohols Benzyl alcohol and phenylethanol	*Rosa centifolia* *R. damascena*
	Phenylpropanoid aldehydes *para*-anisaldehyde Benzaldehyde Cinnamaldehyde Vanillin	*Prunus amygdalus* var. *amara* *Cinnamomum zeylanicum* *Styrax benzoin* *Vanilla planifolia*
	Phenylpropanoid esters Benzyl acetate Benzyl benzoate Eugenyl acetate Methyl benzoate Methyl salicylate Methyl jasmonate	*Betula lenta* (methyl salicylate) *Cananga odorata* var. *genuina*, *Gaultheria procumbens* (methyl salicylate) *Jasminum officinale* (benzyl acetate, methyl benzoate, methyl jasmonate) *Polyanthes tuberosa* (methyl benzoate, benzyl benzoate, methyl salicylate)
	Phenolic ethers *trans*-anethole Dill apiol Parsley apiol Elemicin Estragole (methyl chavicol) Chavicol Methyl-ß-phenylethyl ether Methyl-*para*-cresol Myristicin Safrole and *iso*-safrole	*Anethum graveolens* (dill apiol) *Artemisia dracunculus* (estragole) *Cananga odorata* (methyl-*para*-cresol) *Canarium luzonicum* (elemicin) *Foeniculum vulgare* var. *dulce* (*trans*-anethole) *Illicium verum* (*trans*-anethole) *Myristica fragrans* (myristicin) *Ocimum basilicum* (estragole) *Petroselinium sativum* (parsley apiol and myristicin) *Pimpinella anisum* (*trans*-anethole) *Sassafras albidum* (safrole)

Table A12 Carboxylic acids

Key points	Examples
• Functional group is the carboxyl group (-COOH) • Generally low volatility • Not common essential oil constituents, usually not dominant • May be found in resinoids and absolutes • Aliphatic and aromatic structures	Alantic acid Anisic acid Benzoic acid Cinnamic acid Citronellic acid Hydrocyanic (prussic) acid Phenylacetic acid Valerenic acid

Table A13 Furanocoumarins

Key points	Examples
• Belong to the large chemical family of coumarins – over 1000 exist in nature • Coumarin itself is a cyclic ester (lactone) with the distinctive odour of new-mown hay • The related furanocoumarins are found in the botanical families Rutaceae and Umbelliferae • Sometimes called psoralens, after a derivative of the coumarins • Non-volatile, too large to be distilled, so found in cold pressed oils and absolutes • Some furanocoumarins are phototoxic agents	Bergapten (5-methoxy psoralen, 5-MOP) Bergaptol (non-phototoxic) Bergamottin (bergaptyl geranyl ether; questionable phototoxicity) Citropten Oxypeucedanin Xanthotoxin

Table A14 Fatty aldehydes

Key points	Examples
• Related to the naturally occurring fats • Found as minor and trace components of essential oils, notably citrus oils • Fatty aldehydes are hydrocarbons with 7–12 carbon atoms arranged in chains • They are readily oxidised to fatty acids (carboxylic acids), which have a very unpleasant odour	Octanal (aldehyde C_8) Nonanal (aldehyde C_9) Decanal (aldehyde C_{10})

Table A15 Nitrogen-containing compounds

Key points	Examples
• The amine functional group, -NH$_2$ • Amines occur as esters, derived from anthranilic acid • The imine functional group, -NH • Imines exist in a cyclic form • Not common essential oil constituents. • Found in trace amounts • In pure form, the amines and imines possess unpleasant, powerful fishy and faecal odours, respectively	*Amines* The aromatic esters Methyl anthranilate (*Citrus sinensis, C. limon, C. reticulata, C. aurantium* var. *amara* flos. (neroli), *Cananga odorata, Jasminum officinale*) Methyl N-methyl anthranilate (*C. reticulata*) *Imines* Indole (*Citrus aurantium* var. *amara* flos. (neroli) and *Jasminum officinale*)

Table A16 Sulphur-containing compounds

Key points	Examples
• These occur as sulphides, disulphides, trisulphides and esters • Generally, the presence of sulphur in a compound imparts a powerful, diffusive, unpleasant odour • Present in trace amounts in a few oils and in more significant amounts in some oils of the Liliaceae family, e.g. garlic (*Allium sativum* var. *sativum*) and onion (*Allium cepa*) essential oils	Allyl isothiocyanate Allylpropyl disulphide Dimethyl sulphide Dimethyl disulphide Diallyl disulphide Diallylthiosulphate Diisopropyl disulphide 3,4-dimethylthiophene Methyl allyl trisulphide Phenylethyl isothiocyanate

Essential Oil Constituents

Odour and Therapeutic Potential

Dominant chemical constituent(s)	Typical odour	Essential oil	Properties
Monoterpenes			
d- and *l*-limonene	Fresh, weak, citrus	Citrus (except bergamot)	Bile stimulant
α- and β-pinene	Resinous, woody, pine	Pine Frankincense Juniperberry	Diuretic, analgesic
Camphene	Camphoraceous	Sweet marjoram	Analgesic
β-myrcene, α- and γ-terpinene	Sweet, light, balsamic		
Monoterpene alcohols			
Citronellol	Sweet, rosy, light	Geranium	Anti-infectious
Geraniol	Sweet, rose-like	Palmarosa	Analgesic
Linalool (*d-* and *l-*)	Light, floral, woody	Rosewood	
d-linalool	Lily of the valley	Coriander seed	
l-linalool	Light, floral, woody	Lavender	Sedative, anti-infectious, analgesic
Menthol	Fresh, cool, minty	Peppermint	Antispasmodic Analgesic (*l*-menthol)
α-terpineol	Lilac-like	Tea tree	Anti-infectious, analgesic (activates monocytes?)
Terpinen-4-ol	Mild, spicy, peppery	Tea tree	
Monoterpene aldehydes			
Citral (geranial and neral)	Powerful, harsh, lemon	Lemongrass	Sedative, anti-infectious, antifungal, anti-inflammatory
Citronellal	Harsh citrus, rose-like	*Eucalyptus citriodora*	

cont.

Dominant chemical constituent(s)	Typical odour	Essential oil	Properties
Monoterpene ketones Neurotoxic effects*			
Camphor	Fresh, warm	Camphor*	Vasodilation
Thujone	Powerful, herbaceous, camphoraceous, minty	Sage*	
Pinocamphone	Camphoraceous, herbal	Hyssop*	Mucolytic, wound healing, possibly antiviral
l-carvone	Minty, herbal, fresh	Spearmint	
d-carvone	Warm, herbal, spicy	Caraway	
Italidiones	Honey-like	Everlasting	Anti-haematomal
Terpenoid esters			
Iso-amyl angelate and tiglate	Herbal, fruity	Roman chamomile	Most esters – antispasmodic and sedative
Linalyl acetate	Fresh, light, herbal, fruity	Lavender	
Geranyl acetate	Rose-like and fruity	Geranium	
Neryl acetate	Floral, sweet, rose, fruity	Immortelle	
Bornyl acetate	Camphoraceous, pine	Rosemary	Useful for respiratory system
Monoterpene oxides			
1,8-cineole	'Cineolic' – eucalyptus-like, fresh	Eucalyptus blue gum	Will increase absorption of other constituents. Expectorant, anti-inflammatory, antispasmodic, increase cerebral blood flow
Monoterpene phenols			
Thymol	Powerful, medicated, herbaceous	Thyme	Rubefacient, anti-infectious (irritant)
Carvacrol	Powerful, tar-like, herbal, spicy	Thyme	

Sesquiterpenes			
Chamazulene	Odourless; blue colour	German chamomile	Most are anti-inflammatory
α- and β-caryophyllene	Woody, spicy, 'dry'	Black pepper	
α-cedrene	Woody, cedar-like, camphoraceous	Virginian cedarwood	
Zingiberene	Sweet, warm, spicy, woody	Ginger	
Sesquiterpene alcohols			
α- and β-santalol	Mild, persistent woody	Sandalwood	Some sesquiterpene alcohols may be anti-inflammatory (e.g. α-bisabolol, although this is not significantly linked to the odour of German chamomile), and the scented santalols in sandalwood are thought to be antiviral. Generally, therapeutic effects are attributed to the essential oil rather than just their sesquiterpene alcohols
Norpatchoulenol	Herbal, patchouli-like	Patchouli	
Vetiverol	Sweet, warm, earthy, persistent	Vetivert	
Phenylpropanoid phenols			
Eugenol	Warm, spicy, clove-like	Clove bud	Antibacterial, analgesic (irritant), anti-inflammatory (low doses only)
Phenylpropanoid alcohols			
Phenylethanol	Mild, floral, rose and hyacinth notes	Rose absolute Hyacinth absolute	Psychotropic (mood-altering)
Phenylpropanoid aldehydes			
Cinnamic aldehyde	Sweet, balsamic, cinnamon-like	Cinnamon leaf	Anti-infectious
Vanillin	Sweet, balsamic, vanilla-like	Benzoin Vanilla absolute	Mood altering

cont.

Dominant chemical constituent(s)	Typical odour	Essential oil	Properties
Phenylpropanoid esters			
Benzyl acetate	Floral, fruity, jasmine-like	Jasmine absolute	Antispasmodic
Methyl benzoate	Sweet, floral, slightly medicated	Ylang ylang extra	Antispasmodic
Methyl salicylate	Strong, medicated	Wintergreen	Anti-inflammatory, analgesic, rubefacient
Phenolic ethers			
Trans-anethole	Sweet, aniseed-like	Sweet fennel Star anise	Antispasmodic, analgesic (anaesthetic), psychotropic
Estragole (methyl chavicol)	Sweet, herbaceous, aniseed-like	Exotic basil	
Nitrogen-containing compounds (trace amounts, but contribute to odour)			
Pyrazines	Very powerful, penetrating odours; green, sharp – like green peppers, peas in the pod	Galbanum	None noted
Anthranilates	Floral, fruity, some have a fishy note	Mandarin	

APPENDIX C

Prescribing Essential Oils Using the Molecular Approach

Essential oil prescriptions for inflammation

How might they work?

1. By inhibition of prostaglandin synthesis. (Prostaglandins can sensitise nociceptors to inflammatory mediators such as bradykinin.)

2. By antioxidant activity, which may help prevent the release of, or mop up, chemicals known as free radicals, which are produced by leucocytes as part of the inflammatory process. These substances are antimicrobial, but can also damage normal cells, causing further tissue damage.

3. By action on the adrenal–pituitary axis, stimulating the adrenal glands, and so stimulating the secretion of cortisol.

4. By inhibition of enzymes such as 5-lipoxyoxygenase, which start a cascade of reactions resulting in the formation of pro-leukotrienes (which cause inflammation).

How could we enhance their action?

- Enhance skin penetration by including 1,8-cineole and monoterpenes in the essential oil prescription.

- Use 'frictions' over the adrenal glands with pine and spruce.

- Consider the use of anti-inflammatory and antipruritic carriers.

- Consider using essential oils containing constituents that have anti-inflammatory effects in combinations, so that the final blend is high in the active ingredients (especially some aldehydes, some sesquiterpenes, eugenol, menthol, thymol, 1,8-cineole, β-caryophyllene, α-bisabolol, chamazulene, α- and β-pinene, δ-3-carene).

- Consider the optimum concentration for alleviating inflammation. Sometimes less is best – for example, clove bud is best used at a level of just one drop in 20 ml.

- Consider the terrain too, when planning the aromatherapy treatment.

Applications for inflammation

- Acute stage, superficial injury – cold compress; contrast heat/cold; heat (Ayurveda).

- Aloe vera gel application (lower concentration, as relatively quick penetration).

- Lotions and creams for local application (higher concentrations can be used, up to 10%).

- Oils for localised massage if appropriate, e.g. chronic conditions (up to 5%).

- Frictions (light rubbing) over adrenals with neat *Picea mariana* and *Pinus sylvestris* (black spruce and pine) Schnaubelt (1995).

Useful essential oils for inflammation

Black pepper, cinnamon leaf, clove bud, *Eucalyptus* spp., German chamomile, ginger, helichrysum, laurel, lavender (true and spike), lemon verbena, may chang, myrrh, niaouli, nutmeg, oregano, peppermint, plai, poplar abs., ravintsara, tea tree.

Useful carrier oils for inflammation

Avocado, borage, *Centella asiatica*, comfrey, jojoba wax, kukui nut, marigold, passionflower, St. John's wort, tamanu.

Essential oil prescriptions for tissue healing

How might they work?

1. By reducing inflammation and inflammatory exudates, thus reducing scarring.

2. By promoting cell regeneration, possibly by stimulating fibroblasts/collagen production.

3. By preventing/controlling infection, in the case of wounds.

How could we enhance their action?

- Enhance skin penetration by including 1,8-cineole and monoterpenes in the essential oil prescription.

- Consider the use of anti-inflammatory and regenerating carriers.

- Consider using essential oils containing constituents that have cicatrising, regenerating, circulation-enhancing, phlebotonic, anti-inflammatory effects in combinations, so that the final blend is high in the active ingredients (especially some ketones, some sesquiterpenes, sesquiterpenoids).

- Consider the terrain too, when planning the aromatherapy treatment.

- Applications to accelerate tissue healing.

- Aloe vera gel application (lower concentration, as relatively quick penetration).

- Creams for local application (higher concentrations can be used, up to 10%).

- Carriers with tissue-regenerating properties.

- If skin healing is the issue, inclusion of oils that have slow skin penetration, so that these oils stay in contact with the superficial tissues for longer.

- Inclusion of oils containing 1,8-cineole to enhance skin penetration.

- Apply oils directly to dressings for wound care (will also need to include antimicrobial oils).

- Concentrations up to 12 per cent.

Useful essential oils for tissue healing

Bergamot, *Eucalyptus*, frankincense, geranium, helichrysum, lavender (true, spike), myrrh, niaouli, patchouli, peppermint, sage spp., sandalwood, spearmint, vetivert.

Useful carrier oils for tissue healing

Borage, camellia, *Centella asiatica*, comfrey, evening primrose, kukui nut, marigold, rosehip seed, sesame, tamanu, wild carrot.

Essential oil prescriptions for pain

How might they work?

1. By reducing inflammation.

2. By reducing spasm.

3. By acting as counter-irritants (causing hyperaemia, e.g. clove bud, cinnamon leaf, *Cinnamomum cassia*, *Eucalyptus* spp., wintergreen, camphor).

4. By interrupting the pain impulse at the spinal or supraspinal level (the gate control mechanism).

5. By peripheral mechanisms that inhibit the influx of nociceptive impulses.

How could we enhance their action?

- Enhance skin penetration by including 1,8-cineole and monoterpenes in the essential oil prescription.

- Consider the use of anti-inflammatory and analgesic carriers.

- Consider using essential oils containing constituents that have analgesic, circulation-enhancing, anti-inflammatory, anti-spasmodic effects in combinations, so that the final blend is high in the active ingredients.

- Constituents that have *analgesic* potential include 1,8-cineole, camphor, eugenol, linalool, myrcene, menthol, *para*-cymene, phenols (hyperaemia).

- *Esters* that have *antispasmodic* potential are the esters bornyl acetate,* eugenyl acetate, linalyl acetate,* myrtenyl acetate* and the aromatic ester methyl salicylate (also anti-inflammatory, analgesic and rubefacient).

- *Phenolic ethers* that have *antispasmodic* potential are methyl chavicol, trans-anethole, myristicin and elemicin.

- Consider the terrain too, when planning the aromatherapy treatment.

* Asterisks denote potential use in respiratory spasm.

Applications to promote pain relief

- Include 1,8-cineole to enhance penetration.
- Aloe vera gel application (lower concentration, as relatively quick penetration).
- Creams for local application (higher concentrations can be used, up to 10%).
- Carriers with analgesic properties.
- If using counter-irritants, use an oil or cream base rather than an aqueous base.
- Compresses – heat, cold, contrast.
- Aromatic frictions.

Useful essential oils for pain relief

Basil, bay laurel, bay (West Indian), black pepper, cajuput, clary sage, clove bud, cinnamon leaf, *Eucalyptus* spp., geranium, juniperberry, lavender (true, spike), lemongrass, nutmeg, sweet fennel, sweet marjoram, peppermint, pine, Roman chamomile, rosemary CT 1,8-cineole and CT camphor, spearmint, tarragon (antispasmodic), thyme CT thymol, wintergreen, yarrow.

Useful carrier oils for pain

Comfrey, olive, St. John's wort, tamanu.

Essential oil prescriptions for infection

How might they work?

1. By altering the growth environment in the tissues, making it unsuitable or less hospitable to microbial proliferation.

2. By disrupting the transport properties of the microbial cell wall and underlying membrane, thus causing lysis and cell death (suffi '-cidal'), or by increasing the permeability of the membranes, disrupting cellular metabolism, thus either inhibiting growth (suffix '-static') or killing the cells.

3. In the case of viruses, by affecting the envelope, or preventing replication, or inactivating extracellular viruses, or reducing infectivity.

4. Some essential oil constituents are thought to stimulate the activity of leucocytes, e.g. terpinen-4-ol in tea tree.

How could we enhance their action?

*   Enhance skin penetration by including 1,8-cineole and monoterpenes in the essential oil prescription.

*   Try to establish what type of infection you are dealing with, in broad terms, i.e. bacterial, fungal (including yeast) or viral, because this will influence your choice of oils and mode of application.

*   Ensure that the final blend is high in the active ingredients.

*   Consider the terrain, especially the immune system, when planning the aromatherapy treatment.

Applications for antimicrobial effects

*   Aloe vera gel application (lower concentration, as relatively quick penetration).

*   Creams for local application (higher concentrations can be used, up to 10%).

*   Aromasticks for upper respiratory tract infection.

*   If acute infection, use a higher dose for a short period – do not persist for long periods of time.

*   If chronic infection, e.g. fungal infection of toenail, use lower dose for a more prolonged period.

*   Roller ball applicators for application to small areas, e.g. boils, cold sores, shingles lesions.

*   If skin infection is the issue, include oils that have slow skin penetration, so that these oils stay in contact with the superficial tissues for longer, e.g. use sandalwood

as a carrier for antifungal oils for application in cases of dermatomycoses (aka 'Tinea').

- Include oils containing 1,8-cineole to enhance skin penetration.

- Concentrations from 1–10 per cent. Specific doses have not been established, but always consider the potential effects on the tissues as well as the microbial pathogens.

Note: The *aromatogram* (see page 18) depends to some extent on the water-solubility of essential oil components (agar is an aqueous medium), so this is why, in this type of test, the more hydrophilic essential oil constituents perform better than the more lipophilic ones. Therefore we find that phenols, monoterpene alcohols (especially terpinen-4-ol, α-terpineol, linalool) and the phenolic ether, eugenol, all perform relatively well in this environment. It does not mean that other components are inactive.

Useful essential oils and their active components

Antibacterial

- *Phenols – skin and mucous membrane irritants:*
    - thyme CT thymol/carvacrol
    - oregano (thymol)
    - summer savory (carvacrol)
    - ajowan (thymol).

- *Monoterpene alcohols – well tolerated on the skin:*
    - tea tree (terpinen-4-ol, α-terpineol)
    - lavender (linalool)
    - thyme CT linalool
    - *Eucalyptus citriodora* (citronellol with citronellal).

- *Phenolic ethers – 'all or nothing' effect:*
    - clove bud (eugenol).

- *Others:*
    - cinnamon (cinnamic aldehyde, carbonyl group)
    - manuka (leptospermone)
    - niaouli (1,8-cineole, viridiflorol)
    - cajuput (1,8-cineole, α-terpineol).

Antifungal

- *Aldehydes – skin and mucous membrane irritation possible:*
  - cinnamon (cinnamic aldehyde, carbonyl group)
  - lemongrass (citral)
  - melissa (citral)
  - may chang (citral)
  - *Eucalyptus citriodora* (citronellal)
  - citronella (citronellal).
- *Monoterpene alcohols – well tolerated by the skin and mucous membranes:*
  - tea tree (terpinen-4-ol, α-terpineol)
  - geranium (geraniol and geranial, citronellol).

Antiviral

(*Note:* Depends on viral load; some research *in vitro* only.)

- *Herpes simplex Type 1 (cold sores); (Type 2 (genital herpes) – do not attempt to treat):*
  - sandalwood
  - thuja (caution)
  - Greek sage
  - 1,8-cineole-rich essential oils
  - borneol, *iso*-borneol and bornyl acetate-containing essential oils
  - *Santolina insularis*
  - tea tree
  - eucalyptus (1,8-cineole types)
  - melissa
  - may chang
  - bergamot
  - geranium
  - *Eucalyptus citriodora.*
- *Rhinovirus (common cold):*
  - *Eucalyptus globulus*
  - *Eucalyptus polybractea* CT cryptone

- ○ *Eucalyptus radiata*
- ○ *Eucalyptus smithii*
- ○ ginger (β-sesquiphellandrene, α-curcumene,
- ○ α-zingiberene, β-bisabolene)
- ○ ravintsara
- ○ niaouli (1,8-cineole, viridiflorol)
- ○ cajuput
- ○ spike lavender
- ○ black pepper
- ○ thyme CT thujanol.
- *Influenza:*
  - ○ *Eucalyptus globulus*
  - ○ *Eucalyptus polybractea* CT cryptone
  - ○ *Eucalyptus radiata*
  - ○ *Eucalyptus smithii*
  - ○ ravintsara
  - ○ niaouli (1,8-cineole, viridiflorol)
  - ○ cajuput
  - ○ spike lavender
  - ○ black pepper
  - ○ thyme CT thujanol.
- *Human papilloma virus (viral warts and verrucae):*
  - ○ thuja (*thujone, caution*)
  - ○ *Eucalyptus citriodora*
  - ○ Greek, Dalmatian and Cretan sage.
- *Varicella-zoster virus (chickenpox, shingles):*
  - ○ ravintsara with tamanu (50:50 applied to lesions; can use a roller ball applicator).

Carrier Oils Used in Aromatherapy

In aromatherapy practice, the essential oils are diluted in carrier oils – fixed plant and macerated herbal oils. These have a wide variety of textures and absorbency rates, so that they can be selected in relation to the recipient's skin type and condition. They also have therapeutic properties in their own right, and if selected carefully will become part of the integral synergy of the essential oil prescription.

Carrier oil	Characteristics and properties
Almond (sweet almond)	Fairly thick, not rapidly absorbed. Moisturising and emollient; soothing, antipruritic
Apricot kernel	Light texture, readily absorbed. For dry and sensitive skins; emollient and antipruritic
Avocado	Fairly thick; good skin penetration and feel. Promotes cell regeneration; can increase skin hydration; indicated for sun damage, inflammation, ageing skin
Borage	Use at up to 10 per cent with other carriers. Soothing, moisturising, regenerating and firming
Camellia	Light texture, readily absorbed, good slippage for massage. Skin restructuring and moisturising properties, helps reduce appearance of scars, or prevent scarring
Centella asiatica	Dermatitis and the healing of superficial wounds, including surgical wounds and burns. It may improve circulation. Stimulates skin regeneration and helps with loss of elasticity
Coconut (several products, including fractionated, light)	Unrefined product is solid at cool temperature, gives good lubrication and leaves a slightly greasy film on the skin. The fractionated product is a slightly viscous liquid and has skin softening properties. Unrefined product has skin and hair coating properties; soothing, moisturising
Comfrey	Anti-inflammatory; traditionally used for fractures and sprains
Evening primrose	Unsuitable as a lubricant on its own, but useful in combination with other carriers at up to 20 per cent. Treatment of eczema and psoriasis. Useful on dry, scaly skin. May improve skin elasticity and accelerate healing
Grapeseed	Good slippage. Prevents moisture loss, emollient

cont.

Carrier oil	Characteristics and properties
Hazelnut	Good lubricant, very good penetration and skin feel. Nourishing to the skin, slightly astringent, stimulates circulation. Emollient, restructuring properties, and also prevents dehydration. Potential sun filter
Hemp seed	Good skin feel, rapidly absorbed. Indicated for dry skin conditions and eczema. Possibly anti-inflammatory and analgesic
Jojoba	Very compatible with the skin, temperature sensitive (wax when cold). Good slippage/skin feel. Protective, anti-inflammatory, treatment for eczema, dandruff, sun damage and acne. In aromatherapy, used on both 'dry' and 'oily' skins (sebum 'control')
Kukui nut	Very well absorbed and excellent skin feel. Possibly one of the most useful carriers. Treatment of superficial skin injuries and burns; slows down moisture loss; emollient (treatment of psoriasis and eczema). Antipruritic. Also used in cancer care (radiation treatment). Possibly anti-ageing
Lime blossom	Emollient and antipruritic; used for wrinkles
Macadamia nut	Good penetration and slippage. Nourishing, moisturising and restructuring. Useful on mature skin
Marigold (*Calendula officinalis*)	Anti-inflammatory and vulnerary. Can be used for broken capillaries, varicose veins, bruises and eczema
Olive	Heavy and sticky, pronounced odour. Soothing, anti-inflammatory and emollient – used on burns, sprains, bruises, dermatitis and insect bites
Passionflower/seed	Light texture, readily absorbed, not 'greasy'. Moisturising and emollient; used in treatment of burns; anti-inflammatory. Said to be relaxing
Peach kernel	Light texture, but more body than apricot kernel oil. Moisturising, emollient and antipruritic; used for skin protection and regeneration; anti-ageing. Skin protection, antipruritic
Rosehip seed oil	Too 'rich' for massage, but good in combination at 10–50 per cent. Skin regeneration – used on scarring. May also help burns, wounds and eczema heal. Tissue regeneration – also improves skin texture and discolouration. Useful on wrinkles. Very effective in combination with *Centella asiatica* (Kusmirek 2002)
Safflower	Inexpensive and light, but poor keeping qualities. Emollient, moisturising
Sesame	Sticky skin feel – however, suitable in combinations at up to 20 per cent. Skin restructuring, moisturising and emollient. Improves resilience and skin integrity. Free radical scavenger

St. John's wort	Anti-inflammatory – useful if nerve pain e.g. sciatica, neuralgia. Antispasmodic. Also used on bruises and cuts. Phototoxic – avoid direct sunlight
Sunflower	Sticky skin feel, but reasonable slippage. Emollient and moisturising
Tamanu (*Calophylum inophyllum*)	Thick and sticky with strong odour, so not very suitable for massage unless in combination. Healing and protective; analgesic, anti-inflammatory and cicatrisant. Increases local blood circulation. Not suitable for massage but topical applications are very effective – especially for relieving the pain of shingles (50:50 tamanu with ravintsara). Tamanu stimulates phagocytosis (Schnaubelt 1999)
Walnut	Excellent, medium weight, good texture and skin feel for massage, fairly slow rate of absorption. Highly emollient, reduces moisture loss; regenerative and anti-ageing qualities. Used in treatment of eczema
Wheatgerm	Thick, sticky, strong odour, not suitable for massage unless with other carriers at 5–10 per cent. Useful for mature or damaged skins
Wild carrot	Tonic, cicatrisant and antipruritic. Treatment of eczema and psoriasis

Compiled and adapted from Price (1998), Schnaubelt (1999) and Kusmirek (2002).

Essential Oils, Absolutes and Resinoids in Aromatherapy

Indications and Actions

Angelica root: an expectorant and antispasmodic for the respiratory system, supports the muscular skeletal system's circulation, indicated for toxic accumulations, the digestive system, anorexia, and fatigue and stress/tension. *Caution:* phototoxicity with root oil (not with seed oil).

Basil CT linalool: stress, clears the head, used for headaches, muscular aches and pains, digestion.

Bay (West Indian): tonic oil; an analgesic for muscle and joint pains, neuralgia; also for poor circulation.

Benzoin resinoid: has a calming, comforting scent. The resinoid is useful for stress-related problems, for skin problems and respiratory problems. It has sensitisation potential. It was found to be one of the best aromatic extracts for inhibiting a lipoxyoxygenase enzyme (5-LOX), it therefore has good anti-inflammatory potential. It can also inhibit HLE, therefore may counteract sun damage to the skin.

Bergamot: many uses, especially noted for its uplifting and relaxing scent; also antibacterial, antiviral, antiseptic, possibly antipruritic, antispasmodic and sedative; used on the skin (wounds, acne, eczema, psoriasis), and for relief of tension and stress, insomnia; also for those prone to respiratory and genito-urinary infections.

Bitter orange peel: has a more subtle and green aroma than sweet orange; uses are similar. Especially noted for its relaxing effects and ability to promote cheerful feelings and counteract feelings of anger and frustration.

Black pepper: a grounding oil; rubefacient, useful for joint and muscle pain, indicated for colds, flu and infections, and for digestive complaints such as diarrhoea, flatulence, constipation, colic, loss of appetite and nausea.

Cajuput: stimulating on the senses; antimicrobial, expectorant and analgesic; has been used for respiratory infections and genito-urinary infections.

Cannabis: essential oil is 'legal' but can be difficult to obtain; analgesic and anti-inflammatory properties; potential uses on inflammatory skin conditions.

Caraway: infrequently used to support the respiratory and digestive systems.

Cardamom: a tonic, stimulating oil that is of use in mental fatigue and nervous strain; also antispasmodic and supportive of the digestive system (anorexia, colic, cramp, dyspepsia, flatulence); anticatarrhal and expectorant properties benefit the respiratory system.

Carnation abs.: fragrance may impart feelings of comfort, joy and freedom from cares.

Cassia: Chinese cinnamon, unsuitable for aromatherapeutic use.

Cassie abs.: with spicy and floral notes; the psychotherapeutic actions have not been documented; it might have anti-inflammatory potential.

Cedar (Atlas, Himalayan): the scent, which is sweeter and woodier than some other conifers, can help ground and calm the mind; analgesic, antispasmodic and anti-inflammatory potential; useful for the respiratory and musculoskeletal systems; antipruritic, mucolytic and a lymphatic stimulant.

Champaca abs.: the scent might impart a relaxing, euphoric effect, perhaps similar to that of jasmine or neroli.

Cinnamon leaf: warming on the body and emotions, useful for the circulation, digestion, aches and pains and debility.

Citronella: said to be sedative, analgesic, anti-inflammatory and antispasmodic, thought to be antifungal; used in skin care, and to support the immune system.

Clary sage: versatile – antidepressant, anxiolytic oil with uses for stress, musculoskeletal pain and tension (analgesic and antispasmodic), PMS, digestive (spasm), and also useful for spasmodic coughs and asthma. Interesting fragrance.

Clove bud: a warming oil for the senses; useful as an analgesic for rheumatoid arthritis and neuralgia, as an antiseptic in many situations, as an anti-inflammatory (low concentration of 1 drop in 20 ml) and antispasmodic (especially for the digestive system), as an immunostimulant, and for debility and fatigue. Eugenol content – suggest caution.

Coriander seed: euphoric; antiseptic for the respiratory and urinary tract; antispasmodic, stomachic and carminative properties for the digestive system, indicated for anorexia; an analgesic for osteoarthritis and rheumatic pain.

Cumin seed: rarely used; strongly phototoxic; distinctive scent not usually desired in context of aromatherapy massage.

Cypress: a tonic oil, useful for debility; a phlebotonic, venous and lymphatic decongestant with astringent action, useful for broken capillaries, oedema, varicose veins. Antispasmodic properties aid the respiratory system; diuretic action aids the urinary system. Scent helps in times of difficult transitions.

Dill seed: digestive system support (colic, dyspepsia, flatulence and indigestion).

Douglas fir: the scent can counteract mental and emotional confusion, promoting a still mind and calm vitality.

Eucalyptus (1,8-cineole types): depends on individual species, but generally cephalic, analgesic, anti-inflammatory and expectorant; used for pain, including headaches, muscular aches; immune support and respiratory congestion.

Everlasting: see helichrysum.

Fir, silver and Canadian balsam: The scent of the true firs can impart mental clarity; useful for depression; other applications are for the respiratory, musculoskeletal and immune systems.

Fragonia: versatile oil used for skin care, immune support, pain relief; it probably has anti-inflammatory, analgesic, antiseptic and expectorant properties; soothing on the emotions. Said to be similar in actions to tea tree, but without associated toxicity and has a more acceptable aroma.

Frangipani abs.: rich, exotic, heady floral aroma can allay fear and anxiety; used to treat tremors and insomnia; can bring comfort, impart inner peace and release tension; it has been used in terminal care.

Frankincense: a calming oil, useful for respiratory congestion associated with asthma and bronchitis; for those with compromised immune systems; for alleviating anxiety and depression.

Galbanum: a general tonic; cicatrisant, anti-inflammatory and antiseptic qualities can aid the skin; analgesic, circulatory stimulant properties; useful for the musculoskeletal system; expectorant and antispasmodic properties for the respiratory system. Powerful, diffusive, green odour.

Genet abs.: no reported uses – explore...

Geranium: analgesic and anti-inflammatory, with many applications, especially on the skin, well tolerated even at 100 per cent (post-herpetic pain); possibly antifungal; very good anxiolytic, balancing mood swings, PMS. For best scent, use Réunion or French oil, Egyptian also nice aroma.

German chamomile: a useful anti-inflammatory oil, antipruritic, with anti-allergenic potential; possibly antifungal; calming and sedative properties, useful for tension headaches and migraine. Powerful odour.

Ginger: a tonic oil; an analgesic, possibly anti-inflammatory, a digestive tonic, and a bronchodilator and expectorant. Can reduce nausea and vomiting, and supports the immune system. Powerful odour, potential irritant.

Grapefruit: an activating, uplifting scent; good antiseptic; many uses, including skin care (for acne, oily skin, and for toning the skin), for stiffness and fluid retention, depression, headaches, nervous exhaustion and performance stress.

Helichrysum: anti-allergenic, wound healing, antiseptic, phlebotonic, for trauma to soft tissues – this is a very useful oil with a beautiful scent.

Hyacinth abs.: scent may invoke happiness, sensuality, relaxation and stimulation, while decreasing feelings of apathy, irritation, stress and depression.

Hyssop: good expectorant and mucolytic; see profile for cautions.

Immortelle: see helichrysum.

Inula: see sweet inula.

Jasmine abs.: the scent may counteract depression, stress and lack of confidence, regulate mood, enhance alertness, reduce anxiety and improve hand–eye coordination. The absolute has free radical scavenging ability, it could protect against UV-B damage on human keratinocytes.

Juniperberry: analgesic, rubefacient and depurative qualities suggest applications for muscle and joint pain; it is antiseptic and possibly diuretic and may help those prone to cystitis and oedema; also used for skin problems such as acne and weeping eczema.

Kaffir lime peel: a stimulating, activating oil; may be useful for alleviating depression and stress.

Kewda abs.: this powerful, sweet, lilac, green, honey-like fragrance has not been explored or documented for potential aroma-psycho-therapeutic use.

Laurel leaf (bay laurel): a fortifying oil, useful analgesic, anti-inflammatory; also for upper respiratory tract infections and low immunity.

Lavandin: possibly does not have the sedative actions of true lavender, and is best used as a mucolytic/expectorant or for pain relief. Caution due to camphor – variable content.

Lavender: well investigated, with a strong evidence base for its stress-relieving, calming, relaxing, sedative actions; also analgesic, anti-inflammatory and anti-allergenic properties, cicatrising, well tolerated by the skin. For the best scent, use lavender 50/52.

Lemon: well known for its uplifting, antidepressant effects, also a good antiseptic (skin, respiratory) and digestive stimulant.

Lemongrass: skin care (acne, athlete's foot); for poor circulation, joint and muscle pain, the digestive system, headaches, nervous exhaustion and stress.

Lemon-scented eucalyptus: anti-inflammatory and antimicrobial.

Lemon-scented tea tree: antimicrobial, potential use against MRSA.

Lime: no phototoxicity risk. In massage it is sedative, anti-inflammatory, anticoagulant and antispasmodic; it is indicated for anxiety and stress and for inflammatory and spasmodic problems of the digestive system.

Linden blossom abs.: has a green-herbaceous aroma; indicated for cramps, indigestion and headaches; may also have the ability to counteract sun damage on the skin, and anti-ageing potential.

Lotus (pink) abs.: a rich, sweet floral heart, fruity/leathery notes and a powdery, spicy dryout – the psychotherapeutic and other uses have not been documented; it symbolises patience, calm and transcendence; maybe the fragrance will carry the message.

Mandarin/tangerine: an uplifting yet calming scent; particularly useful for insomnia and agitation, tension; thought to be antispasmodic; also used in skin care (acne, oily skin, scars, stretch marks) and for digestive support. Tangerine may have a better fragrance, but this depends on the source.

Manuka: antimicrobial, also anti-inflammatory and analgesic. Can help prevent the diffusion of toxins (e.g. venom) in the tissues. Often used with kanuka oil.

May chang: a relaxing oil used for alleviating stress; it may be anti-inflammatory and a digestive aid.

Melissa: calming, reduces agitation.

Mimosa abs.: the powerful, green-floral odour is suggested for anxiety, stress, tension and oversensitivity.

Myrrh: used in skin and wound healing, as an expectorant and antiseptic (genito-urinary system). The absolute has anti-inflammatory and anti-ageing potential.

Myrtle: expectorant qualities, of value in asthma, bronchitis, catarrh and chronic coughs. It also has applications for skin care, colds and influenza.

Narcissus abs.: in dilution, the earthy floral scent may be narcotic, relaxing.

Neroli: antidepressant and calming, sedative; useful for fatigue, to aid sleep and to redress sympathetic nervous system imbalance, stress and tension. Also widely used in skin care.

Niaouli: expectorant, anti-allergenic and anti-asthmatic; potential protection against radiation burns. The best oil for hygienic massage practice.

Nutmeg: this has analgesic potential, and may find use in diarrhoea, hypertension, rheumatoid arthritis, anxiety, depression and sleep disorders.

Ocimum gratissimum: wound healing, antiseptic, acne (best in hydrophilic base).

Orange blossom abs.: very calming, can aid sleep and counteract stress and tension; anti-inflammatory potential.

Osmanthus abs.: the fragrance has stimulating and happy qualities, and it may counteract apathy and depression; the absolute may also enhance collagen formation, soothe skin sensitivity and help restore and refine the skin.

Palmarosa: for skin care (acne, dermatitis, and infections), nervous exhaustion and stress, immune support.

Patchouli: a relaxing, uplifting fragrance, very useful on the skin – inflammation, redness, healing, acne; for alleviating stress, and also a phlebotonic. Beautiful, complex, persistent, evocative odour.

Peppermint: stimulating on the senses, excellent analgesic (headache), antipruritic (skin, wound healing), respiratory decongestant. May aid digestion, IBS. *Caution:* children and babies.

Pimento berry: has been recommended for muscle and joint pain, poor circulation, chills, bronchitis and nervous exhaustion. *Caution:* see profile.

Pine, Scots: mucolytic, but also may be irritating to the respiratory tract, so use with caution on those who suffer from asthma; also rubefacient and analgesic, useful for muscle and joint pain; possibly an adrenal tonic/stimulant.

Plai: a cooling action; a powerful anti-inflammatory, ability to reduce oedema and pain has been used for treating post-operative swelling. Might reduce the intensity of exercise- or allergy-induced asthma. Also recommended for IBS and menstrual cramps.

Poplar bud abs.: tenacious, sweet, cinnamon-like, balsamic odour, with resinous and coumarinic undertones; the psychotherapeutic potential has not been documented. Found to have a very high capacity to inhibit 5-LOX; it therefore has good anti-inflammatory potential.

Ravintsara: a bronchodilator useful for asthma; for immune system, debility and shingles. Sedative rather than stimulating, has been used for insomnia.

Roman chamomile: calming, sedative action, useful for insomnia. Also useful for muscular aches/pains/spasm, especially tension-related. Powerful odour.

Rosalina: similar uses to tea tree; toxicity does not appear to be a problem and it could be considered to have a more acceptable odour, especially in massage.

Rose: a relaxing, uplifting oil; antibacterial, astringent, anti-inflammatory and cicatrisant actions, used to help the skin. Also used to support the female reproductive system, including PMS and menopause. The aroma is said to be antidepressant and aphrodisiac.

Rose abs.: its scent is often described as relaxing and euphoric, calming and gentle; useful for regulating moods, stress and tension.

Rosemary CT 1,8-cineole: a stimulating oil that promotes alertness; it is analgesic, useful for fatigue and stress, also useful for the respiratory system.

Rosewood: tonic oil that is said to support the immune system.

Sage, Dalmatian: use only with caution, and sparingly; possible uses for female reproductive system and pain.

Sage, Spanish: might improve mood and cognition, potential applications for dementia.

Sandalwood: a general tonic, and as a sedative; its antimicrobial properties are indicated for genito-urinary tract infections, and bronchodilatory actions indicate its use in respiratory infections. Used in skin care for maintaining skin health and alleviating acne, dermatitis and eczema. Possibly a diuretic, and a lymphatic and venous decongestant.

Spearmint: uses similar to peppermint, less well investigated, possibly less hazardous for children.

Spike lavender: a more stimulating oil than true lavender, has uses as an expectorant and analgesic; caution due to camphor content.

Spikenard: a calming oil useful for emotional support in times of transition, stress, tension, insomnia; also used in skin care (allergies and inflammation).

Star anise: has antispasmodic and anaesthetic effects, used for muscular aches and pains, colic and cramp. Also used for the respiratory system for its expectorant properties. See profile for cautions.

Sweet fennel: many uses, some well researched; inhalation can decrease mental stress, fatigue; antifungal (fungal nail infections), analgesic/antispasmodic for dysmenorrhea, digestive system; bronchodilatory actions. See profile for cautions.

Sweet inula: a notable mucolytic, use by diffusion for bronchitis, catarrh, sinusitis.

Sweet marjoram: well tolerated on the skin; analgesic (muscular, joint pain), soft tissue trauma; stress, calming.

Sweet orange: uplifting, can promote cheerfulness and vigour, used for the relief of depression and stress; also a useful antiseptic, a digestive stimulant and circulatory and lymphatic system stimulant.

Tagetes: strongly phototoxic, so care needed with dermal use; interesting scent.

Tarragon: use with care, for pain and spasm, and as a respiratory decongestant.

Tea tree: a well-investigated antimicrobial, also analgesic. Potential toxicity if ingested, children are more susceptible; best avoided in pet care, especially with dogs and cats.

Thuja: best avoided due to toxicity; unproven antiviral action on warts.

Thyme: generally stimulating and warming on the senses; depends on the species or chemotype, but generally used for muscular aches and pains, debility, fatigue, respiratory congestion/coughs and low immunity.

Tuberose abs.: the heavy, honey-floral scent is narcotic and sleep-inducing.

Tulsi (holy basil): can be used in the treatment of acne; it is antiseptic and may help prevent scarring.

Vanilla abs.: some find the scent soothing and comforting; the psychotherapeutic uses are not well documented, although apparently it was used in a short-lived sensory product designed for appetite reduction (presumably the sweet/food/confectionery/chocolate associations satiated the appetite centre in the brain?).

Vetivert: a relaxing oil with many uses related to its anti-inflammatory and healing qualities, such as in skincare for acne, cuts, wounds, oily skin and eczema; for arthritis, muscular pain, rheumatism, sprains and stiffness. Also useful for debility, depression, insomnia and nervous tension. Said to be immunostimulant.

Violet leaf abs.: strong, green odour; indicated for stress, insomnia and headache; the absolute showed the ability to inhibit the enzyme HLE, so may have applications on sun-damaged skin, and as an anti-ageing absolute.

Virginian cedar: the scent can anchor the emotions and focus the mind; possibly analgesic and anti-inflammatory, useful for muscular and joint pain; also supportive of the respiratory system.

West Indian bay: see bay.

White ginger lily: warm, sweet, honey-like, exotic floral notes and a spicy, fruity, balsamic undertone; could be useful for relaxation and stress relief, possibly pain relief, and to aid sleep.

Wintergreen: use with caution; a powerful counterirritant that is useful for muscular aches and pains and sciatica.

Wormwood: possibly best avoided in aromatherapy, although it is interesting to experience its fragrance.

Yarrow: musculoskeletal pain and inflammation; varicose veins and ulcers. Avoid camphor CT; yarrow has been used successfully for insomnia and stress too.

Ylang ylang: for relaxation, harmonising effect (stress, tension, frustration and insomnia); skin care; muscular aches and cramp. Use ylang ylang extra for its scent.

References

Adorjan, B. and Buchbauer, G. (2010) 'Biological properties of essential oils: an updated review.' *Flavour and Fragrance Journal 25*, 407–426.

Aftel, M. (2008) *Essence and Alchemy.* Layton: Gibbs Smith.

Akutsu, H., Kikusui, T., Takeuchi, Y., Sano, K. *et al.* (2002) 'Alleviating effects of plant-derived fragrances on stress-induced hyperthermia in rats.' *Physiology and Behaviour 75*, 355–360.

Alaoui-Ismaïli, O., Vernet-Maury, E., Dittmar, A., Delhomme, G. and Chanel, J. (1997) 'Odor hedonics: connection with emotional response estimated by autonomic parameters.' *Chemical Senses 22*, 237–248.

Alifano, P., Del Giudice, L., Talà, A., De Stefano, M. and Maffei, M.E. (2010) 'Microbes at work in perfumery: the microbial community of vetivert root and its involvement in essential oil biogenesis.' *Flavour and Fragrance Journal 25*, 121–122.

Amoore, J.E. (1963) 'The stereochemical theory of olfaction.' *Nature 198*, 271–272. Cited in J.C. Leffingwell. and Associates (1999) *Olfaction – A Review.* Accessed on 28 December 2011 at www.leffingwell.com/olfaction.htm

Angelo, J. (1997) *Hands-on Healing.* Rochester: Healing Arts Press.

Arctander, S. (1960) *Perfume and Flavour Materials of Natural Origin.* Elizabeth, NJ: Steffen Arctander. Cited in Lawless, J. (1992) *The Encyclopaedia of Essential Oils.* Shaftesbury: Element Books.

Arroyo, S. (1975) *Astrology, Psychology and the Four Elements: an Energy Approach to Astrology and its use in the Counselling Arts.* Reno, NE: CRCS Publications.

Baerheim Svendsen, A. and Scheffer, J.J.C. (eds) (1985) *Essential Oils and Aromatic Plants. Proceedings of the 15th International Symposium on Essential Oils.* The Netherlands: Dr. W. Junk Publishers and Martinus Nijhoff.

Balacs, T. (1995) 'The psychopharmacology of essential oils.' *Aroma '95 Conference Proceedings.* Brighton: Aromatherapy Publications.

Balacs, T. (1997) 'Cineole-rich Eucalyptus.' *International Journal of Aromatherapy 8*, 2, 15–21.

Balacs, T. (1998/1999) 'Research reports.' *International Journal of Aromatherapy 9*, 2, 86–88.

Baldovini, N., Delasalle, C. and Joulain, D. (2011) 'Phytochemistry of the heartwood from fragrant *Santalum* species: a review.' *Fragrance and Flavour Journal 26*, 7–26.

Ballard, C.G., O'Brien, C.T., Reichelt, K., and Perry, E.K. (2002) 'Aromatherapy as a safe and effective treatment for the management of agitation in severe dementia: The results of a double-blind, placebo-controlled trial with melissa.' *Journal of Clinical Psychiatry 63*, 553–558. Cited in Elliot, M.S.J., Abuhamdah, S., Howes, M-J.R., Lees *et al.* (2007) 'The essential oils from *Melissa officinalis* L. and *Lavandula angustifolia* Mill. as potential treatment for agitation in people with severe dementia.' *International Journal of Essential Oil Therapeutics 1*, 4, 143–152.

Bartram, T. (1995) *Encyclopaedia of Herbal Medicine.* Christchurch: Grace. Cited in Price, S. and Price, L (1999) *Aromatherapy for Health Professionals.* (2nd edition.) Edinburgh: Churchill Livingstone.

Baumann, L.S. (2007a) 'German chamomile and cutaneous benefits.' *Journal of Drugs in Dermatology 6*, 11, 1084–1085.

Baumann, L.S. (2007b) 'Less-known botanical cosmeceuticals.' *Dermatologic Therapy 20*, 330–342.

Baylac, S. and Racine, P. (2003) 'Inhibition of 5-lipoxygenase by essential oils and other natural fragrant extracts.' *International Journal of Aromatherapy 13*, 2/3, 138–142.

Baylac, S. and Racine, P. (2004) 'Inhibition of human leukocyte elastase by natural fragrant extracts of aromatic plants.' *International Journal of Aromatherapy 14*, 4, 179–182.

Beckstrom-Sternberg, S.M. and Duke, J.A. (1996) *CRC Handbook of Medicinal Mints.* Boca Raton, FL: CRC Press. Cited in Price, S. and Price, L. (1999) *Aromatherapy for Health Professionals.* (2nd edition.) Edinburgh: Churchill Livingstone.

Behra, O., Rakotoarison, C. and Harris, R. (2001) 'Ravintsara vs. ravensara: a taxonomic clarification.' *International Journal of Aromatherapy 11*, 1, 4–7.

Belaiche, P. (1979) *Traite de Phytothérapie et d'Aromathérapie vols 1–3.* Paris: Maloine Editeur.

Bensouilah, J. (2005) 'The history and development of modern British aromatherapy.' *International Journal of Aromatherapy 15*, 3, 134–140.

Bensouilah, J. and Buck, P. (2006) *Aromadermatology.* Oxford: Radcliffe Publishing Ltd.

Bhagwan Dash, V. (1989) *Fundamentals of Ayurvedic Medicine.* Seattle, WA: Konark Publishers.

Bischoff, K. and Guale, F. (1998) 'Australian tea tree (*Melaleuca alternifolia*) oil poisoning in three purebred cats.' *Journal of Veterinary Diagnostic Investigation 10,* 208–210.

Bowles, E.J. (2003) *The Chemistry of Aromatherapeutic Oils.* (3rd edition.) Crows Nest, NSW: Allen and Unwin.

Boyd, E.M. and Pearson, G.L. (1946) 'The expectorant action of volatile oils.' *American Journal of Medical Science 211,* 602–610. Cited in S. Van Toller and G.H. Dodd (eds) (1988) *Perfumery: the Psychology and Biology of Fragrance.* London: Chapman and Hall.

Bronaugh, R.L., Webster, R.C., Bucks, D., Maibach, H.I. and Sarason, R. (1990) '*In vivo* percutaneous absorption of fragrance ingredients in rhesus monkeys and humans.' *Food and Chemical Toxicology 28,* 5, 369–373. Cited in Tisserand, R. and Balacs, T. (1995) *Essential Oil Safety – A Guide for Health Care Professionals.* London: Churchill Livingstone.

Brophy, J.J. and Doran, J.C. (2004) 'Geographic variation in oil characteristics in *Melaleuca ericifolia.*' *Journal of Essential Oil Research,* January/February.

Brownfield, A. (1998) 'Aromatherapy in arthritis: a study.' *Nursing Times 13,* 5.

Brud, W.S. and Ogyanov, I. (1995) 'Zdravetz.' *International Journal of Aromatherapy 7,* 1, 10–11.

Brudnak, M. (2000) 'Cancer-preventing properties of essential oil monoterpenes *d*-limonene and perillyl alcohol.' *Positive Health* 23–25.

Buchbauer, G. (1993) 'Biological effects and modes of action of essential oils.' *International Journal of Aromatherapy 5,* 1, 11–14.

Buchbauer, G. (1996) 'Methods in aromatherapy research.' *Perfumer and Flavorist 21,* 31–36.

Buchbauer, G., Dietrich, H., Karamat, E., Jirovetz, L. *et al.* (1991a) 'Aromatherapy: evidence for sedative effects of the essential oil of lavender after inhalation.' *Journal of Biosciences 46,* 1067–1072.

Buchbauer, G., Jäger, W., Jirovetz, L., Dietrich, H. and Plank, C. (1991b) In: *Zeitschrift Naturforschaft 46,* 1067–1072. Cited in Bowles, E.J. (2003) *The Chemistry of Aromatherapeutic Oils.* Crows Nest, NSW: Allen and Unwin.

Buchbauer, G., Jirovetz, L., Jäger, W., Plank, C. and Dietrich, H. (1993) 'Fragrance compounds and essential oils with sedative effects upon inhalation.' *Journal of Pharmaceutical Sciences 82,* 6, 660–664.

Buchbauer, G., Jirovetz, L., Jäger, W., Ilmeberger, J. and Dietrich, H. (1993) In: Teranchi *et al.* (eds) *Bioactive Volatile Compounds from Plants.* ACS Symposium Series 525. Cited in Price, S. and Price, L. (1999) *Aromatherapy for Health Professionals.* (2nd edition.) Edinburgh: Churchill Livingstone.

Buck, P. (2004) 'Skin barrier function: effect of age, race and inflammatory disease.' *International Journal of Aromatherapy 14,* 2, 70–75.

Buckle, J. (2003) *Clinical Aromatherapy – Essential Oils in Practice.* (2nd edition.) Edinburgh: Churchill Livingstone.

Budhiraja, S.S., Cullum, M.E., Sioutis, S.S., Evangelista L. and Habanova, S.T (1999) 'Biological activity of *Melaleuca alternifolia* (tea tree) oil component, terpinen-4-ol, in human myelocytic cell line HL-60.' *Journal of Manipulative Physiological Therapies 22,* 7, 47–53. Cited in Bowles, E.J. (2003) *The Chemistry of Aromatherapeutic Oils.* Crows Nest, NSW: Allen and Unwin.

Burfield, T. (2002) 'Cedarwood oils.' *The Cropwatch Series.* Accessed on 31 November 2011 at www.cropwatch.org

Burfield, T. (2004) 'Rosewood sustainability: Critical assessment of the May and Barata paper.' *The Cropwatch Series.* Accessed on 30 November 2011 at www.cropwatch.org/cropwatch6.htm

Caelli, M., Porteus, J., Carson, C.F., Heller, R. and Riley, T.V. (2001) 'Tea tree oil as an alternative topical decolonisation agent for methicillin-resistant *Staphylococcus aureus.*' *International Journal of Aromatherapy 11,* 2, 97–99.

Caldecott, T. (2006) *Ayurveda the Divine Science of Life.* London: Mosby Elsevier.

Calkin, R.R. and Jellinek, J.S. (1994) *Perfumery: Practice and Principles.* New York: John Wiley and Sons, Inc.

Caplin, J.L., Allan, I. and Hanlon, G.W. (2009) 'Enhancing the *in vitro* activity of *Thymus* essential oils against *Staphylococcus aureus* by blending oils from specific cultivars.' *International Journal of Essential Oil Therapeutics 3,* 1, 35–39.

Cappello, G., Spezzaferro, M., Grossi, L., Manzoli, L. and Marzio, L. (2007) 'Peppermint oil (Mintoil) in the treatment of irritable bowel syndrome: a prospective double-blind placebo-controlled randomized trial.' *Digestive and Liver Disease 39,* 6, 530–536.

Carson, C. (2006) Personal communication. Cited in Turnock, S. (2006) 'Potent oil.' *Nova*, January 2006, 29–36.

Carson, C.F. and Riley, T.V. (1995) 'Antimicrobial activity of the major components of the essential oil of *Melaleuca alternifolia*.' *Journal of Applied Bacteriology 78*, 3, 264–269. Cited in Bowles, E.J. (2003) *The Chemistry of Aromatherapeutic Oils*. Crows Nest, NSW: Allen and Unwin.

Carson, C.F., Hammer, K.A. and Riley, T.V. (1995) 'Broth microdilution method for determining the susceptibility of *Escherichia coli* and *Staphylococcus aureus* to the essential oil of *Melaleuca alternifolia* (tea tree oil).' *Microbios 82*, 332, 181–185. Cited in Price, S. and Price, L (1999) *Aromatherapy for Health Professionals*. (2nd edition.) Edinburgh: Churchill Livingstone.

Carson, C.F., Cookson, B.D., Farrelly, H.D. and Riley, T.V. (1995) 'Susceptibility of methicillin-resistant *Staphylococcus aureus* to the essential oil of *Melaleuca alternifolia*.' *Journal of Antimicrobial Chemotherapy 35*, 421–424. Cited in Price, S. and Price, L. (1999) *Aromatherapy for Health Professionals*. (2nd edition.) Edinburgh: Churchill Livingstone.

Cavalieri, E., Mariotto, S., Fabrizi, C., de Prati, A.C. *et al.* (2004) 'α-Bisabolol, a non-toxic natural compound, strongly induces apoptosis in glioma cells.' *Biochemical and Biophysical Research Communications 315*, 589–594.

Chen, H., Chan, K.K. and Budd, T. (1998) 'Pharmacokinetics of *d*-limonene in the rat by GC-MS assay.' *Journal of Pharmaceutical and Biomedical Analysis 17*, 631–640.

Chrea, C., Grandjean, D., Delplanque, S., Cayeux, I. *et al.* (2009) 'Mapping the semantic space for the subjective experience of emotional responses to odours.' *Chemical Senses 34*, 49–62.

Chu, S. (2008) 'Olfactory conditioning of positive performance in humans.' *Chemical Senses 33*, 65–71.

Classen, C., Howes, D. and Synnott, A. (1994) *Aroma. The Cultural History of Smell*. London: Routledge.

Clerc, O. (1995) 'Portraits in oils.' *International Journal of Aromatherapy 7*, 1, 15–17.

Cornwall, P.A. and Barry, B.W. (1994) '456 sesquiterpene components of volatile oils as skin penetration enhancers for the hydrophilic permeant 5 fluorouracil.' *Journal of Pharmacy and Pharmacology 46*, 4, 261–269. Cited in Price, S. and Price, L (2007) *Aromatherapy for Health Professionals*. (3rd edition.) Edinburgh: Churchill Livingstone.

Davies, S.J., Harding, L.M. and Baranowski, A.P. (2002) 'A novel treatment for postherpetic neuralgia using peppermint oil.' *Clinical Journal of Pain 18*, 3, 200–202.

Davis, P. (1991) *Subtle Aromatherapy*. Saffron Walden: The C.W. Daniel Company Ltd.

Day, S. (1996) 'The sweet smell of death.' *New Scientist,* 7 September, 28–31.

de Domenico, G. and Wood, E.C. (1997) *Beard's Massage*. London: W.B. Saunders Company.

de Medici, D., Pieretti, S. and Salvatore, G. (1992) 'Chemical analysis of essential oils from Malgasy medicinal plants by gas chromatography and NMR spectroscopy.' *Flavor and Fragrance Journal 7*, 275–281. Cited in Behra, O., Rakotoarison, C. and Harris, R. (2001) 'Ravintsara vs ravensara: a taxonomic clarification.' *International Journal of Aromatherapy 11*, 1, 4–7.

de Pradier, E. (2006) 'A trial of a mixture of three essential oils in the treatment of postoperative nausea and vomiting.' *International Journal of Aromatherapy 16*, 1, 15–20.

Diego, M.A., Jones, N.A., Field, F., Hernandez-Reif, M. *et al.* (1998) 'Aromatherapy positively affects mood, EEG patterns of alertness and math computations.' *International Journal of Neuroscience 96*, 217–224.

Dobetsberger, C. and Buchbauer, G. (2011) 'Actions of essential oils on the central nervous system: an updated review.' *Flavour and Fragrance Journal 26*, 5, 300–316.

Dodd, G.H. (1988) 'The Molecular Dimension in Perfumery'. In S. Van Toller and G.H. Dodd (eds) *Perfumery: the Psychology and Biology of Fragrance*. London: Chapman and Hall.

Donoyama, N. and Ichiman, Y. (2006) 'Which essential oil is better for hygienic massage practice?' *International Journal of Aromatherapy 16*, 3, 175–179.

Douek, E. (1988) 'Foreword – Abnormalities of Smell'. In S. Van Toller and G.H. Dodd (eds) *Perfumery: the Psychology and Biology of Fragrance*. London: Chapman and Hall.

Duraffourd, P. (1982) *En forme tous les jours*. Perigny: La Vie Claire. Cited in Price, S. and Price, L (2007) *Aromatherapy for Health Professionals*. (3rd edition.) Edinburgh: Churchill Livingstone.

Duraffourd, P. and Lapraz, J.-C. (1995) 'The application of clinical phytotherapy in terrain medicine.' *British Journal of Phytotherapy 3*, 3.

Dyson, G.M. (1938) 'The scientific basis of odour.' *Chem. Ind. 57*, 222–238. Cited in J.C. Leffingwell and Associates (1999) *Olfaction – A Review*. Accessed on 28 December 2011 at www.leffingwell.com/olfaction.htm

Elliot, M.S.J., Abuhamdah, S., Howes, M-J.R., Lees, G. *et al.* (2007) 'The essential oils from *Melissa officinalis* L. and *Lavandula angustifolia* Mill as potential treatment for agitation in people with severe dementia.' *International Journal of Essential Oil Therapeutics 1*, 4, 143–152.

Emamghoreishi, M, Khasaki, M. and Aazam, M.F. (2005) '*C. sativum*: evaluation of its anxiolytic effects in the elevated plus-maze.' *Journal of Ethnopharmacology 96*, 365–370.

Engen, T. (1988) 'The Acquisition of Odour Hedonics'. In S. Van Toller and G.H. Dodd (eds) *Perfumery: the Psychology and Biology of Fragrance.* London: Chapman and Hall.

Erligmann, A. (2001) 'Sandalwood oils.' *International Journal of Aromatherapy 11*, 4, 186–192.

Evans, W.C. (1989) *Trease and Evans' Pharmacognosy.* (13th edition.) London: Ballière Tindall.

Faiyazuddin, Md., Baboota, S., Ali, J. and Ahmad, S. (2009) 'Characterisation and *in vitro* bioactive studies of lemongrass oil phytonanoemulsion system in the treatment of acne vulgaris.' *International Journal of Essential Oil Therapeutics 3*, 1, 13–21.

Faiyazuddin, Md., Suri, S., Mustafa, G., Iqbal, Z. *et al.* (2009) 'Phytotherapeutic potential of tea tree essential oil *in vitro* and emerging vistas in the skincare industry: a comprehensive review.' *International Journal of Essential Oil Therapeutics 3*, 2–3, 84–90.

Falk-Filipsson, A., Löf, A., Hagberg, M., Hjelm, E.W. and Wang, Z. (1993) '*d*-Limonene exposure to humans by inhalation: uptake, distribution, elimination, and effects on the pulmonary function.' *Journal of Toxicology and Environmental Health 38*, 1, 77–88.

Fewell, F., McVicar, A., Gransby, R. and Morgan, P. (2007) 'Blood concentration and uptake of *d*-limonene during aromatherapy massage with sweet orange oil: a pilot study.' *International Journal of Essential Oil Therapeutics 1*, 97–102.

Forster, S. (2009) 'Ancient wisdom for today's therapists.' *In Essence 8*, 3, 24–26.

Franchomme, P. (1985) *Phytoguide 1.* La Courtête: International Phytomedical Foundation. Cited in Lawless, J. (1992) *The Encyclopaedia of Essential Oils.* Shaftesbury: Element Books.

Franchomme, P. and Pénoël, D. (1990) *L'Aromathérapie exactement.* Limoges: Jallois.

Frasnelli, J., Lundström, J.N., Boyle, J.A., Katsarkas, A. and Jones-Gotman, M. (2011) 'The vomeronasal organ is not involved in the perception of endogenous odors.' *Human Brain Mapping 32*, 450–460.

Frawley, D., and Lad, V. (1986) *The Yoga Of Herbs.* Twin Lakes, WI: Lotus Press.

Fuchs, N., Jäger, W., Lenhardt, A. Bohm, L. *et al.* (1997) 'Systemic absorption of topically applied carvone: Influence of massage technique.' *Journal of the Society Cosmetic Chemists 48*, 277–282. Cited in Buck, P. (2004) 'Skin barrier function: effect of age, race and inflammatory disease.' *International Journal of Aromatherapy 14*, 2, 70–75.

Gattefossé, M. (1992) 'René-Maurice Gattefossé – the father of modern aromatherapy.' *International Journal of Aromatherapy 4*, 2, 18–22.

Geiger, J.L. (2005) 'The essential oil of ginger, *Zingiber officinalis*, and anaesthesia.' *International Journal of Aromatherapy 15*, 1, 7–14.

Gimelli, S.P. (2001) *Aroma Science.* Weymouth: Micelle Press.

Gobel, H., Schmidt, G., Dworschak, M., Stolze, H. and Heuss, D. (1995) 'Essential plant oils and headache mechanisms.' *Phytomedicine 2*, 2, 93–102.

Goerner, S.J. (1999) *After the Clockwork Universe.* Edinburgh: Floris Books.

Goode, J.A. (2000) 'Sending out an SOS: semiochemicals in nature.' *Biologist 47*, 5, 247–250.

Gordon, L. (1980) *A Country Herbal.* Devon: Webb and Bower Publishers Ltd.

Greenway, F.L., Frome, B.M., Engels, T.M. and McLellan, A. (2003) 'Temporary relief of postherpetic neuralgia pain with topical geranium oil.' *American Journal of Medicine 115*, 7, 586–587.

Grieve, M. (1992 [1931]) *A Modern Herbal.* London: Tiger Books International.

Hadji-Mingalou, F. and Bolcato, O. (2005) 'The potential role of specific essential oils in the replacement of dermacorticoid drugs.' *International Journal of Aromatherapy 15*, 2, 66–73.

Harris, B. (2003) Editorial. *International Journal of Aromatherapy 13*, 2/3, 57.

Harris, R. (2002) 'Synergism in the essential oil world.' *International Journal of Aromatherapy 12*, 4, 179–186.

Harris, R. (2003) 'Anglo-Saxon aromatherapy: its evolution and current situation.' *International Journal of Aromatherapy 13*, 1, 9–17.

Harris, R. (2005) 'Research reports.' *International Journal of Aromatherapy 15*, 207–210.

Harris, R. (2009) 'Lionel's combat – using essential oils to increase physical and mental endurance: a case study.' *International Journal of Clinical Aromatherapy 6*, 2, 27–32.

Harvala, C., Menounos, P. and Argyriadou, N. (1987) 'Essential oil from *Silva triloba*.' *Fitoterapia 58*, 5, 353–356.

Heuberger, E., Hongratanaworakit, T. and Buchbauer, G. (2006) 'East Indian sandalwood and α-santalol odor increase physiological and self-rated arousal in humans.' *Planta Medica 72*, 9, 792–800.

Heuberger, E., Hongratanaworakit, T., Bohm, C., Weber, R. and Buchbauer, G. (2001) 'Effects of chiral fragrances on human autonomic nervous system parameters and self-evaluation.' *Chemical Senses 26*, 281–292.

Hicks, A., Hicks, J., and Mole, P. (2011) *Five Element Constitutional Acupuncture.* London: Elsevier.

Hirsch, A., Ye, Y., Lu, Y. and Choe, M. (2007) 'The effects of the aroma of jasmine on bowling score.' *International Journal of Essential Oil Therapeutics 1*, 79–82.

Hirsch, A.R., Hoogeveen, J.R., Busse, A.M. and Allen, E.T. (2007) 'The effects of odour on weight perception.' *International Journal of Essential Oil Therapeutics 1*, 21–28.

Holland, R.W., Hendriks, M. and Aarts, H. (2005) 'Smells like clean spirit: nonconscious effects of scent on cognition and behaviour.' *Psychological Science 16*, 9, 689–693.

Holmes, P. (1997) *Fragrance Energetics: a Working Model of Holistic Aromapharmacology.* Presentation at Aroma 97 Seminar, Warwick University. Brighton: Aromatherapy Publications.

Holmes, P. (1998a) 'Jasmine – queen of the night.' *International Journal of Aromatherapy 8*, 4, 8–12.

Holmes, P. (1998b) 'Energy medicine – aromatherapy past and present.' *International Journal of Aromatherapy 9*, 2, 53–56.

Holmes, P. (2001) *Clinical Aromatherapy.* Boulder, CO: Tigerlily Press Inc.

Hongratanaworakit, T. (2009) 'Relaxing effects of rose on humans.' *Natural Products Communications 4*, 2, 291.

Hongratanaworakit, T. (2011) 'Aroma-therapeutic effects of massage blended essential oils on humans.' *Natural Product Communications 6*, 8, 1199.

Hongratanaworakit, T. and Buchbauer, G. (2004) 'Evaluation of the harmonizing effect of ylang ylang on humans after inhalation.' *Planta Medica 70*, 7, 632–636.

Hongratanaworakit, T. and Buchbauer, G. (2006) 'Relaxing effect of ylang ylang on humans after transdermal absorption.' *Phytotherapy Research 20*, 9, 758–763.

Hongratanaworakit, T. and Buchbauer, G. (2007) 'Autonomic and emotional responses after transdermal absorption of sweet orange oil in humans: placebo controlled trial.' *International Journal of Essential Oil Therapeutics 1*, 29–34.

Hongratanaworakit, T., Heuberger, E. and Buchbauer, G. (2004) 'Evaluation of the effects of East Indian sandalwood oil and α-santalol on humans after transdermal absorption.' *Planta Medica 70*, 1, 3–7.

Howard Hughes Medical Institute (2004) www.hhmi.org/research/nobel/buck.html.

Imanishi, J., Kuriyama, H., Shigemori, I., Watanabe, S. *et al.* (2009) 'Anxiolytic effect of aromatherapy massage in patients with breast cancer.' *Evidence Based Complementary and Alternative Medicine 6*, 1, 123–128.

International School of Aromatherapy (1993) *A Safety Guide on the Use of Essential Oils.* London: Natural by Nature Oils Ltd.

Jacob, T. (1999) *Olfaction: a Tutorial on the Sense of Smell.* Accessed on 28 December 2011 at www.cf.ac.uk/biosi/staff/jacob/teaching/sensory/olfact1.html

Jacob, T. (1999) *Human pheromones.* Accessed on 28 December 2011 at www.cf.ac.uk/biosi/staff/jacob/teaching/sensory/pherom.html

Jäger, W., Buchbauer, G., Jirovetz, L. and Fritzer, M. (1992) 'Percutaneous absorption of lavender oil from a massage oil.' *Journal of the Society of Cosmetic Chemists 43*, 1, 49–54. Cited in Tisserand, R. and Balacs, T. (1995) *Essential Oil Safety – a Guide for Health Care Professionals.* London: Churchill Livingstone.

Jäger, W., Buchbauer, G., Jirovetz, L. Dietrich, H. and Plank, C. (1992) In *Journal of Essential Oil Research* 4, 387–394. Cited in Balacs, T. (1995) 'The psychopharmacology of essential oils.' *Aroma '95 Conference Proceedings.* Brighton: Aromatherapy Publications.

Jäger, W., Nasel, B., Nasel, C., Binder, R. *et al.* (1996) 'Pharmacokinetic studies of the fragrance compound 1,8-cineole in humans during inhalation.' *Chemical Senses 21*, 4, 477–480.

Jeannot, V., Roger, B., Chahboun, J. and Baret, P. (2007) 'Ravintsara (*Cinnamomum camphora* (L.) Presl.) essential oil and hydrolat in therapeutics.' *The International Journal of Essential Oil Therapeutics 1*, 35–38.

Jellinek, P. (1959) *The Practice of Modern Perfumery.* London: Leonard Hill.

Jellinek, J.S. (1994) 'Aroma-chology: A status review.' *Perfumer and Flavorist 19*, 25–48.

Jellinek, J.S. (1997) 'Psychodynamic odor effects and their mechanisms.' *Perfumer and Flavorist 22*, 29–41.

Jenkins, S. (2006) 'Modern British aromatherapy – the way forward: education and regulation.' *International Journal of Aromatherapy 16*, 2, 85–88.

Jennings-White, C., Dolberg, D.S. and Berliner, D.L. (1994) 'The human vomeronasal system.' *Psychoneuroendocrinology 19*, 673–686.

Jirovetz, L., Eller, G., Buchbauer, G., Schmidt, E. *et al.* (2006) 'Chemical composition, antimicrobial activities, and odor descriptions of some essential oils with characteristic floral-rosy scent and of their principal aroma compounds.' *Recent Developments in Agronomy and Horticulture 2*, 1–12.

Jouhar, A.J. (ed.) (1991) *Poucher's Perfumes, Cosmetics and Soaps. Volume 1: The Raw Materials of Perfumery.* (9th edition.) London: Chapman and Hall.

Juergens, U.R., Stöber, M. and Vetter, H. (1998) 'Inhibition of the cytokine production and arachidonic acid metabolism by eucalyptol (1,8-cineole) on human blood monocytes *in vitro*.' *European Journal of Medical Research 3*, 508–510. Cited in Jeannot, V., Roger, B., Chahboun, J. and Baret, P. (2007) 'Ravintsara (*Cinnamomum camphora* (L.) Presl.) essential oil and hydrolat in therapeutics.' *The International Journal of Essential Oil Therapeutics 1*, 35–38.

Kar, K., Puri, V.N., Patnaik, G.K., Sur, R.N. *et al.* (1975) 'Spasmolytic constituents of *Cedrus deodara* (Roxb.) Loud: pharmacological evaluation of himachalol.' *Journal of Pharmaceutical Science 64*, 2, 258–262. Cited in Burfield, T. (2002) 'Cedarwood oils.' *The Cropwatch Series.* Accessed on 31 November 2011 at www.cropwatch.org

Kennedy, D.O., Dodd, F.L., Robertson, B.C., Okello, E.J. *et al.* (2010) 'Monoterpenoid extract of sage (*Salvia lavandulaefolia*) with cholesterinase-inhibiting properties improves cognitive performance and mood in healthy adults.' *Journal of Psychopharmacology 25*, 1088.

Kehrl, W., Sonnemann, U. and Dethlefsen, U. (2004) 'Therapy for acute non-purulent rhinosinusitis with cineole: results of a double blind, randomised, placebo-controlled trial.' *Laryngoscope 114*, 738–742. Cited in Harris, B. (2006) 'Research reports.' *International Journal of Aromatherapy 16*, 3/4, 199–203.

Kim, H.-M. and Cho, S.-H. (1999) 'Lavender oil inhibits immediate-type allergic reaction in mice and rats.' *Journal of Pharmacy and Pharmacology 51*, 221–226. Cited in Balacs, T. (2000) 'Research Reports.' *International Journal of Aromatherapy 10*, 1/2, 68–71.

Kim, T.H., Ito, H., Hatano, T., Hasegawa, T., Akiba, A., Machiguchi, T. and Yoshida, T. (2006) *Tetrahedron 62*, 6981. Cited in Baldovini, N., Delasalle, C. and Joulain, D. (2011) 'Phytochemistry of the heartwood from fragrant *Santalum* species: a review.' *Fragrance and Flavour Journal 26*, 7–26.

King, J.R. (1983) 'Have the scents to relax?' *World Medicine 19*, 29–31.

King, J.R. (1988) 'Anxiety Reduction Using Fragrances'. In *Perfumery: The Psychology and Biology of Fragrance.* S. Van Toller and G.H. Dodd (eds) London: Chapman Hall.

King, J.R. (1994) 'Scientific status of aromatherapy.' *Perspectives on Biological Medicine 37*, 409.

Kirk-Smith, M., Van Toller, S., and Dodd, G.H. (1983) 'Unconscious odour conditioning in human subjects.' *Biological Psychology 17*, 221–231.

Kirk-Smith, M. (1995) *The Physiological and Psychological Effects of Fragrances.* In ISPA Conference Proceedings: Kingston-upon-Hull: ISPA.

Klimes, I. and Lamparsky, D. (1976) 'Vanilla volatiles – a comprehensive analysis.' *International Flavors, Food and Additives 7*, 272–291.

Knasko, S.C. (1997) 'Ambient odour: effects on human behaviour.' *International Journal of Aromatherapy 8*, 3, 28–33.

Komori, T., Matsumoto, T., Yamamoto, M., Motomura, T. *et al.* (2006) 'Application of fragrance in discontinuing the long-term use of hypnotic benzodiazepines.' *International Journal of Aromatherapy 16*, 1, 3–7.

Komori, T. (2009) 'Effects of lemon and valerian inhalation on autonomic nerve activity in depressed and healthy subjects.' *International Journal of Essential Oil Therapeutics 3*, 1, 3–8.

Kuriyama, H., Watanabe, S., Nakaya, T., Shigemori, I. *et al.* (2005) 'Immunological and psychological benefits of aromatherapy massage.' *eCAM 2*, 2, 179–184.

Kuroda, K., Inoue, N., Ito, Y., Kubota, K. *et al.* (2005) 'Sedative effects of jasmine tea odour and l-(-) linalool, one of its major odor components, on autonomic nerve activity and mood states.' *European Journal of Applied Physiology 95*, 107–114.

Kusmirek, J. (2002) *Liquid Sunshine: Vegetable Oils for Aromatherapy.* Glastonbury: Floramicus.

Lachenmeier, D. W. (2008) 'Absinthe.' *Med. Monatsschr. Pharm. 31*, 101. Cited in Dobetsberger, C. and Buchbauer, G. (2011) 'Actions of essential oils on the central nervous system: an updated review.' *Flavour and Fragrance Journal 26*, 5, 300–316.

Lachenmeier, D.W. (2010) 'Wormwood (*Artemisia absinthium* L.) – a curious plant with both neurotoxic and neuroprotective properties?' *Journal of Ethnopharmacology 131*, 1, 224–227.

Lavabre, M. (1990) *Aromatherapy Workbook*. Vermont: Healing Arts Press.

Lawless, J. (1992) *The Encyclopaedia of Essential Oils*. Shaftesbury: Element Books.

Lawless, J. (1994) *Aromatherapy and the Mind*. London: Thorsons.

Lawless, J. (1995) *The Illustrated Encyclopaedia of Essential Oils*. Shaftesbury: Element Books.

Lawless, J. (1996) *The Illustrated Encyclopaedia of Essential Oils*. Shaftesbury: Element Books.

Lederman, E. (1997) *Fundamentals of Manual Therapy*. London: Churchill Livingstone.

Leelarungrayub, D. and Suttagit, M. (2009) 'Potential antioxidant and anti-inflammatory activities of Thai plai (*Zingiber cassumunar* Roxb.) essential oil.' *International Journal of Essential Oil Therapeutics 3*, 1, 25–30.

Leffingwell, J.C. and Associates (1999) *Olfaction – A Review*. Accessed on 28 November 2011 at www.leffingwell.com/olfaction.htm.

Leffingwell, J.C. (2000) *Osmanthus*. Accessed on 4 December 2011 at www.leffingwell.com.html.

Lehrner, J., Marwiski, G., Lehr, S., Johren, P. and Deecke, L. (2005) 'Ambient odours of orange and lavender reduce anxiety and improve mood in a dental office.' *Physiology and Behaviour 86*, 92–95.

Lertsatitthanakorn, P., Taweechaisupapong, S., Aromdee, C. and Khunkitti, W. (2006) '*In vitro* bioactivities of essential oils used for acne control.' *International Journal of Aromatherapy 16*, 1, 43–49.

Lind, E.M. (1998) 'Profile of tuberose.' *Aromatherapy Quarterly*, 56, 17–20.

Lis-Balchin, M. (1995) *The Chemistry and Bioactivity of Essential Oils*. Surrey: Amberwood Publishing Ltd.

Livingstone, J. (2010) Personal communication.

Ludvigson, H.W. and Rottman, R. (1989) 'Effects of ambient odours of lavender and cloves on cognition, memory, affect and mood.' *Chemical Senses 14*, 4, 525–536.

Maddocks-Jennings, W., Cavanagh, H.M. and Shillington, D. (2009) 'Evaluating the effects of the essential oils *Leptospermum scoparium* (manuka) and *Kunzea ericoides* (kanuka) on radiotherapy-induced mucositis: a randomised, placebo-controlled feasibility study.' *European Journal of Oncology Nursing 13*, 2, 87.

Maddocks-Jennings, W., Wilkinson, J.M., Shillington D. and Cavanagh, H. (2005) 'A fresh look at manuka and kanuka essential oils from New Zealand.' *International Journal of Aromatherapy 15*, 3, 141–146.

Mahendra, P. and Bischt, S. (2011) 'Anti-anxiety activity of *Coriandrum sativum* assessed using different experimental anxiety models.' *Indian Journal of Pharmacology 43*, 5, 574.

Mailhebiau, P. (1994) *La Nouvelle Aromathérapie*. Lausanne: Editions Jakin.

Mailhebiau, P. (1995a) *Portraits in Oils*. Saffron Walden: C.W. Daniel Co. Ltd.

Mailhebiau, P. (1995b) *La Nouvelle aromathérapie: characterologie des essences et temperaments humaines*. Lausanne: Editions Jakin.

Mailhebiau, P., Goëb, P. and Azémar, J. (1996) 'Properties and indications: *Rosmarinus officinalis*.' *Aromatherapy Records*, 2, 40–45.

Malnic, B., Hirono, J., Sato, T. and Buck, L.B. (1999) 'Combinatorial receptor codes for odours.' *Cell 96*, 5, 713–723.

Martin, G.N. (1996) 'Olfactory remediation: current evidence and possible applications.' *Social Science and Medicine 43*, 1, 63–70.

Maruyama, N., Ishibashi, H., Hu, W., Morofuji, S. and Yamaguchi, H. (2006) 'Suppression of carrageenan- and collagen-induced inflammation in mice by geranium oil.' *Mediators of Inflammation 3*, 1–7.

Matsubara, E., Fukagawa, M., Okamoto, T., Ohnuki, K., Shimizu, K. and Kondo, R. (2011) 'The essential oil of *Abies siberica* (Pinaceae) reduces arousal levels after visual display terminal work.' *Flavour and Fragrance Journal 26*, 204–210.

Maury, M. (1961) *Le Capital 'Jeunesse'*. Paris: Editions de la Table Rondes.

Maury, M. (1964) *The Secret of Life and Youth*. London: McDonald & Co. (Publishers) Ltd.

Maury, M. (1989 [1961]) *Marguerite Maury's Guide to Aromatherapy – the Secret of Life and Youth: A Modern Alchemy*. Saffron Walden: C.W. Daniel Co. Ltd.

McCarthy, M. (1998) 'Skin and touch as intermediates of body experience with reference to gender, culture and clinical experience.' *Journal of Bodywork and Movement Therapies 2*, 3, 175–183.

McMahon, C. (2011a) Monograph: 'Frangipani (*Plumeria alba*).' Accessed on 3 December 2011 at www.whitelotusblog.com/2011/07monograph-frangipani-plumeria-alba.html

McMahon, C. (2011b) Monograph: 'Lotus, Pink (*Nelumbo nucifera*).' Accessed on 3 December 2011 at www.whitelotusblog.com/2011/07monograph-lotus-pink-nelumbo-nucifera.html

McMahon, C. (2011c) Monograph: 'Poplar Bud (*Populus balsamifera*).' Accessed on 3 December 2011 at www.whitelotusblog.com/2011/07monograph-poplar-bud-populus.html

McMahon, C. (2011d) Monograph: 'White Ginger Lily (*Hedychium coronarium*).' Accessed on 3 December 2011 at www.whitelotusblog.com/2011/07monograph-ginger-lily-white-hedychium.html

Mediavilla, V. and Steinemann, J. (1997) 'Essential oil of *Cannabis sativa* L. strains.' *Journal of the International Hemp Association 4*, 2, 80–82. Accessed on 29 November 2011 at www.internationalhempassociation. org.

Mertens, M., Buettner, A. and Kirchoff, E. (2009) 'The volatile constituents of frankincense – a review.' *Flavour and Fragrance Journal 24*, 279–300.

Mertz, D.F. (1994) *New Zealand Coromandel Mountains Tea Tree Oil Company*. (Unpublished report.) Whitianga.

Milinski, M. and Wedekind, C. (2001) 'Evidence for MHC-correlated perfume preferences in humans.' *Behavioural Ecology 12*, 2, 140–149.

Miller, G. (2004) 'Axel and Buck 2004 Nobel Prize.' *Science 306*, 5694, 207.

Mills, S.Y. (1991) *The Essential Book of Herbal Medicine*. Harmondsworth: Penguin Arkada. Cited in Price, S. and Price, L (2007) *Aromatherapy for Health Professionals*. (3rd edition.) Edinburgh: Churchill Livingstone.

Mojay, G. (1996) *Aromatherapy for Healing the Spirit*. London: Gaia Books.

Mojay, G. (1998) 'Fragrant rhythms: the energetics of aroma.' In *Rhythms of Life*. Hinkley: ISPA 1998 Conference Proceedings.

Mojay, G. (1999) *Aromatic Energetics and the Oriental Five Elements*. London: Institute of Traditional Herbal Medicine and Aromatherapy London.

Mojay, G. (2001) Letter. *International Journal of Aromatherapy 11*, 4, 232–233.

Morris, N., Birtwistle, S. and Toms, M. (1995) 'Anxiety reduction.' *International Journal of Aromatherapy 7*, 2, 33–39.

Moss, M., Cook, J. Wesnes, K. and Duckett, P. (2003a) 'Aromas of rosemary and lavender essential oils differentially affect cognition and mood in healthy adults.' *International Journal of Neuroscience 113*, 15–38.

Moss, M., Cook, J., Wesners, K. and Duckett, P. (2003b) 'Aromas of rosemary and lavender essential oils differentially affect cognition and mood in healthy adults.' *International Journal of Neuroscience 113*, 15–38.

Moss, M., Howarth, R., Wilkinson, L., Wesnes, K. (2006) 'Expectancy and the aroma of Roman chamomile influence mood and cognition in healthy volunteers.' *International Journal of Aromatherapy 16*, 2, 63–73.

Moss, M., Hewit, S. and Moss, L. (2008) 'Modulation of cognitive performance and mood by aromas of peppermint and ylang ylang.' *International Journal of Neuroscience 118*, 59–77

Müller, J. (1992) *The Hand Book of Perfume*. Hamburg: Verlagsgesellschaft R. Gloss and Co.

Müller, M. and Buchbauer, G. (2011) 'Essential oil components as pheromones: a review.' *Flavour and Fragrance Journal 26*, 357–377.

Nagai, H., Nakagawa, M., Nakamura, M., Fujii, W. *et al.* (1991) 'Effects of odours on humans (II). Reducing effects of mental stress and fatigue.' *Chemical Senses 16*, 198.

O'Brien, D (1969) *Empedocles' Cosmic Cycle: A Reconstruction from the Fragments and Secondary Sources*. (Cambridge Classical Studies.) Cambridge: Cambridge University Press.

Orafidiya, L.O., Agbani, E.O., Abereoje, B., Awe, T. *et al.* (2003) 'An investigation into the wound healing properties of essential oil of *Ocimum gratissimum* Linn.' *Journal of Wound Care 12*, 9, 331–334.

Orafidiya, L.O., Agbani, E.O., Oyedele, A.O., Babalola, O.O. *et al.* (2004) 'The effect of aloe vera gel on the anti-acne properties of the essential oil of *Ocimum gratissimum* Linn. leaf – a preliminary clinical investigation.' *International Journal of Aromatherapy 14*, 1, 15–21.

Orafidiya, L.O., Adesina, S.K., Igbeneghu, O.A., Akinkunmi, E.O. *et al.* (2006) 'The effect of honey and surfactant type on the antibacterial properties of the leaf essential oil of *Ocimum gratissimum* Linn. against common wound-infecting organisms.' *International Journal of Aromatherapy 16*, 2, 57–62.

Orlandi, F., Serra, D. and Sotgiu, G. (1973) 'Electric stimulation of the olfactory mucosa: a new test for the study of hypothalamic functionality.' *Hormone Research 4*, 141–152. Cited in Kirk-Smith, M. (1995) *The Physiological and Psychological Effects of Fragrances*. In: Kingston-upon-Hull ISPA Conference Proceedings.

Ostad, S.N. *et al.* (2001) 'The effect of fennel essential oil on uterine contraction as a model for dysmenorrhoea, pharmacology and toxicity.' *Journal of Ethnopharmacology 76*, 299–304. Cited in Harris, B. (2001) 'Research reports.' *International Journal of Aromatherapy 11*, 4, 225–228.

Overman, W.H., Boettcher, L., Watterson, L., Walsh, K. (2011) 'Effects of dilemmas and aromas on performance of the Iowa gambling task.' *Behavioural Brain Research* 218, 64–72.

Patil, J.R., Jaiprakasha, G.K., Murthy, K.N.C., Tichy, S.E. *et al.* (2009) 'Apoptosis-mediated proliferation inhibition of human colon cancer cells by volatile principles of *Citrus aurantifolia*.' *Food Chemistry 114*, 1351–1358.

Patnaik, G.K. *et al.* (1977) 'Spasmolytic activity of sesquiterpenes from *Cedrus deodora. Indian Drug Manufacturing Association Bulletin* (VII), 18, 238–242. Cited in Burfield, T. (2002) 'Cedarwood oils.' *The Cropwatch Series.* Accessed on 31 November 2011 at www.cropwatch.org.

Patra, M., Shahi, S.K., Midgley, G. and Dikshit, A. (2002) 'Utilisation of sweet fennel oil as natural antifungal against nail-infective fungi.' *Flavor and Fragrance Journal 17*, 91–94.

Pauli, A. (2006) 'α-Bisabolol from chamomile – a specific ergosterol biosynthesis inhibitor?' *International Journal of Aromatherapy 16*, 1, 21–25.

Pénoël, D. (1991) *Médecine aromatique, médicine planetaire.* Limoges: Jallois. Cited in Price, S. and Price, L (1999) *Aromatherapy for Health Professionals.* (2nd edition.) Edinburgh: Churchill Livingstone.

Pénoël, D. (1992) 'Winter shield.' *International Journal of Aromatherapy 4*, 4, 10–12.

Pénoël, D. (1998/1999) 'Medical aromatherapy.' *International Journal of Aromatherapy 9*, 4, 162–165.

Pénoël, D. (2005) 'Fragonia (*Agonis fragrans*).' Newsletter, 15 August. Cited in Turnock, S. (2006) 'Potent oil.' *Nova,* January 2006, 29–36.

Perfumery Education Centre (1995) *Diploma in Perfumery Correspondence Course.* Plymouth: Plymouth Business School.

Pole, S. (2006) *Ayurvedic Medicine: The Principles of Traditional Practice.* Edinburgh: Churchill Livingstone.

Pongprayoon, U (1997) 'Topical anti-inflammatory activity of the major lipophilic constituents of *Zingiber cassumunar.* Part 1: The essential oil.' *Phytomedicine 3*, 4, 319–322.

Porcherot, C., Delplanque, S., Raviot-Deren, S., Le Calvé, B. *et al.* (2010) 'How do you feel when you smell this? Optimization of a verbal measurement of odour-elicited emotions.' *Food Quality and Preference 21*, 938–947.

Prabhu, K.S., Lobo, R., Shirwaikar, A.A. and Shirwaikar, A. (2009) '*Ocimum gratissimum*: a review of its chemical, pharmacological and ethnomedicinal properties.' *The Open Complementary Medicine Journal 1*, 1–15.

Prashar, A., Locke, I.C. and Evans, C.S. (2004) 'Cytotoxicity of lavender oil and its major components to human skin cells.' *Skin Proliferation 37*, 221–229. Cited in L.S. Baumann (2007) 'Less-known botanical cosmeceuticals.' *Dermatologic Therapy 20*, 330–342.

Prehn-Kristensen, A., Wiesner, C., Bergmann, T.O., Wolff *et al.* (2009) 'Induction of empathy by the smell of anxiety.' *PloS ONE 4*, 6, e5987.

Price, L. (1998) 'Oils from the Myrtaceae family.' *Aromatherapy World.* Harvesting Issue, 20–21.

Price, L. (1999) *Carrier Oils for Aromatherapy and Massage.* Stratford-upon-Avon: Riverhead.

Price, S. and Price, L (1999) *Aromatherapy for Health Professionals.* (2nd edition.) Edinburgh: Churchill Livingstone.

Price, S. and Price, L (2007) *Aromatherapy for Health Professionals.* (3rd edition.) Edinburgh: Churchill Livingstone.

Quéry, S. (2009) 'Aromatherapy in sports therapy: interview with Stéphane Query.' *International Journal of Clinical Aromatherapy* I, 2, 24–26.

Reynolds, J.E.F. (ed.) (1972) *Martindale: the Extra Pharmacopoeia.* (29th edition.) London: Pharmaceutical Press. Cited in Price, S. and Price, L (1999) *Aromatherapy for Health Professionals.* (2nd edition.) Edinburgh: Churchill Livingstone.

Rhind, J. and Greig, J. (2002) *Riddle's Anatomy and Physiology Applied to Health Professionals.* (7th edition.) Edinburgh: Churchill Livingstone.

Rhind, J. (2009) *Essential Oils: a Handbook for Aromatherapy Practice.* Edinburgh: Edinburgh Napier University.

Robbins, G. and Broughan, C. (2007) 'The effects of manipulating participant expectations of an essential oil on memory through verbal suggestion.' *International Journal of Essential Oil Therapeutics 1*, 2, 56–60.

Rose, J. (1999) *375 Essential Oils and Hydrosols.* Berkeley, CA: Frog Ltd.

Ryman, D. (1989 [1961]) 'Preface.' In Maury, M. (1989) *Marguerite Maury's Guide to Aromatherapy – the Secret of Life and Youth: a Modern Alchemy.* Saffron Walden: C.W. Daniel Co. Ltd.

Sacks, O. (1985) *The Man who Mistook His Wife for a Hat.* London: Picador.

Safayhi, H., Sabieraj, J., Sailer, E.R. and Ammon (1994) 'Chamazulene: an antioxidant-type inhibitor of leukotriene B 4 formation.' *Planta Medica 60*, 5, 410–413. Cited in Bowles, E.J. (2003) *The Chemistry of Aromatherapeutic Oils.* (3rd edition.) Crows Nest, NSW: Allen and Unwin.

Saiyudthong, S., Ausavarungnirun, R., Jiwajinda, S. and Turakitwanakan, W. (2009) 'Effects of aromatherapy massage with lime essential oil on stress.' *International Journal of Essential Oil Therapeutics 3*, 2, 76–80.

Saladin, K.S. (2001) *Anatomy and Physiology: the Unity of Form and Function.* Boston, MA: McGraw-Hill.

Salvo, S. (1999) *Massage Therapy: Principles and Practice.* Philadelphia, PA: W.B. Saunders Co.

Salvo, S. (2003) *Massage Therapy: Principles and Practice, 2nd Edition.* Philadelphia, PA: W.B. Saunders Co.

Sanderson, H., Harrison, J. and Price, S. (1991) *Massage and Aromatherapy for People with Learning Difficulties.* Birmingham: Hands On Publications.

Santana, A.S., Ohashi, L. de Rosa and Green, C.L. (1997) 'Brazilian rosewood oil.' *International Journal of Aromatherapy 8*, 3, 16–20.

Satou, T., Matsuura, M., Takahashi, M., Umezu, T., Hayashi, S., Sadamoto, K. and Koike, K. (2011) 'Anxiolytic-like effect of essential oil extracted from *Abies sachalinensis.*' *Flavour and Fragrance Journal 26*, 416–420.

Sayyah, M., Saroukhani, G., Peirovi and A., Kamaladinejad, M. (2003) 'Analgesic and anti-inflammatory activity of the leaf essential oil of *Laurus nobilis* Linn.' *Phytotherapy Research 17*, 733–736.

Schinde, U.A., Kulkarni, K.R., Phadke, A.S., Nair, A.M. *et al.* (1999a) 'Mast cell stabilising and lipoxygenase inhibitory activity of *Cedrus deodara* (Roxb.) Loud. wood oil.' *Indian Journal of Experimental Biology 37*, 3, 258–261. Cited in Burfield, T. (2002) 'Cedarwood oils.' *The Cropwatch Series.* Accessed on 31 November 2011 at www.cropwatch.org

Schinde, U.A., Phadke, A.S., Nair, A.M., Mungantiwar, A.A. *et al.* (1999b) 'Studies on the anti-inflammatory and analgesic activity of *Cedrus deodara* (Roxb.) Loud. wood oil.' *Journal of Ethnopharmacology 65*, 1, 21–27. Cited in Burfield, T. (2002) 'Cedarwood oils.' *The Cropwatch Series.* Accessed on 31 November 2011 at www.cropwatch.org

Schmiderer, C., Grassi, P., Novak, J., Weber, M. and Franz, C. (2008) 'Diversity of essential oil glands of clary sage (*Salvia sclarea* L., Lamiaceae).' *Plant Biology 10*, 433–440.

Schmidt, G., Romero, A.L., Sartoretto, J.L., Caparroz-Assef, S.M., Bersani-Amado, C.A., Cuman, R.K. (2009) 'Immunomodulatory activity of *Zingiber officinalis* Roscoe, *Salvia officinalis* L. and *Syzygium aromaticum* L. essential oils: evidence for humor- and cell-mediated responses.' *Journal of Pharmacy and Pharmacology 61*, 7, 961–967.

Schnaubelt, K. (1995) *Advanced Aromatherapy.* Rochester, VT: Healing Arts Press.

Schnaubelt, K. (1999) *Medical Aromatherapy: Healing with Essential Oils.* Berkeley, CA: Frog Ltd.

Schnaubelt, K. (2000) 'Functional group therapy.' *International Journal of Aromatherapy 10*, 1/2, 62–63.

Schnaubelt, K. (2003) 'Theory and practice in aromatherapy.' *In Essence 2*, 1, 8–10.

Seol, G.H., Shim, H.S., Kim, P-J., Li, K.H. *et al.* (2010) 'Antidepressant-like activity of *Salvia sclarea* is explained by modulation of dopamine activities in rats.' *Journal of Ethnopharmacology 130*, 1, 187–190.

Seth, G., Kokate, C.K. and Varma, K.C. (1976) 'Effect of essential oil of *Cymbopogon citratus* Stapf. on the central nervous system.' *Indian Journal of Experimental Biology 14*, 3, 370–371.

Sharafzadeh, S. and Zare, M. (2011) 'Influence of growth regulators on growth and secondary metabolites of some medicinal plants from Lamiaceae family.' *Advances in Environmental Biology 5*, 8 2296–2302.

Shawe, K. (1996) 'Essential oils and their biological roles.' *Aromatherapy Quarterly 50*, 3, 23–27.

Sheen, J. and Stevens, J. (2001) 'Self-perceived effects of sandalwood.' *International Journal of Aromatherapy 11*, 4, 213–219.

Shen, J., Niijima, A., Tanida, M., Horii, Y. *et al.* (2005a) 'Olfactory stimulation with scent of grapefruit oil affects autonomic nerves, lipolysis and appetite in rats.' *Neuroscience Letters 380*, 289–294. Cited in Harris, B. (2005) 'Research Reports.' *International Journal of Aromatherapy 15*, 4, 207–210.

Shen, J., Niijima, A., Tanida, M., Horri, Y. *et al.* (2005b) 'Olfactory stimulation with scent of lavender affects autonomic nerves, lipolysis and appetite in rats.' *Neuroscience Letters 383*, 188–193. Cited in Harris, B. (2006) 'Research Reports.' *International Journal of Aromatherapy 16*, 1, 51–54.

Shiffman, S.S. and Siebert, J.M. (1991) 'New frontiers in fragrance use.' *Cosmetics and Toiletries 106*, 6, 39–45. Cited in Kirk-Smith, M. (1995) *The Physiological and Psychological Effects of Fragrances.* In: Kingston-upon-Hull: ISPA Conference Proceedings.

Silva, J., Abebe, W., Sousa, S.M., Duarte, V.G. *et al.* (2003) 'Analgesic and anti-inflammatory effects of essential oils of eucalyptus.' *Journal of Ethnopharmacology 89*, 277–283.

Sorensen, J.M. (2000) 'Melissa officinalis.' *International Journal of Aromatherapy 10*, 1/2, 7–15.

Soulier, J.M. (1995) 'The Thymus genus.' *Aromatherapy Records 1*, 38–56.

Soulier, J.M. (1996) 'The Rosmarinus genus.' *Aromatherapy Records 2*, 29–35.

Stoddart, D.M. (1988) 'Human odour culture: a zoological perspective'. In S. Van Toller and G.H. Dodd (eds) *Perfumery: The Psychology and Biology of Fragrance.* London: Chapman Hall.

Svoboda, K. (1996) 'The biology of fragrance: how plants produce essential oils.' *Aromatherapy Quarterly 48*, 1, 33–37.

Svoboda, K.P. and Greenaway, R.I. (2003) 'Lemon-scented plants.' *International Journal of Aromatherapy 13*, 1, 23–32.

Svoboda, K., Hampson, J. and Hunter, T. (1999) 'Secretory tissues: storage and chemical variation of essential oils in secretory tissues of higher plants and their bioactivity.' *International Journal of Aromatherapy 9*, 3, 124–131.

Svoboda, K.P., Svoboda, T.G. and Syred, A.D. (2000) *Secretory Structures of Aromatic and Medicinal Plants: a Review And Atlas of Micrographs.* Powis: Microscopix Publications.

Svoboda, R.E. (1984) *Prakruti: Your Ayurvedic Constitution.* Albuquerque, NM: Geocom.

Svoboda, R.E. (2004) *Ayurveda: Life, Health and Longevity.* Albuquerque, NM: The Ayurvedic Press.

Takayama, K. and Nagai, T. (1994) 'Limonene and related compounds as potential skin penetration promoters.' *Drug Development and Industrial Pharmacy 20*, 4, 677–684. Cited in Price, S. and Price, L (2007) *Aromatherapy for Health Professionals.* (3rd edition.) Edinburgh: Churchill Livingstone.

Takakai, I., Bersani-Amado, L.E., Vendruscolo, A., Sartoretto, S.M. *et al.* (2008) 'Anti-inflammatory and antinociceptive effects of *Rosmarinus officinalis* L. essential oil in experimental animal models.' *Journal of Medicinal Food 11*, 4, 741–746.

Tester-Dalderup, C.B.M. (1980) 'Drugs Used In Bronchial Asthma And Cough.' In *Meyler's Side Effects of Drugs.* (9th edition.) Dukes M.N.G. (ed.) Amsterdam: Excerpta Medica. Cited in Price, S. and Price, L. (1999) *Aromatherapy for Health Professionals* (3rd edition). Edinburgh: Churchill Livingstone.

Tisserand, R. (1977) *The Art of Aromatherapy.* Saffron Walden: C.W. Daniels Co. Ltd.

Tisserand, R. (1988) 'Essential oils as therapeutic agents'. In S. Van Toller and G.H. Dodd (eds) *Perfumery: the Psychology and Biology of Fragrance.* London: Chapman Hall.

Tisserand, R. (ed.) (1993) *Gattefossé's Aromatherapy.* Saffron Walden: C.W. Daniels Co. Ltd.

Tisserand, R. and Balacs, T. (1994) 'Nutmeg.' *International Journal of Aromatherapy 6*, 4, 28–38.

Tisserand, R. and Balacs, T. (1995) *Essential Oil Safety: a Guide for Health Care Professionals.* London: Churchill Livingstone.

Tubaro, A., Giangaspero, A., Sosa, S., Negri, R., Grassi, G., Casano, S., Della Loggia, R and Appendino, G. (2010) 'Comparative topical anti-inflammatory activity of cannabinoids and cannabivarins.' *Fitoterapia 81*, 816–819.

Turin, L. (1996) 'A spectroscopic mechanism for primary olfactory reception.' *Chemical Senses 21*, 773–791.

Turin, L. (2006) *The Secret of Scent.* London: Faber and Faber.

Turin, L. and Sanchez, T. (2009) *Perfumes: the A–Z Guide.* London: Profile Books Ltd.

Turner, R. (1993) 'Absinthe – the green fairy.' *International Journal of Aromatherapy 5*, 2, 24–26.

Turnock, S. (2006) 'Potent oil.' *Nova,* January 2006, 29–36.

Ubukata, Y., Hanafusa, M., Hayashi, S., Hashimoto, S. *et al.* (2002) 'Essential Oil Constituents of the Ukon-no-Tachibana (*Citrus tachibana*) in Heian-Jingu Shrine.' In *International Symposium on the Chemistry of Essential Oils, Terpenes and Aromatics, Tokushima, Japan 1*, 3, 8–9. Cited in Svoboda, K.P. and Greenaway, R.I. (2003) 'Lemon-scented plants.' *International Journal of Aromatherapy 13*, 1, 23–32.

Valder, C., Neugebauer, M., Meier, M., Kohlenberg, B. (2003) 'Western Australian sandalwood oil – new constituents of *Santalum spicatum* (R.Br.) A. DC. (Santalaceae).' *Journal of Essential Oil Research,* May/June.

Valnet, J. (1982) *The Practice of Aromatherapy.* Saffron Walden: The C.W. Daniel Company Ltd (English translation. First published in 1964 under the title *Aromathérapie,* Paris: Librairie Maloine).

Voinchet, V. and Giraud-Robert, A.-M. (2007) 'Utilisation de l'huile essentielle d'hélichryse italienne et de l'huile végétale de rose musquée après intervention de chirurgie plastique réparatrice et esthétique.' *Phytothérapie 2*, 67–72.

Warren, C and Warrenburg, S. (1993) 'Mood benefits of fragrance.' *International Journal of Aromatherapy 5*, 2, 12–16.

Watson, L. (1999) *Jacobson's Organ.* Harmondsworth: The Penguin Press.

Weiss, E.A. (1997) *Essential Oil Crops.* Wallingford: CAB International.

Weiss, E.A. (2000) *Spice Crops.* Wallingford: CAB International.

Weiss, E.A. (2002) *Spice Crops.* Wallingford: CAB International.

Wells, C. (2003) 'Plai.' *Essentially Oils Newsletter,* March 2003. Oxfordshire: Essentially Oils.

Wheeler, J.R., Marchant, N.G., Robinson, C.J. (2001) '*Agonis fragrans* (Myrtaceae), a new species from Western Australia.' *Nuytsia 13,* 3, 567–570.

Williams, A.C and Barry, B.W. (2004) In *Advanced Drug Delivery Review 56,* 603. Cited in Adorjan, B. and Buchbauer, G. (2010) 'Biological properties of essential oils: an updated review.' *Flavor and Fragrance Journal 25,* 407–426.

Williams, D.G. (1996) *The Chemistry of Essential Oils.* Dorset: Micelle Press.

Williams, D.G. (2000) *Lecture Notes on Essential Oils.* (2nd edition.) London: Eve Taylor London Ltd.

Williams, L.R., Stockley, J.K., Yan, W. and Home, V.N. (1998) 'Essential oils with high antimicrobial activity for therapeutic use.' *International Journal of Aromatherapy 8,* 4, 30–40.

Xu, F., Uebaba, K., Ogawa, H., Tatsuse, T. *et al.* (2008) 'Pharmaco-physio-psychologic effect of Ayurvedic oil-dripping treatment using an essential oil from *Lavandula angustifolia.*' *Journal of Alternative and Complementary Medicine 14,* 947–956.

Zaidia, S.M.A., Pathan, S.A., Singh, S., Jamil, S.S. *et al.* (2009) 'Chemical composition, neurotoxicity and anticonvulsant profile of *Lavandula stoechas* L. essential oil.' *The International Journal of Essential Oil Therapeutics 3,* 4, 136–141.

Further Reading

Benson, S.G. and Dundis, S.P. (2003) 'Understanding and motivating health care employees: integrating Maslow's hierarchy of needs, training and technology.' *Journal of Nursing Management 11*, 315–320.

Blackwell, R. and Smith, M. (1995) 'Aromatograms International.' *Journal of Aromatherapy 7*, 1, 22–27.

Capon, B. (2005) *Botany for Gardeners.* Oregon: Timber Press.

Capra, F. (2000) *The Tao of Physics: an Exploration of the Parallels Between Modern Physics and Eastern Mysticism.* (25th edition.) London: Flamingo.

Fritz, S., Paholski K., Grosenbach, M.J. (1998) *Mosby's Basic Science for Soft Tissue and Movement Therapies.* London: Mosby Lifeline.

Gilbert, A. (2008) *What the Nose Knows.* New York: Crown Publishers.

Goerner, S.J. (1999) *After the Clockwork Universe.* Edinburgh: Floris Books.

Goswami, A. (2004) *The Quantum Doctor: A Quantum Physicist Explains the Healing Power of Integral Medicine.* Newburyport, MA: Hampton Roads Publishing Co.

Goswami, A., Reed R.E. and Goswami, M. (1995) *The Self-Aware Universe: How Consciousness Creates the Material World.* New York: Putnam Books.

Hicks, A. and Hicks, J. (1999) *Healing your Emotions.* London: Thorsons.

Lavabre, M. (1990) *Aromatherapy Workbook.* Vermont: Healing Arts Press.

Lawless, A. (2009) *Artisan Perfumery or Being Led by the Nose.* Stroud: Boronia Souk Ltd.

Micozzi, M. (2011) *Vital Healing.* London: Singing Dragon.

Mojay, G. (1996) *Aromatherapy for Healing the Spirit.* London: Gaia Books.

Nissen, L., Zatta, A., Stefanini, I., Grandi, S., Sgorbati, B., Biavati, B. and Monti, A. (2010) 'Characterisation and antimicrobial activity of essential oils of industrial hemp varieties (*Cannabis sativa* L.).' *Fitoterapia 81*, 413–419.

Pert, C. (1997) *Molecules of Emotion: Why You Feel the Way You Feel.* London: Simon and Schuster.

Sacks, O. (1985) 'The dog beneath the skin' in *The Man who mistook his Wife for a Hat.* London: Picador.

Schnaubelt, K. (1999) *Medical Aromatherapy.* Berkley: Frog Ltd.

Svoboda, K.P., Svoboda, T.G. and Syred, A.D. (2000) *Secretory Structures of Aromatic and Medicinal Plants: A Review and Atlas of Micrographs.* Powis: Microscopix Publications.

Tisserand, R. (1977) *The Art of Aromatherapy.* Saffron Walden: C.W. Daniel Co. Ltd.

Tisserand, R. (ed.) (1993) *Gattefossé's Aromatherapy.* Saffron Walden: C.W. Daniels Co. Ltd.

Turin, L. (2006) *The Secret of Scent.* London: Faber and Faber Ltd.

Watson, L. (1999) *Jacobson's Organ and the remarkable nature of smell.* London: Allen Lane, The Penguin Press.

Essential Oils Index

Subject Index

Author Index